ASK MI

Mike Pearson

chipmunkapublishing
the mental health publisher

Mike Pearson

All rights reserved, no part of this publication may be reproduced by any means, electronic, mechanical photocopying, documentary, film or in any other format without prior written permission of the publisher.

> Published by
> Chipmunkapublishing
> PO Box 6872
> Brentwood
> Essex CM13 1ZT
> United Kingdom

http://www.chipmunkapublishing.com

Copyright © Mike Pearson 2009

Chipmunkapublishing gratefully acknowledge the support of Arts Council England.

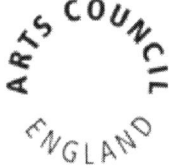

ASK ME NOW

'Life gets you,' came from the window; 'sooner or later it gets you all the same.'
'I don't know what it's for, why or who wants it. It seems so unnecessary, useless, even silly. And yet I cannot think that it's all in vain. There must be - perhaps a larger pattern somewhere in which all these futilities, these shifting congruities are somehow reconciled. But shall we know? Shall we ever know the reason?

William Gerhardie : 'Futility'

For MMD and FCP

Mike Pearson

ASK ME NOW

THE BRIGHT ELUSIVE BUTTERFLY OF LOVE

Alan looked through the window as another cadaver passed by and reflected that the dead really did go on before you if your office overlooked the hospital mortuary. Further on, pale October sun surprised the last leaves of fed up trees stuck in the car park as an off grey Fiesta came to a stop and a storm tossed vision in purple work boots and ankle length coat came out backwards struggling to supervise a pile of unruly buff folders. At least one official looking piece of paper managed to discharge itself from the pile to drift gracefully down to a loose group of leaves. There could have been more but Alan thought they were more likely to be stray sheets of Kleenex from the bunched up clump on her dashboard.

The woman's hennaed hair caught the same gust of strong wind which took the leaves and paper off to a distant corner of the car park, she pushed it away from her face with one hand, dumped the files back into the car then let the breeze buoy her in a north-easterly direction. With the hood lifting from the back of her coat she resembled somebody out of an advert for Scottish financial services. He watched with a kind of muted concern as the purple Doc Martens disappeared into the bushes where lovers tarried and dogs went for heroic bowel movements. When she hadn't re-emerged after about five minutes he felt he should go out and offer to help, however, a silent presence off to his left proffered a mug with a picture of Count Basie on it. As the grinning bandleader was full of warm tea and as Alan hadn't had any since he left home half an hour ago, he stayed where he was. The matter was settled by the two porters returning from the mortuary with their trolley. He could tell it was empty because the drab curtain material lay flat on the barrow where before there had been signs of former life in the lumps and valleys beneath the material. Everyone knew this went on but did they have to see it? He was beginning to accept that what you didn't know couldn't bother you, so why go on looking?

Was this what the Staff Development Unit meant by critical reflection and evaluation? Perhaps he should ask Mandy, who had been known to crack a joke - something to do with the area director, an emergency admission and a drug rep. He couldn't recall structure, outcome, what it was about or anything beyond it being funny. He did recall noticing that she was fanciable too, so what on Earth was she doing at SDU with Ivor, Ross and Bimmy? They tended to treat jokes as symptoms of a deeper problem which the teller might want to discuss and, while he knew what they meant, Alan, on reflection, thought them a set of tossers. And what that said about him, he'd rather not know.

The bushes were showing signs of new life, the Scottish Widow was reversing from darkness into the light, her boots looked unsmeared but her hands were empty. Pulling her coat about her and shaking her hair into the weather she turned back towards the building and meandered carwards where she slid into the passengers seat to relight a three-quarters smoked roll up. After a couple of industrial strength lung fulls she flicked it out into the car park, lumbered through and out of the drivers side with the pile of files clamped to her breast and came towards reception with her head down. The Consultant Psychiatrist had arrived for work.

'What's so interesting out there this morning Dickie?'

'I was just watching Dr. Wallace arrive, it's incredible really.'

'What is?'

'Oh, you know, she seems so disorganized but the clinics seem to run all the same.'

'A lot of that is down to the med secs.'

ASK ME NOW

'Yes but they don't do the clinical work. Lucy told me she saw twenty-five outpatients last week - and that's on top of three assessments, a ward round and that bloody faff on with Benny The Ball down the cop shop. They reckoned to have him on a 136 but when we got down there he'd been arrested for a breach of the peace. Of course he'd started to come out with all sorts of stuff - the microchip in his penis, the penis in his brain, the asteroid in his underpants. He tried to offend her but she just kept asking him to tell her more so he clammed up. Apparently he's known as Dick Head down there.'

'No imagination, at least we acknowledge his uniqueness and respect his individuality by using his proper surname.'

'What was he christened though?'

'Alan.'

'You're kidding.'
'No, his Dad was a footie fan and Benny came along in 1966.'

He's getting on a bit now, what do they think's wrong with him? He's been in enough times.'

'Wallace reckons he's a borderline personality disorder who has learned how to reproduce pseudo-psychotic symptoms under stress.'

'Hmm, sounds about right. Didn't they used to think he was schizophrenic?'

'God, that was old Dr. Patel. You won't remember him - he was that one they effed off back to the Punjab before Woodbine Winnie came. I'm not being racist but he was useless, used to get the medications mixed up and forget patient's names.

Mike Pearson

There was another one - Singh or Bindi or something, she was another one who didn't know where her ...'

'But he'd been assessed a good few times though.'

'Oh not much, it was funny how his diagnosis began to change. Bally came in once, he'd been on the ward a couple of days and went missing for a few hours. Guess where they found him?'

'Go on.'

'On the Geriatric ward. He'd gone there with a white coat he'd got hold of on the sly, told one of the nursing auxiliaries he was 'the new doctor' and managed to get one of the patients to undress so's he could examine her before anyone cottoned on. After that he was seen to be suffering from the kind of enduring personality disorder that was best treated in the community. I believe that nurse is now a sister; she was from India or Pakistan, or somewhere. Huddersfield probably.'

Alan objected to Graham Dixon's racism and felt he should say so. He had done once and been advised to spend less time 'with those wankers in Training' and didn't he recognize a joke? After all he would never talk to 'them' like that, it was just that they got 'affirmativeness' stuffed down their throats all the time in this job. The Dixon view was that people would get along much better if they were left alone, that you couldn't force these things. Alan knew he wasn't daft, not by a long way, and he had been really impressed by Grahams approach to an old Pakistani they'd assessed together once. He just seemed to carry this chip, being told what to do generally set things off, then it seemed to bring out the Norman Tebbit in him. He also liked to annoy people with it and it cut him off from them. They sometimes met socially and Alan had been to Grahams' house where he had been

ASK ME NOW

surprised to learn that his friend also liked Julie Burchill and didn't, as Alan did, hide this. He was glad when Graham spoke first.

'Look lively, Ina's on her way.'

'Shit, it's referrals this morning. I can't pick anything up this week.'

'Well don't then.'

'Have you seen how long the waiting list is now?'

'Not our problem.'

'No, but ...'

'Look, it isn't your responsibility. Your trouble is you want to be everybody's mate and you can't be. Start saying no and other people will have to start saying yes. You might not be so popular then, after all everyone loves a mug. Start saying no for your own good.'

'No.'

'Yes.'

'Right.'

An empty Count Basie joined the communal tea tray next to Homer Simpson, a rare first edition commemorative mug from the British Association of Social Workers (BASW) conference of 1978, two more functional vessels from a drug company, and a bone china affair from Whitby displaying a jolly sailor with an eating disorder. By the time the referrals meeting came around at ten it would be time for a refill. Both men took to their desks to do some social work. This task was mainly discharged by purposefully picking up some pieces of paper, aimlessly putting down others, arranging them into piles, rustling diary pages with an air of desperate vagueness and much recourse to charged emotionality on the telephone. Graham was talking. 'What? No, yes, - I mean when - but he only went there last week, his benefits still haven't been sorted out. But you can't do that, where's he supposed to go now? No he can't, she's nearly eighty. Look ... He's put the phone down on me, he's late for a review - at quarter past nine on a Monday ... the bastard. What's he expect me to do?'

'Sounds like somebody needs a coffee.' Cindy appeared smoothly, carrying a satchel of weathered leather and a tired smile. 'If you wash up I'll make them. Fancy a cup Alan?'

He affected a complex tussle with an awkward file leaving just enough energy to nod a heroic yes- you're-a life-saver look, which he knew would do. Graham beetled off with the pots as Cindy placed her bag on a chair by her desk and began to look meaningfully at Alan's back. He knew this was happening and cranked up his rate of administration ('if only they'd let us get on with our jobs') to a higher level. Cindy narrowed her eyes, pursed her lips and picked up a phone. She continued looking at her colleague as she slid up to perch on the edge of the desk and punch in a set of digits. A plausible scene of effective teamwork thus offered itself to the team manager as she came in followed by Graham bearing washed crockery and an offer of coffee he claimed shameless credit for.

'No thanks mate, I've not long since had one. Alan looks as if he could do with one though.'

She turned to head off to her own office across the corridor followed by Graham. 'Oh, Val - I need to have a word about Dave Harris, Stagework want him out.'

ASK ME NOW

'He's only just gone there hasn't he? God, they're a right shower there, talk about putting on a performance - it's always the same song and dance with them whenever there's a difficulty there, you'd better come in.'

Val Meatings' door edged across the carpet in an irregular stalking movement towards the door frame as she pushed away a rubber wedge with her green court shoe. Dixons scuffed deck loafers followed on and as their voices faded two of the community psychiatric nurses passed along the corridor. The female CPN waved to Cindy as Alan replaced another telephone. Cindy had finished her own call and stood blankly with the air of a woman kept waiting. Alan said 'hi' but she didn't react. Alan thought he'd best show willing. 'You want to talk about the Jessup thing?'

'That's right.'

'Well, she's at home today. I guess you'll be seeing her at some point.'

'So I gather, and don't be a prat - it's her being at home I wanted to talk about. I spent most of my last week preparing the ground for an admission, you've read the risk assessment, you know what she's like. Her daughter threatened to complain if something wasn't done - she's an accident waiting to happen. What on Earth were you doing?'

'Because I didn't get her in?'

'Yes you prat. She'd have gone informally, now it'll have to be a section, probably a section four and it won't be you that gets lumbered.'

'Not necessarily.'

'What, are you offering to do it?'

'No, it may not come to an admission - she wasn't that bad. I saw her twice last week and Dr. Wallace came the second time, she got a pretty thorough looking at.'

'Tell me.' Cindy said flatly.

'There should be a copy of Lyns' letter to the GP in your tray. Honestly we've known her to be worse, much worse. There was food in, she hadn't nailed up the door - the daughter had been round and she wasn't that bothered.'

'She told you that did she?'

'No but Ruth told us her daughter was happy with her and we could ask her directly if we liked. Lyn Wallace gave her a pretty good going over, you couldn't fault...'

'So you didn't speak to the daughter?'

'Look, it was hell on wheels here last week, you were off, the CPN's been off a fortnight and probably for another week now. There weren't any beds available - it was a risk we felt able to take. Ina knew all about it.'

'Yeah, I'm sure she did and she knows you call her that .... Dickie.'

Even someone as speculative about detail and as creative regarding evaluation as Alan Durite had taken pains to keep his manager fully informed about 'the Jessup thing'. The old lass was going off it again but she wasn't that bad yet and her hip meant she couldn't get out to cause too much mayhem, the consultant hadn't thought we should act at this point and there were no female beds anyway. Cindy would be back next week. It was agreed that it would keep till then.

'We decided to leave things, the daughter would be going in

ASK ME NOW

over the weekend ...'

'And I'd be back on Monday.'

'Look, what did you expect us to do? Bang her up just like that when there's a real chance she could be kept in the community. If we get the adult care lot involved and some day care sorted out ... I know she's a bit iffy about taking her tablets but Lyn could look at that.'

Cindy sighed as she slid back off the desk. Alan held his tongue and found himself pondering a parched tradascantia that had also been left unattended during Cindy Watson's week off. Count Basie grinned right back at him. 'Look Alan, you can forget all that long suffering stuff - and I don't like having to nag you either, the truth is you didn't want to be bothered and I'll bet Dr. Wallace only heard half the tale to begin with. She's two sheets to the wind herself these days, you know she's having to cover at Westbrook while Yellow Pages is suspended? Was she playing Val Doonican?'

'Dr. Wallace?'

'No you idiot - Ruth Jessup.'

'There was some music playing, something about a light and lucid something or other and don't be afraid no ones going to hurt you. Is that Val Doonican?'

Sounds like it. Anyway, it's a bad sign if it was - one of her fixed delusions is that Val Doonican is her son. Once she sat herself outside the house in a rocking chair importuning passers by.'

Alan failed to quell a snigger. 'What for?'

'It really isn't funny. She asks people when he's coming

home, it's awful because she's normally such a polite, reserved old dear. That's one reason why getting her into hospital sooner rather than later is important.'

'And another is that you didn't want to be bothered with the hassle.'

'Exactly.'

Well, reflected Alan, that made two of them. Then Becky from reception came in with a yellow sheet of A4 bearing a message. 'This came in first thing marked urgent, it's for you Cind.' She took in the gist of it and favored Alan with an expression suggestive of sexual abandon and indigestion. 'It's from Ruth Jessup's' daughter wanting to speak to someone urgently. Apparently she tried three times on Friday.'

He engineered a fleet departure as Cindy's' phone started chirruping, meeting Graham in the corridor. 'I'm off for a slash, come on you can tell me all about it in the bogs Dick.'

As the fire door swished behind them Val Meating crossed the corridor to see Cindy in the team room. Her conversation with Graham Dixon had confirmed two things, things which she'd always known really; that he was an experienced and insightful practitioner, capable of promoting and enabling his clients self-determination and that he was also a devious sod who would drop his colleagues in it as soon as look at them. Which caused her to reflect that as predicted, Alan Durite was nowhere to be seen though his flashers Mac and beret were so no 'urgent visits' had transpired. She looked again at his ill judged outfit - he obviously thought it lent him some of the understated élan of a Parisian saxophonist but most people felt it looked daft. More Frank Spencer than Hank Mobley, no wonder they called him Dickie. Cindy looked a bit frayed already; she couldn't help admiring her just for sharing an office with the pair of them. 'Did you have a good break then?'

ASK ME NOW

'Yeah.... it was nice. Mum was a bit brighter so I was able to get away on my own for a couple of days.'

'Anywhere nice?'

'Over to Southport actually, I've not been there before - it was very erm.... unexpected – sands like a muddy Sahara. All a bit cut off and left alone if you know what I mean.'

'I think so, maybe a bit like Monkseaton without tears.'

'Yes maybe, that's near Hartlepool isn't it?'

'Yes, stick to the North West if you can.'

Val hoped that their little exchange might suggest that Cindy had met someone - a man ideally, all that heavy stuff wasn't Cindy's thing really. What she needed was a good bloke, there were some somewhere. She'd read about them. 'I'm afraid that Jessup business blew up while you were away. Alan went in last week with Dr. Wallace but they didn't think they could do anything at that point.'

'I know, Alan said he went in to see her twice.'

'Oh, he couldn't get in the first time - it was all a bit hectic here last week, anyway it'll need picking up today.

'I've just spoken to her daughter, she can't get in and there's music blaring out. The neighbors are kicking up already.'

'Right, well it looks as if it's going to end up in an admission, you'd better nab the consultant after the referral meeting.'

'I thought that was tomorrow.'

'No, it's been switched because she's having to go over to Westbrook on Tuesdays now. It's due to start at ten in the group room.'
'What? It's five to now.'

'I know. Becky can take any messages.'

Alan and Graham were sitting in the group room laughing with Nav and Estelle, two of the CPN's. Nav had been at Westbrook before coming over to Northside. 'You do know why they call him Yellow Pages don't you?'

Graham smirked but Alan had an idea. 'Because he likes to tout for private work.'

Nav perfuffed scornfully. 'They wouldn't suspend him for that. No, it was because he couldn't stop his fingers doing the walking.'

Estelle rolled her eyes, Alan looked shocked and Graham laughed out loud. 'Haven't you heard about him - Dr. Snoddie, early onset penile dementia. They should get him to assess Bally.'

Estelle cut in. 'You can laugh, at one time he was eyeing up Cindy - just when she was splitting up with Dave as well. I'm sure he knew that, probably felt it would cheer her up. The big concern is has he been abusing the patients?'

Alan was appalled. 'Do you really think he could have?'

'Why not? Cindy saw him coming but the bastard could tell she was vulnerable. Powerless patients would be just up his street - he's horrible as well, nose fungus and green teeth.'
Nav took a sudden interest in his diary but Graham joined the debate. 'It could all be bollocks.'

Estelle bit. 'That's exactly what it is.'

ASK ME NOW

'No, I mean we've been taking the piss but what if there's nothing to it? What if the Trust sacks him? What about his family? And what about us? It'll mean trouble here if Wallace is daft enough to cover long term. This lot won't be in a hurry to get a replacement. How did it all start anyway?'

'I assume someone complained.' Said Estelle.

'Right, you assume. What does anyone actually know?'

It was time for Alan to take sides. He'd liked Estelle ever since they'd done a joint assessment and she'd asked his opinion on psychosocial interventions, being as how social workers were more experienced in that way of working. He also recognized Grahams tone of belligerent affront, the we-can-be-victims-too bit that could end in beers before bedtime and more of same for the next few days. People were beginning to talk about him and he wondered if his mate had acquired a nickname. Perhaps if he kept in with Estelle she'd tell him. 'All I know is that he's been called Yellow Pages for ages and, like I said, I thought it was a dig at him moonlighting. Now I think about it there was something a few years ago about a female SHO leaving his team abruptly, she was a real looker apparently.'

'Oh well that settles it. a real looker.' Estelle hadn't quite caught Alan's supportive intent. 'I suppose he just couldn't help himself, she should have made herself down a bit.'

Nav suddenly remembered a referral form he needed and left them to it. Alan hoped he hadn't offended him because the concupiscent consultant was Indian too, he could have some fun with Graham though - was his colleague suggesting that there might be a racist perspective to Dr. Snoddie's troubles? The doughty libertarian might struggle to locate his personal value base on this one. He'd see how things were likely to go first.

'You surprise me Alan.' Estelle's remark bypassed the third party smiling to himself as Alan dug himself in a bit more with some half hearted stuff about simply reporting what he'd heard. She then turned to Graham, it was clear she felt rattled. 'And what does the Daily Male think about this?' So that was it.

Before he could answer footfalls followed stifled conversation along the corridor and into the room. A dozen or so more or less respectable looking public servants entered and found themselves seats in a rough circle, Nav and Dr. Wallace came in last talking about 'non-compliance' and 'probably needs to come in'. Cindy and Val Meating were nowhere to be seen and Alan thought this was bad news. A high risk situation almost certainly to do with Mrs. Jessup whose circumstances were fraught with hazard and vulnerability. Thanks to him.

Dr. Wallace balanced an unruly roll call of blue files on the green chair beside her and cast a tight business like smile about the group. The weekly referrals meeting of the Northfield's Multi-disciplinary Community Mental Health Team had begun. There were five new cases, twelve on the waiting list and something that had just come in. Dr. Wallace caught Alan's eye as she shared the last item with the group and he therefore spent the bulk of the meeting in a study of the variety of avoidance strategies on view. Generally, the more seasoned members of the CMHT did better at not picking anything up - Clinical Psychology being in a league of their own - but one of the new CPN's surprised him by shamelessly quoting a recent policy guideline no one else had heard about and going on to cite the lack of assertive outreach services. She then looked blandly over to the representative from Rehab. - an old hand himself at this sort of thing but who soon found himself in the path of some assertive eye contact from the consultant. So he duly caved in and took the referral. Alan thought she'd need watching but with that sort of talent she'd be a sector manager in six months anyway. He showed willing when a depressed plumber came up. If he had a specialism it was probably working with people who were depressed and as the GP had started the chap on lustral directly but delayed the referral, he'd be on the mend by the time Alan saw him. Supportive counseling sometimes worked that way. Only one more referral made it through - one of the Occupational Therapists took it to assess for anger management, so that meant two more for the waiting list, which didn't get looked at as Dr. Wallace 'needed to speak to one of the social workers'.

As there was only one of the social workers available Alan made the best of it and offered to come along to her office where he met Nav, which threw him a bit because he had expected Cindy.

The consultant put down a drug card. 'Yes, Alan. Thanks for joining us, it looks like we're going to need an admission this morning.'

He looked at Nav who asked him if he remembered a man called Bill Clayton. 'I think so, was he the guy with the cross bow?'

'It wasn't a cross bow but someone said it was so we had to get the Police involved and the family kicked up about it afterwards. His neighbors got a petition up too and the council moved them eventually, a right carry on - totally over the top, he wouldn't hurt anyone.'

'So what's been happening then?'

Dr. Wallace swiveled in her chair as she rolled a yellow post-it into a thin funnel. 'This chaps got a pretty well defined bi-polar condition, pretty well managed but every so often he takes a unilateral decision to have a drug holiday. We normally manage to head him off at the pass but with Nav doing his course and no one in to cover it's got out of hand again. His wife went away last week - to his daughters was it Nav?'

'Yes, she's over at Sheffield, went for a week. When she got back he'd bought her a camper van and repainted the whole of the downstairs without moving the furniture. Went ballistic when she didn't jump for joy.'

'Hadn't she noticed anything before she went away?' Asked Alan.

Nav smiled sadly and shook his head. 'No, it seems as if he might have been planning the whole thing as a surprise. Her trip had been arranged for some time so I think he managed to keep the lid on things till she'd gone. It's a bugger because he's been all right for years - turned up for his lithium bloods, no problem about seeing people in the community. He's a nice bloke, all that stuff about a cross bow was cobblers. He's long since retired.'

'What did he do?'

Dr. Wallace leafed backwards through the notes. 'Ah, here it is, my report for his Mental Health Review Tribunal last time he was in - which he got by the way - yes he was still working at that point for the RSPCA. An Inspector - stressful job, give me cruelty to people anytime. He was good at it apparently.'

It was at times like this that he warmed to Lyn Wallace. One received view of medics. was that they saw the symptoms which indicated the diagnosis which determined the treatment. It then followed that if a patient heeded the excellent advice dispensed with their prescriptions they stood a fighting chance. He could see that despite Stalinist work loads and third world facilities she really wasn't like that. She'd told him once that Psychiatry wasn't really a science.

ASK ME NOW

He'd remembered that recently on a course when someone he had lunch with kept banging on about social work being a profession. They'd been looking at recognizing the individual behind the label and like most of these things it had been well intentioned but stultifying. His new friend had opined that some of the paradigms on offer needed tweaking, and Alan had thought so do you mate. But what did he believe? It was too easy to mock some of this stuff, for all the risible berks he'd met over the years was his own set-piece cynicism just a front, and for what? A leaky bran tub holding some warmed over notions of individual liberty, the right to help with dignity and an expectation of effective agencies resting on a chipped and shifty value base. He often found himself involved in this kind of reflective practice when there was work to be done and he found that he'd missed some of what had been said but managed to come in on cue. 'It sounds as if we need to get out there this morning, is there a bed available if it comes to it?'

'I'll phone the ward now if Nav brings you up to date, I'll also try to get the GP teed up. We might as well do it in one go, he could take off in his doormobile.'

Within ten minutes Alan had learned of Mrs. Clayton's agitated phone call, a ripple of concern from the people next door (who'd heard about the cross-bow, which had in the event turned out to be a garbled version of cross-bun, an industrial quantity of which had been baked by Mr. Clayton at the time, but these things stick) and had a look at the nursing notes. Nav's file looked right enough with its tightly knit care plan, detailed risk assessment and smart green treasury tags. So what had happened? Nav rehashed the unfortunate break in contact and talked about the need for some review of the community services with a meaningful look at Alan. He felt that he shouldn't come out on the assessment because it would mean there would be too many people, which was fair, and that his involvement would compromise his relationship with the Clayton's, which was bollocks.

Alan's agitation began to simmer; it was all right for CPN's, all they did was go out and check the medication - or not in this case - and push it over to the social workers when things got nasty. Why hadn't the stupid old sod swallowed his pills anyway? Why had Dixon taken himself off? He thought about his little sermon to Cindy about hasty measures and authoritarian ways and was again pulled back to the business at hand. This time by controlled squawk from Dr. Wallace, some silence, then a further outburst of high expressed emotion down the telephone. 'When? Oh come on he can't have, I gave him enough acuphase to take him off his feet for a week - look, organize a side room, report him missing and get the Police involved directly. What? - I know that means the new admission will have no - eh? Well that can't be helped - all right, look once they get Darren back he's going to need constant obs. till we can move him. Well how on Earth can we....? Just notify the ward manager and I'll face that when I come in to see the new admission tonight.' She put the phone down calmly and turned to Alan. 'Talk about Bedlam, any way has Nav brought you up to date with Bill Clayton?

'More or less. He decided to give himself a drug holiday without telling anyone and has swung up quite high. It sounds as if he's been all right since his last admission which was a while ago.'

'He had and we lost sight of him and as we're about to be reorganized into an assertive outreach type service you can draw your own conclusions.'
'What's happening on the ward, it sounds a bit lively?'

'Oh Darren Willis managed to get one of his mates to bring him some wiz in. He'd been a handful but I thought we'd managed to contain him. The lad's a worry really but the drugs team say his main problem is mental illness and his

ASK ME NOW

Probation Worker wants to play that line when the soft youth finally gets into court. Darren just thinks it's a big joke, when the Magistrates adjourned for reports he told them Beelzebub had a devil in reserve for him. It's not funny though, he's upset a few of the patients so I'm afraid the ward is not much of a sanctuary today. I see from his notes that when he was in before one of the things this chap complained of was the noise on the unit. If Darren Willis had any gumption he might abscond properly.'

'Are we sure this will result in an admission?'

'Well it sounds like it doesn't it? What do you think?'

'Well we obviously need to assess but we might be able to hold it at home.'

'We might, we'll have to see. I'll talk to the GP now but we need to look sharp, I've got a clinic all afternoon, including two new patients. I'll come and find you when I've got a time from him.'

'Who is it?'

'He's registered with Dr. Jobling but he's retired. The practice has been filling in with locums so who knows. I'll come and find you as soon as I know whets happening.'

Alan knew a friendly pop off for now when he heard one and left the consultants office. Just along the corridor he came upon Graham Dixon holding forth with knowledge and authority about the National Service Framework plans for integrated and proactive mental health resources to the new CPN who had so effectively marked her card in the referral meeting. His mind furred over every time he thought about this particular issue but his mate appeared to have comfortably grasped some of the basic premises and already delineated the implications for local services, if what he could overhear was anything to go by. The only bit Alan could confidently beat his gums about was the Thought Through Finance Network and that was only because it made him think about Jimmy Young. Graham was dressed for the outdoors in a shapeless green car coat with matching fleece cap, with brief case about him and car keys to hand he was possibly destined for work. How had this happened?

Alan approached as the nurse concluded her remarks about pump priming and the ballpark. How on earth did Graham listen to this stuff? 'How on earth can you take that seriously? What does it mean?'

'That last bit? I know what I'd like it to mean, I could put myself up for a steering group there without too many problems.'

'You're a right case you are; she obviously thinks you're interested in service reformulation. You lying get.'

'I am interested, a bit, sometimes and don't call me nasty names I've just had a bollocking from Ina - all honeyed words and caveats aplenty but a good one nonetheless. I think she's got a bit of a thing about me actually.'

Why did he play the fool like this? People took him at face value, he'd walked into a room recently where Lyn Wallace had been saying something about ... 'probably a high functioning borderline personality disorder' to Val Meating then promptly shut up. As it can't have been him it must have been Graham they were discussing and as for his queer notions regarding their managers favors he really was in disorder. Val was in a formidably committed tryst with an arthritic Airedale terrier called Cal - named, apparently, after a dead American poet who had written of his own mental illness. As far as was known the dog was not given to confessional versifying or barber shop quartets so his appeal

ASK ME NOW

would have to be the pretty as- a- picture-daft-as-a-brush variety. Which might mean there was something in Graham's strange musings after all.

'Gray, what's your position on rats?'

'You what? Can't be doing with them since you ask - is it important? Mrs. Jessup hasn't got them has she?'

'You're off there then?'

'Yeah - meeting Cinders at Wood Street, the daughter reckons she can get us in. Ina reckons it's a two person job, which is right but also my punishment for the cock-up at Todgers.'

The Lindens group home was managed by Claire Todgers who'd taken firmly against Graham, and any of his known associates, after he'd persisted in calling her Mrs. Todgers even though she knew that he knew her partner was called Pauline. She was also a mate of Cindy's, so any placement there had to be tightly wrapped and Grahams last one hadn't been. He'd somehow forgotten to tell them that the socially handicapped and deeply traumatized chancer he'd swung a place for was also an arsonist with at least one documented incident on file and a tendency to drink when under stress. Like the stress of moving to a new home. Fortunately the waste paper basket had had some cider in it so had taken some time to get going, and the battery in the smoke alarm had been changed that week. Otherwise it didn't bear thinking about. Val had decided to field this herself after calling Dixon something very like an arsonist.

Alan was shocked at his friends devil-may-care attitude. 'They'll kick up over this, it could have been horrendous.'

'I know, the more I think about it the worse it gets. You could hardly call him an arsonist though.'

'They will now.'

'And it's all my fault.'

'Well largely you must admit.'

Graham said the only thing he could say. 'Just fuck off, Dickie.'
The two compadres went their separate ways and as Alan passed through the fire doors back into the eastern side of the buildings H-block he overheard the medical secretaries conferring over a missing prescription. The tail end of a sentence about 'forever losing things these days' diminished as a door closed and Val Meating emerged from her office. 'I gather you've picked up an assessment.'

'Yes, a chap called Bill Clayton, he's known to the CPN's. I'm phoning the nearest relative and Lyn's getting on to the GP. Come through and I'll fill you in.'

'I've not got time, I need to speak to Claire - she's on her way over from The Lindens, in fact I think I can hear her now. Graham's left hasn't he?'

'Gone to meet Cindy at Mrs. Jessup's.'

'Good. I'll catch you later Alan.'
At this point Alan caught sight of Claire Todgers in the corridor, with her face turned away from them, in conversation with someone going the other way. As she paused to finish what she was saying - which seemed to be something cross with a fair amount of emphatic gesture and mutual exasperation involved - Alan nipped back into the team room and picked up a phone, deftly punching some numbers with his thumb. With his free hand in his pocket and the line ringing in his ear he was thus pre-occupied enough to miss her baleful glance in passing.

ASK ME NOW

The line was still ringing as Alan wondered how to do this. If Mr. Clayton answered he'd play it straight - Nav away, no contact for a while, important to get up to date and clarify things. If Mrs. then straighter; they were on their way. It was Mr. - of course he could come round, bring some friends if he liked, he'd just let Mrs. Clayton know. Silence, a dull thudish sound then the distant but familiar tones of a significant other at wits end. 'Hello? Oh, thank goodness, the doctor told me to phone you first. Yes, that's all right, he's just gone out - what have I to do? You wouldn't believe the mess he's made.'

'I'll be visiting with Dr. Wallace and his GP as soon as we can. Has he seen anyone from the surgery recently?'

'Dr. Trunnion saw him last week when he cut his thumb but that was the first time she's seen him.'

'What happened to his thumb?'

'Oh he took it into his head to cut down a sycamore to let more light into our back, got halfway through with an old rusty saw and nearly sliced his thumb off. If I try to say anything it just sets him off shouting - it's horrible, he's not like that at all really. Sometimes he looks terrible but then he just goes even faster. Heaven help us if he gets behind the wheel of that damn van - he says we can't get in it till he's got enough supplies in. That's where he's gone now, he's spending money we haven't got ......'

'Mrs. Clayton try not to worry, I'm sure we can sort this out. How do you think he'll react if we all arrive together? You say he's shouted .....'

'Look, he'd never hurt a fly, all that rubbish about
dangerous weapons wants sorting out while you're about it - that last time was a proper performance, Easter it was so he

bakes me some hot crosses because he knows I like them. Next thing the Police are here and Bill's the mad axe man, it took him so long to get over that. He's not sleeping hardly, won't eat a thing, put his name down for a darts team when he barely drinks - you've heard about this caravan caper and the decorating .....'

'So all this behavior is not normal for him?'

'What time did you say you were coming?'

Dr. Wallace was hovering. 'Beth Trunnion can meet us there at eleven.'

'Is eleven 'o clock OK Mrs. Clayton?'

'Yes, fine, soon as you like. Will he have to go into hospital?'

'Let's see how we go when we see him. I think that whatever happens there's every chance we can help him through this.' As poor Mrs. Clayton seemed to take some sustenance from Alan's assurances he put down the receiver and readied himself for some inter disciplinary planning.

'Got your section forms to hand Alan? With the best will in the world it's not looking too clever for the old boy, a manic episode like this is very bad news for someone his age. Once he crashes there'll be an almost certain deep depression, guilt, shame - he's just the type to take his life. There's a bed reserved anyway.'
Alan managed to agree with all of this without speaking. He also thought there was very little in the way of alternatives he could come up with at this stage. Maybe the day unit but that would be expecting a lot of his wife and a shed load of insight from him. Not a good idea and besides day therapy services were under 'review' being thought to be too expensive and not 'effective' enough according to research looking at alternatives to 'on site facilities'. People wondered how

ASK ME NOW

disinterested said research was as it had been funded by 'the industry' - which meant a drug company. Alan could afford to come on like Ken Barlow but he wondered how Lyn Wallace coped, lucky to get an SHO every six months, even luckier if they were any good, over worked, overly relied on but slagged off like a withholding mummy, no private life with those hours. Alan had made her laugh a couple of times and noticed how nice she looked, a sort of storm tossed Emma Thompson. But flirting with her was just asking for it so he was therefore pleased when her car wouldn't go and they had to travel together. He blithely informed her she could smoke if she wanted ('I like the smell of rollies').

As they pulled out of the car park she frowned to herself when they passed the bushes and stretched back to see behind Alan's head. He looked forward as she let out a gentle sigh through her nose. 'Anyway, lets hope Beth Trunnion knows her onions.'

'She's knew at Hill Street isn't she?'

'Mmm, I don't know how much psychiatry she's done. Old Walter Norris has been trying to run the practice himself so she's probably had a crash course in anxiety disorders already - forget I said that.'

'He would have known Mr. Clayton from before though?'

'I should think so, I'll just have another look at the notes ..... that last admission sounds like a nightmare.'

Alan threaded his way down Lancaster Road and out past the industrial estate towards the by-pass. The late morning light was lovely; washed and vivid it shot through mobile cloud to brighten antique brick. Supersonic pigeons wheeled up and away from the engineering works as the sun hit the fire escape. The redemptive transcendence of all this vanished like light from a gable when he accidentally cut up a passing fork lift and was called a cunt for his troubles. He knows I'm a social worker thought Alan, he rebukes me because I don't do a real job, because I've been to college but can't find my own arse. I'm a soggy broadsheet to his rolled up tabloid, the swarthy brute laughs in my face. Another fork lift turned to face them, horns scraping the ground like a hostile dinosaur of restricted growth.

'Is there another way Alan, we shouldn't get lost?'

'Yes, just down here past the weighbridge, this way we can miss the road works at the station.'

His passenger pulled on her rollie and said nothing, offering further thought when they were within sight of the Riverside Estate. 'You know the wards really quite lively at the moment, I've been on at the trust for ages about getting a proper unit sorted out for PD's - basically the Darrens of this world - it's hopeless housing them on an admissions ward, they just skew the culture of the place. I'm sending people out on leave and even discharging them before I should just to give the rest a break.'

' So, if we do admit this chap it would be to somewhere ... lively.'

'Well, not ideal, but we're never going to get that - we have to do the best with what we've got. The unit manager wants to raise it at the next BINS meeting. I think the real problem is a law and order issue, every time some little scamp gets nicked they start taking amphetamines like smarties, raising merry hell and get sent over to us with mental health problems. They don't stay on the ward for long but they don't half make life difficult.'

'It's interesting that wiz seems to mimic a bi-polar process doesn't it, and it's the downer they can't cope with.'

ASK ME NOW

'Yes, it is a bit. I wonder how fast our chap's been speeding, which house are we looking for?'

'It's number fifteen, that's probably it where the white camper van's parked.'

Alan pulled in a couple of spaces behind the camper and switched off the engine without unclipping his belt. 'Doesn't look as if the GP's here yet.'

'We should go straight in, she can join us. I haven't a lot of time today at all.'

The Claytons lived in the right hand half of a pre-war semi. A Clematis climbed the masonry by the door and behind a hedge ten feet of crew cut lawn told of therapeutic toil. A shape moved behind the thin strip of frosted glass in the front door and Mrs. Clayton appeared before he could knock, she simply stood back with her hand on the handle and Mr. Clayton appeared from the back room. He held in his arms at least seven loaves of bread and as the door behind him fell open, Alan could see the red handle of a supermarket trolley. 'Just in time eh, you'll have a sandwich - go on through, I won't take long.'

'Watch the paintwork and don't sit down just yet.' Mrs. Clayton murmured. 'I'll bring him through as soon as I can.'

Betty Clayton slipped back through to the hall taking care to pull the door to behind her. Another was heard to open and close on muffled voices - Alan was able to pick up a short pitched 'what did you say?' and looked at Dr. Wallace who stood neutrally in front of a wooden fire surround. Above the mantle a large Malaysian looking woman cast a pebbly stare in his direction, all three of them were avoiding the rooms most eye-catching feature - the lime green paint that had been

slapped up. It jarred violently with the existing browns and creams and seemed to be spattered on a lot of the furniture. Dr. Wallace had learned that he'd written to Sarah Beenie and phoned Channel Four that morning to delay her on account of the camping trip. 'I think we'd better get him in Alan.'
'In here you mean?'

'Well, here to begin with, do you want to find out what's happening?'

Alan thought that was a daft one but moved towards the kitchen where the voices were. He heard a kettle click off and a cupboard door being opened so he knocked and went in, his stomach tightened a bit as Mr. Clayton looked at him. It was an awful thing - the man smiled with his mouth in a kind of Hitchcocked parody of hysterical sociability. The rest of his face sent fear into the room. Alan had seen this face before and it was at times like this that he knew for sure how bad mental illness could be. Bill Clayton's eyes were screaming. To rub it cruelly home his poor wife was pottering about in a heartfelt production of the everyday, making tea for the visitors. 'You go through with Mr. Duright - I'll just get a plate for the biscuits.'

He stopped in his tracks. 'Knew I'd forget something - back in a minute.' He was jogging up the side of the house before his wife demurred; she steadied herself and motioned Alan towards the front room.

'Was that Mr. Clayton going out?' Dr. Wallace asked when they went in.

'Forgotten the biscuits, he actually got a catering pack of digestives this morning but I think you're getting the picture.'

Dr. Wallace looked around her. 'Yes, I think so. Nav spoke to me after your phone call this morning, you look shattered.' Mrs. Clayton managed a wan smile and, despite her earlier

ASK ME NOW

caution, sank into a beige wing armchair. Alan noted that the stain on the seat didn't attach itself to her tracksuit bottoms when she suddenly got up to see to the tea. The gentle steamy slush sounded disproportionately loud in the sudden quietness. He'd noticed this before on mental health assessments, how you found yourself in the middle of someone's life, someone's sitting room, a significant others emotional car crash, the most intense angst and confusion and life going on all the same. He felt like sitting back and picking up the paper, normality could ease back into the house and Bill could get better. Alan knew of a poem about this kind of thing, how one person was being tortured at the same time as someone else down the road was washing the windows or talking to the cat. He knew what he was doing though; this was a kind of willful reverie he indulged in during times of stress. The Doctor was watching him, was she reading his mind? She put the wind up him really - it was always women who endured and did the sensible stuff, men just fannyed about and generated problems, forgot the biscuits or went bonkers. 'Do you think your husband will be coming back?'

'Don't worry, he'll be back.'

Alan prided himself on his tact. 'He seems to have been very busy recently.'

'You mean all this? He got it into his head that everything's dark and needs brightening up. This camper van idea, he let it slip this morning where we're supposed to be going - Brighton, where there's a light on. He couldn't stop laughing then he seemed to sag and I thought he was going to cry, then he was off again to the shops, for provisions. It's awful, none of this is Bill, none of it.'

'How long would you say he's been off his medication?' Asked Dr. Wallace.

'I've no idea really, I've been away for a week but he seemed all right before that. It's hard to know with Bill because he doesn't let on much about anything. He told me he'd have a surprise for me when I got back but I didn't think..... it's years since he's been like this, I don't understand it.' She looked into the middle distance and even the painted lady couldn't meet her gaze. Alan felt the tension harden and remembered why they were here, they needed to take charge and Lyn Wallace's alert neutrality seemed like the right line. He was formulating a set of queries about sleep patterns; weight loss and household economics when outside doors banged in unison and Bill Clayton reappeared.

'I'll get that, she's come to change my bandage, she's had a wasted journey - it's better in double quick time. Come in anyway, you're lucky to catch us. Do you like custard creams, I can do you a kit-kat if you'd prefer - you look as if you need a good feeding up.' He then took himself off again leaving a rather startled GP on the front doorstep. Dr. Wallace gave Mrs. Clayton a rueful smile and went to rescue her colleague. Mr. Clayton then darted back in with several plates and a twelve-pack of penguins.

This was were he had to steer them forward, establish some rapport the better to involve the service user in a decision making process, earn his money. He wondered if he should ask them if they came here often. 'I think you've met Dr. Trunnion recently, this is Dr. Wallace and my name is Alan Duright, I'm a social worker.'

Mr. Clayton had been staring at Alan throughout without moving or otherwise indicating emotion, then he switched on his mad smile and waiting five seconds before speaking. 'Two Doctors to look at a cut, well sit down then, you'll need fortifying for this job. Pick up a penguin while you're at it. I once had to pick up a real penguin and a seal who was green at the gills - what do you think ....'

ASK ME NOW

'Bill, this gentleman and the Doctors have come to talk to you about ....'

'I know, if you'd stop interrupting I was telling them.'

'They don't want to hear about penguins.'

'How do you know what they want to know if you wont let anyone get a word in?'

Here we go thought Alan. 'Mr. Clayton we've come to talk to you about your mental health, Dr. Wallace is a psychiatrist and Dr. Trunnion has come too because there is a lot of concern from people who know you best.' And the good Dr. can take it from here, give her something to do other than look at me.

Mr. Clayton turned directly away from Alan to Dr. Trunnion who looked at Dr. Wallace who looked back at Mr. Clayton, who said. 'That seal could have done with a social worker.'

She smiled quite naturally and looked around the room. 'I see you've had the decorators in.'

'Decorators? You must be joking - I did this, the place had become very dull. We all need more brightness these days - it's hard to live in a world without light. The plants wont grow the butterflies fall flat, I wanted green light.'

'Does the weather affect your mood?' Asked Dr. Trunnion.

'It's the other way round with me - I need to keep my pecker up so the sun will come out. All this rain, it's not right for people.'

'Do you blame yourself for the weather?' Dr. Wallace seemed quite keen on this point.

'Well someone's at fault aren't they, we should be doing better than this.'

'But you can't blame yourself for the weather, it's out of our control surely?'

This appeared to puzzle him and as he turned to his wife she discreetly took his hand then, completely without warning, the clouds broke and he wept. Great wet sobs, which seemed to pull down his head and shoulders like a daffodil in a downpour. She reached up to hold him then helped them both into the two seater settee, motioning the rest of the group to sit too. Again a bizarre equilibrium hovered as Betty Clayton comforted her husband and Alan felt like settling himself more comfortably in his chair. Dr. Wallace simply waited, her manner as unbudgebly calm as it had been since they arrived. Dr. Trunnion looked shocked. The safe feeling seemed to attach itself to Dr. Wallace who was safe enough with it. 'Mr. Clayton, I think we need to ask you some things about how you came to cut yourself, and how you've been feeling lately. You are obviously most upset about something.'

'Bill love, talk to the Doctor. We can't go on like this, you're not right are you - all this painting, what were you thinking of?' She held on to his good hand and got him sitting straight but he wouldn't look at anyone or say anything.

Alan felt the impetus coming his way. 'You're planning a trip Mr. Clayton, judging by the stuff you've bought you must be planning to be away for a while.' Why didn't he tell them where to go? And why had he come back from the shops, did he, at some level, want what was going to happen to happen? 'Do you feel that you need to get away?'

'Instead of being put away you mean?'

Bill Clayton's tone had a dull vinegary flavour and his

ASK ME NOW

demeanour conveyed thwarted rage. The overall effect was to render him childlike but old, persecuted by inverted hostility. It was powerful and awful and everyone in the room wanted to stop it for him. Dr. Wallace led off. 'I think it's fair to say that you've suffered a relapse of your condition and that you really need some care and treatment. I'm clear in my own mind that if we leave things as they are you will only become more poorly.'

Betty Clayton took it from there. 'Do you remember when you took ill before love? It's not as bad as it was then but I think they're right, best do what they say.'

Before handing back to the consultant. 'I'd like to get you into hospital Mr. Clayton to have a proper look at you and get you better again, the sooner the better really. We're all concerned that you've been making decisions and doing things you wouldn't normally and putting yourself at risk.' She waited a bit but Bill just sat like a penitent two year old looking at her with a horrible glazed over guilt. 'We know what kind of illness you're enduring and how to treat it, I'm confident that we can get you well again, in the right setting.'

Nothing happened for an eternal twenty seconds then he clapped both knees and got purposefully to his feet. Turning to his wife he said. 'We need to pack.' Then they left together.

The visitors were left to talk amongst themselves as feet shuffled overhead and floorboards creaked. Alan heard a drawer being pulled open. Dr. Trunnion spoke first. 'What do you think he's packing for, do you think he'll come voluntarily?'

'We'll soon find out. What do you think Alan, can we swing it informally?'

'It's hard to see any way we can keep him out the way things are, I'm worried about him taking off in that van, also I agree he could become suicidal and his wife is pretty stretched. Let's try to avoid sectioning him if we can.'

'You're treating him for manic-depression aren't you?' Asked Dr. Trunnion.

'Yes and in many ways he's text book material, very well maintained on an effective mood stabilizer and generally compliant. God knows what's happened this time. He is very labile right now and I'd guess just about ready to dip into a depression, which is very dangerous. He'll be full of guilt and remorse at what he's been up to and he's just the type to harm himself.'

Dr. Trunnion looked even more alarmed. 'Well shouldn't we be sectioning him then for his own good?'

Alan glanced at the consultant who batted it his way with a knowing smile. 'Well, I think he needs to be in a safe place and that it's expecting too much of his nearest relative to care for him as things stand. I also think he's making a choice to go along with what's happening, I mean, why hasn't he voted with his feet - we couldn't stop him?'

The GP looked at him doubtfully. 'Is that the same as agreeing?'

'All the act says is that 'the patient be not unwilling' for an informal admission to be legal. Anyway, we might have no choice and even if he does go in informally, there's always the danger that he'll kick up on the ward and end up detained there.'

'One way or the other that's a fair degree of coercion.' She reflected.

ASK ME NOW

'You do agree he's very poorly though, a danger to himself and others, unlikely to go along with the treatment he needs if we leave him alone?' Dr. Wallace just about managed to make this sound like a question.

'Oh yes, certainly, but is he really a danger? He seems like a decent bloke and when he's well this kind of thing would be anathema to him.'

'That's really the point.' Chimed in Alan. 'What we're seeing is so far from normal for this guy that we need to step in now, I think as I said that there's a glimmer of insight but it's fleeting and reliant on his wife's input. She's the key to getting him in smoothly. Imagine him bombing about in that van - he could have done worse with that hacksaw too.' The GP looked at him, he hoped he hadn't gone too far.

Dr. Wallace cocked her head and lowered her voice. 'I think he might be borderline psychotic as well.'

'He seemed so normal when I saw him in surgery.'

'It's very hard to spot sometimes but I think we may have caught him just in time, it's only just beginning to break through. All this business about his mood regulating the weather - grandiose, flight of ideas, disordered thinking. We really need him in .... I think they're coming down.'

Alan smiled at Dr. Trunnion in a speculative what-a-caper-eh sort of way but she blanked him and looked at the consultant with her bottom lip sucked in. Alan reckoned that she would be ready for a fag by now, she had been known to light up during assessments before but it was obvious the Clayton's were non-smokers. The door opened and Betty Clayton shuffled in wearing immaculate white trainers and he felt a pang of sadness at this; the track suit and jogging shoes were an investment in something worth staying fit for - she'd stay the course through all this and help him back up the hill, might even write a note of thanks to the team for 'all its help'. And he knew as well as Lyn Wallace that this could have been avoided, that care plans and patient's charters weren't worth the reams of paper they consumed if there weren't people in post to do the work. The Claytons were from the last batch of that thinning generation that felt a measure of respect for public servants - Bill had been one himself - and took the view that things you saw in the paper were often more complicated than they seemed. Sometimes they were but thank God she'd phoned when she did. Betty Clayton joined them with an ambiguous 'we're all packed' and, courtly but insistent, ushered her husband into the room. In the hall Alan spotted a single suitcase. She seemed to be directing events. 'I think if we all go together then I can stay at the hospital for a bit, would you be able to take us Mr. Duright?

'Yes, of course.' And, given his impromptu risk assessment of the route down fuck-off avenue definitely by the by-pass. 'Could I just phone the ward to let them know we're on our way?' To his surprise Bill Clayton nodded towards the hall and indicated the new mobile in its handset.

When he'd finished his call Dr. Wallace joined Alan. 'Well, this looks pretty straightforward, Beth can give me a lift back if you finish off here and I can brief the ward - I think we'd better have him on close obs. for the first week.' Alan could hear Dr. Trunnion making her good-byes then the two medics left the house, as the front door drifted shut he caught the tail end of Dr. Wallaces remarks..... 'classic scenario' 'poor old soul'.

So that left the three of them, Bill sat down again. He must be exhausted, would their daughter come over to stay? 'Shall we go now or would you prefer to wait a bit?'

'Bill's very tired, can we have a bit sit?'

ASK ME NOW

'Of course, once we get you on the ward and settled they can give you something to help you sleep if you like, I think they've been able to give you a room of your own.'

'Is it a room with a view then?'

Christ, don't say he's going off on one again, he might get to see the recreation ground beyond the laundry but that would be it. 'Well, it's hardly Florence but the main thing is that you'll have some privacy and rest, which is the main thing you need right now.'

'I might have a good long rest.'

Alan didn't like the sound of that, nor did Betty Clayton when he caught her eye. They sat for what Alan estimated was a bit then he became focused and professional - amiable but decisive, keen to get things running along the lines that had been agreed on. 'Shall we get going then? Is there anything else you need?'

Mr. Clayton just sat where he was, seemingly out of steam too. Again, it felt so easy to sit with them and let the firm comfort of old furniture and domestic routine fix him in a daydream. They could stay like figures in an Edwardian oil painting for as long as it took for Bill Clayton to pull through. Then he looked again at the mad green walls and remembered why he was there, also, Bill had begun to cry again, quietly this time, sitting very still while the tears slipped down his cheeks like rain on a train windows, some of them making it all the way to his chin. Betty looked lost, worn out by the effort of getting this far. If Alan couldn't get things moving again it would need to get more formal and assertive with pink forms, expensive ambulances and hot cross consultants. 'Are you ready to go Mr. Clayton?'

'Just about. You're coming with us then?'

Alan felt a bit foolish then decided he didn't really understand what Bill Clayton had meant. 'We're all going together, in my car, to the hospital. As we agreed with the Doctors.'

The man simply turned to his wife, fished some keys out of his pocket and said. 'Here, you load up while I have a last check round - he can give you a hand.' On his way upstairs he added that it looked like a good day for a run.

Alan decided to take things as they came. 'He expects us to go in the van doesn't he - where on earth does he think we're headed for?'

'The hospital, like we agreed. It's the only way he'll go - he's set his heart on driving off down the street for a break in his new van. He's told the people next door, I'll bring us back in it.'

'And he'll drive us there?'

'Look, just do it shall we? Have you got any better ideas? I know as well as you do what will happen if it doesn't come off. I know Bill - he deserves a chance.'

He sat in the long front seat with Betty while Bill locked up, he could have passed for their nephew. A man was fiddling with an upturned bike in the garden next door and they exchanged a few friendly looking words as Bill moved past him. An old tyre hung high in a tree by the van. 'Ready for the off then.' He said as he swung himself up into the drivers seat and Alan marvelled at the effort he was making - if they hadn't known they wouldn't have guessed, but that was one of depressions quieter cruelties. In the middle of the most dreadful torment people could still put on a convincing show. For a bit. Not for the first time in his life Alan reflected that if

ASK ME NOW

there was a God he was a comedian.

The vehicle started second time and they pulled off past Alan's car towards the town, he noted that the tank was full and Bill switched on the digital radio, which needed tuning in. They went straight on through two sets of traffic lights then took a right turn down Selby Street towards the ring road. Bill hadn't spoken at all so it was a relief when Betty got on to the local station in time to catch the end of The Human League doing 'Don't You Want Me?' then inane hospital radio twaddle from someone who wasn't in Jimmy Young's league. His theme for the day seemed to be 'the power of lurve in all its many forms' and this was to be demonstrated by 'the power of music'. Alan wondered if they'd be getting Celine Dion or Hughey Lewis and the News but the DJ started to wax on about comfortable cardies, rocking chairs and 'seductive Celtic charm'. Apparently Saturday evenings had never been the same since this particular songbird had fallen off his perch. Did we remember this?

And Alan did. He'd heard it at Mrs. Jessup's - the sound of someone moving past a window ..... across my dreams with necks (nets?) of wonder I chase the bright elusive butterfly of love. Val Doonican; aural nembutal. The record ran on and Alan wished he wasn't such a musical snob. The John Coltrane Quartet weren't everybody's cup of cocoa after all, and hadn't somebody else sung about love being like a butterfly? For some reason he thought of Wendy Craig but it had been a long day already. Most likely Robert Wyatt.

The Clayton's seemed to recognize the song and exchanged glances, as they neared the by-pass Bill looked halfway towards Alan and said. 'The hospital's just out past Hampsons Textiles on the estate?'

'Yes, I should go round the estate rather than through, they looked very busy earlier.'

This meant a winding arterial road affording a grand tour of mucky industrial units, larger mysterious looking buildings with no windows and blank oily stretches of abandoned land where bizarre weeds flourished. At one point they needed to stop to let a lorry back into space. When the driver gave Bill the thumbs up he nodded back. All pretty normal - one man on his way to the psychiatric hospital as another collects some deliveries.

'If you go left here and head for the roundabout, the hospital is signposted on the next to last exit.'

Bill followed the route as indicated and they were soon, too soon it seemed to Alan, turning in to the car park and past the bushes. He thought he saw something or body rooting in the undergrowth but couldn't see for sure. They pulled into one of the disabled spaces by the main entrance and the driver switched off and sat back. 'Right I've got us all here in one piece, I'm all yours now.'

ASK ME NOW

OUT TO LUNCH

A stray dog sniffed along the line of a wall along Sepoy Street as a palsied warble from behind the high red brick could be heard inquiring peevishly for the whereabouts of Lord Salisbury. The dog reached the corner and turned left into the grounds of an institutional setting. The building and its environs resembled something from a 1950's Soviet Bloc as might have been designed for Postman Pat. A small concrete bridge carried the dog beyond an ornamental pond and past some fiercely symmetrical flowerbeds to the main entrance. From behind the frosted glass a small figure could be seen shuffling in and out of focus as a more distant voice asserted that the key could not be reached. The dog skittered off along the gravel and disappeared behind a hedge.

Beyond the glass a little old lady was marking time in decreasing loops of arthritic anxiety. She came to a stand still as a much younger woman appeared to lead her off gently like a clapped out lamb, faded and wooly in a porridge colored cardie. The process had a familiar, peaceful quality to it - something that was benign and essential to the life of the building as if, behind the high wall and ambiguous glass, more malleable and contingent forces were held in play. As the two women passed slowly down a long hall another couple came towards them. As their paths met and passed sudden brightness from a window lit up four women moving through the light in a study of faint abstraction. The place could host a perpetual slow dance of people deep in a dream of loss and diminishing returns. Viewed like this the fly on the wall nearby had its own beauty and redemptive power. Viewed like this, without the sounds and the smells, the baggy mess of sentience and the tang of piss, a well meaning but soft minded fly might decide that growing old and losing your marbles wouldn't be so bad. That if you got there you could, within limits, pretty much please yourself.

'When you've settled the old lass could you get that can of Bee-No Alison. There seem to be a few flies hanging about the landing. They unsettle Mr. Page since that Jeff Goldblume film he saw at his Grandsons.' The Manageress passed on to the meat order and left the care workers a clear path.

'Okay, no he's not arriving today Rita but we can look at the times if you like.' The young woman looked to her colleague by way of explanation. 'They're coming back from the war this week apparently.'

'Which one'?

'Don't know, they're coming by rail so it must be ... well, anyway.'

'But they've had railways since eighteen something.'

'Does it matter?'

'Monte Casino.' An older voice, chesty but emphatic.

'What is it Clarice ... Monty knows?'

'She said Monte Casino - Second World War, Italian campaign. We're on familiar territory.'
'Let's hope he was.'

The younger women went their separate ways with their charges and 'the old lass' was settled in a chair by a window while Clarice and her carer made a close reading of the bus timetable. It was finally understood that the train bearing her husband home would arrive at five, by which time the drugs trolley would have departed having stamped Clarice's ticket for a different journey. So that was her done for the day.

The other two spent a bit longer together. Alison thought that Mrs. Watson could be about to say something and didn't want

ASK ME NOW

to leave without being sure so she sat down in the chair next to her. At one point Mrs. Watson looked intently in her direction but nothing came and Alison found herself regarding a china dog on top of the telly. It was modeled on 'Nipper' the HMV listening terrier, his near side brown ear was missing and the way he cocked his head suggested that it had just dropped off. She settled into the high backed chair and began to loose her self in the narcotic bustle of institutional care. Growing old might not be so bad she thought, it wouldn't bother her.

'Ah, there you are. I need to talk to you about the new admission - are you doing anything at the moment?'

Mrs. Watson was disinclined to come to Alison's rescue and stared ahead as she picked at her terelyne tabard. 'We can talk now if you like Mrs. Charles.'

'In the office I think Alison. Good morning Mrs. Watson.'
Alison looked back as she left the sitting room. The older lady's eyes followed her but the rest of her stayed still. She'd had this experience before; sitting with them convinced there was nothing happening apart from the antique plumbing running its leaky course, their hair wisping outwards like that green furzy stuff by the bypass in summer. Then there'd be a glance, sometimes a grin but usually something else and it would seem that they knew. Alison thought that this was why everyone preferred them all the way round the bend, once they'd settled on the idea that the world and its works ended at the back door you could persuade yourself it wasn't that bad.

This was after all the Sweethaven way, medicated acceptance, regulated autonomy. What was the point of convincing Mrs. Windsor that she wasn't Queen Victoria? A well-meaning volunteer had tried this and she'd taken to her bed for a week. The only way they'd managed to avoid a hospital admission had been to get Mr. Blunket to pretend he was Disraeli and get him to visit so that he could tell her the country was missing her and that some had even come to believe she had perished. Fortunately those residents capable of reasoned reflection had reassured themselves when news came through that she had inspired a ceremony in the day room. Mrs. Charles had permitted a brass band CD but drawn the line at Ahmed getting himself up as an emissary from Calcutta. It was felt that you could take things too far.

Alison followed Mrs. Charles to the office where the tacky scent of burning sandalwood obscured the other stuff. 'Have a seat Alison, are you all right to meet this gentleman this morning?'

'Our new resident?'

'Well ... yes. My understanding is that he thinks he's coming for a look round and, if he likes it, for a few days - but its up to us to make him feel welcome, obviously. But you know what I mean, it's not anticipated he'll be going home.'

Alison thought she probably did and wondered just how welcoming they might need to be. 'Where is he coming from, his family?'

'His daughter virtually moved in with Mr. Prince about eighteen months ago after his wife died. As far as I know there hadn't been a lot of contact prior to this and, as his wife seemed to have done everything no one knew how far gone he was. This last year has been pretty bad apparently. He's only sixty four.'

'What do they think's wrong?'

'Alzheimer's and bad - he's pretty lively too.'

'Have they tried him in day care or anything?'

ASK ME NOW

'No, the picture I'm getting is that the daughters own health has broken down and the team over at Northfield got straight in with them both. Anyway, Alan Duright's coming along at eleven with him so we'll hear more then.'

On her way back to the large day room Alison looked into a smaller space called the 'Ladies Lounge'. It was edged on each side by eight easy chairs - she had wondered what tricky ones were like - and at that moment held two elderly men staring stupefied at the previous evenings episode of 'Where The Heart Is'. As a district nurse simpered to camera one of the viewers observed in hurt tones that he thought she'd gone to Home Base. His companion seemed to think it was Do-It-All, then they fell into a comfortable and familiar riff around the way we live now and nothing being as it was. Whole mornings would pass like that.

'Morning lads, have you scared off the ladies again?'

'Gone to work at Home Base.' Said one.

'It's B &Q.' Said the other.

Alison considered pointing out that the actress in question had made her name in a show about men behaving badly but decided there was enough blurring of the wafer thin membrane separating reality from fantasy in these parts. You didn't have to be sane to work at Sweethaven but it did help. Mr. Rhule and his mate Mr. Rocket were two of the 'higher functioning' residents of the place and this had helped build a touching bond between them. Like star crossed lovers in a Russian play they would spend parts of each day struggling through the diurnal mayhem of the Sweethaven experience to share affirmative moments chuntering on about Leslie Ash. And if an unforeseen caprice in a distant and rarely visited part of the building kept them apart then Alison or one of the others would generally find time to bring them together. Today there was some catching up to be done. Harold Rocket had spent most of yesterday pinioned by a voluble relative in the pavilion before Ahmed had pointed out to the visitor that it was getting near bedtime. Even the guests were nonconformists, Bob Rhules son was another inclined to linger leaving his old Dad all talked out and tattered. His wife would have to clap her knees in a business like fashion and bark 'home Rhule'. Mrs. Windsor had taken exemption to this once and been heard to cry 'God blast Mr. Gladstone' as they took their leave. No one had minded. Free now of importuning relatives or affronted Empresses the old men fell to an impassioned if fragmentary debate about the days before Home Base.

'We had to make our own fun then.' Said Bob.

'And our own cabinets.' Said Harry.

Alison thought why not? 'We've got a new gentleman coming to see us today. I wonder if you could tell him a bit about our community.'

'A what?'

'A new gentleman Harry.'

'From Home Base?'

Jesus, did he think they came in flat packs? 'No Mr. Rocket, a new gentleman who might want to come to live here. He's been living with his daughter.'

'What's he want to come here for then?' Asked Harry reasonably enough.

'To have a look.' Persisted Alison.

ASK ME NOW

'Well, there's not much to see is there?'

Alison left it at that and took her leave.

At the same moment five miles away Briony walked into another room where her Father sat in another easy chair looking a television screen. On it there was a woman on a sofa with her feet up looking lewdly at the viewer as half-hearted disco music pumped away gamely in the background. Mr. Prince looked up imploringly at his daughter, tears forming in his eyes, great guilt inducing sobs building in his frail chest and asked her for the fifth time that morning why Bet Lynch was selling sofas.

'It's not Bet Lynch Dad, it's Natalie and she's just doing an advert.'

'Oh does your Mother do adverts now then?' She'd be good - sell Eskimos to fridges she could.'

With an obvious effort Briony tried to quell the chaos threatening without and within them both. 'Mr. Durights coming to see you this morning.'

'He can see my arse.'

She wanted to weep and shout simultaneously. Her soft sweet natured Father had never sworn in front of her until last year. As a child she'd thought he looked like John Lennon, now he'd shrunk away somewhere inside himself and thought her mum was Julie Goodyear.

'Look there she is again the dirty bitch. Look, brassy tart - who's giving you one now?'

'Dad for fucks sake stop it, you know she's dead - I can't

stand anymore.'

'Don't you use language like that in front of me. It's as well.' Then nothing. Briony could almost see the connections falling out inside him as he sat back with a look of fogbound affront that, in it's turn, faded away to leave him pulling absently at his plum colored jumper. So maybe this was the answer; shout at him and you'd get a brief blurt of sense then some peace. Briony breathed more deeply and began to feel better then the adverts finally gave way to a trailer for the evenings highlights. A familiar face showed itself behind the bar at The Rovers. In a surprise twist to the recent three-cornered affair, which had ensnared Jack, Rita and Norris the nations favorite barmaid would be making a surprise 'return'. As she fled the room in tears a triumphant but short winded 'see for yourself'' was followed by further rebukes for a partner who, her daughter was certain, had never committed adultery.

The dope was hidden in her grans old Mazawatee tea caddy. She felt that Old Nandy wouldn't mind given that she was fond of barley wine and Black Cat cigarettes. As she stretched for the caddy Briony felt the stool beneath her wobble slightly and shifted her weight to stabilize the arrangement. It came to her that if she did fall and broke a few bones they'd have to take her in to hospital to look after her - it might not be so bad after the shock and initial pain. She'd broken an ankle at college and it hadn't hurt much although she had been well pissed at the time, she couldn't really do that now. If she got her act together though and took a header off the draining board just as the social worker rang the bell he could call an ambulance then see to her Dad. As they were borne towards opposite ends of the street that would be it. They'd have to keep him then and by the time she was better he'd be used to it anyway. Just some finite pain then the healing stainless purity of hospital linen, far better than the sapping slow-drip misery of what they'd come to.

She consulted the round red wall clock and began to cry

ASK ME NOW

again. It was moulded in plastic and had marked time in the house almost as long as she'd lived, an object of bright lets-do-it fifties technology that had helped measure what had happened to happen. Bought possibly by her Mother on a special trip up the town with her in tow and maybe a younger Nandy, it was like a wedding photo or a faded slice of younger time - the hands moving in one direction but indicating another. The different configurations of the hands suggested firm associations too; four pm was home time in summer and happy, four am the Sylvia Plath hour, ten to nine was late for work and six at tea time was Daddy's home. The news now was that Mr. Duright 'from the social' would be due in five minutes so she'd have to rethink her escape.

She looked again at the clock and recalled the day when there'd been a minor earthquake; afterwards her Dad had gone round painstakingly fixing things. Briony reached back up carefully and unhooked the clock, there were two hairline fractures where the frame had cracked and been glued back together. This started her off again, had she been allowed to help, hold the pieces together for him ? It was just the sort of thing they might have done. She had a clear memory of digging potatoes with him and being encouraged to slice worms with the blade from the garden spade, the two halves writhing in affronted disarray. Her Mum laughing as she told him not to. The clock had outlived its time and carried its history with it. It was the kind of artifact design buffs called iconic and she could see why they might. Without spelling it out everything about it told you it was post-war but pre-sixties, serviceable and discreetly modern. The red plastic fanned out cleverly to make it seem bigger than it was - having this in your home in 1958 stated that you were usefully stylish, smart yet durable. It was nearly time, if her Dad settled at this place maybe he'd like it in his room. She composed herself to look in on him.

He was still in his chair staring slack jawed at the television.

There was a gardening programme on and she could tell he wasn't tuned in to it because at one time he'd have been carping at Alan Titchmarch or pointing at the poinsettias. Now he just looked at it and if you watched him you'd see something wrong behind the eyes, internal agitation like a mad clock whizzing every which way or a stymied windmill with all its works worn away. It was even worse when his mind fell back into place for a bit, she thought he must know then and willed it all to trip back into confusion for him. She tried to make herself believe that without memory torment couldn't root properly.

'The social worker'll be here shortly Dad.'

'Has he found your Mother then?'

Briony pulled in a sharp shaft of air and placed both hands decisively on the chair back facing him. 'Mr. Duright came last week and he's coming back today to take you to see a nursing home called Sweethaven - to see what you think.'

She had become increasingly candid but he surprised her when he regarded her calmly and said. 'I remember.'

'What? Mr. Duright calling?'

'Yes, from the social - shiny shoes.'

Briony couldn't recall this detail and decided he was making it up. The bell buzzed and she steeled herself. Alan smiled tightly as she pulled back the front door with a little mock flourish; he went straight through while she stayed where she was toying with the notion of standing there till she could close it on them both as they left. When she did join them Alan was sitting in the chair facing her Father with one foot resting on his other knee. He had on new Doc. Marten shoes in lustrous ox-blood, the beige rubber soles caught the light sideways as he dangled his foot.

ASK ME NOW

'The social worker's here Dad.'

'Have you seen her.?' Asked Mr. Prince.

'Dad, he's come to take you to Sweethaven. To have a look.' She was just about holding it together and thought that if the kindly almoner didn't start earning his money she would take the dog and leave them to it. Charlie just lay in his basket content to nap away another day as he twitched and grumbled through dreams of wee soaked nettle and unlicensed liberty. His number was nearly up too.

Alan said. 'Shall we go then' and stood up decisively. The older man gave him a look of damp vacancy but pulled himself forward and before she knew what was happening they had passed out of the room and were threading their way down the concrete steps - the social worker a gently solicitous guide - towards a red car missing its offside wheel trims. She hurried after clutching her Fathers smart green jerkin and new cap, arriving just in time to see him strapped safely into the front seat. Alan looked over as he closed his door to say that he would ring her when they got there, indicating that she should shut her door and started the car. Her Father just looked ahead. She stood back on the kerb and they were off, she found herself waiving into space as they disappeared and a little girl on a bike at the other side of the road waived back at her. Briony went back up to the front door, pulled it shut behind her and flopped down in his chair to wait for her call. Cleo Laine pitched up on the screen before her and started belting out 'This Can't Be Love'.

Back across town the two oldsters held on to their seats and fell to talking about the bits of Alison's input that had stuck - enough to register the basic premise. Someone new was coming to stay, a gentleman who hadn't worked at any of the DIY emporiums of the North West. 'They want us to put him right.' Counselled Bert.

'Oh.' Said Harry as he hauled himself towards the television to switch it back on. 'Not her again.' He muttered as the Southeastern songbird segued into 'Green Dolphin Street'.

'Leave it on Harry, she's good she is. Her and her old man - he must be on if she is.'

'Bloody racket.' Harry was not a music lover. 'Her Acker Bilk started it all then that lot came over and took it up, bloody nonsense music.'

'It's not nonsense if you listen Harry and it's Johnny Dankworth. Cleo and Johnny.'

'Might as well be Frankie and Johnny - it's all the same to me.'

Bob gave him a long suffering look then the genial saxophonist joined his melodious chickadee on screen to tell them that it was time to pack away the music until next week and say goodbye from Cleo and 'all the boys in the band'. Then another voice, coarser and less deferential drowned him out and the colour came back as further archive footage of 'Thames Valley Hep Cats' was promised for later. This brief trip down Cleo Lane caused Bob to drift into a reverie of his own. It featured a significant other out with a friend while he had the house to himself at ten thirty on a Saturday morning. His new Nixa extended play record by the Buddy Featherstonehaugh Quintet was spinning forth sounds of poised nobility, his cup of Indian Prince had cooled to the perfect temperature and he was about to ignite a pipeful of Sweet William. He was looking forward to a pint with his mate before they went off to watch Bury play Darlington, both teams 'vying for the right to be crowned overlords of the

ASK ME NOW

Third Division (North)', a pale winter sun was making the cat stretch on the rug - Saturdays; sleep, sport, slippers and se...

'Bloody repeats.' Rasped Harry but he was powerless to get up again now.

There were times when Bob was very nearly happy, Harry too perhaps - he might always have been a prickly and querulous type. Bob had learned that his pal had run an electrical shop prior to his own circuits shorting out and couldn't help wondering what he would have been like with the customers. Maybe what you got when you reached this stage was a craggier unvarnished version of what had always been there. But that didn't explain the rest of it, the animal noises, shit on the carpet, baby talk at teatime. Why were there times when he was almost happy at Sweethaven?

In the 'conservatory' Alison was trying to manoeuvre a woman twice her bulk out of a wheelchair. The object was to transfer her painlessly to a large wicker chair well padded with cushions. The old lady looked up and nodded as Alison held her arms out towards her and smiled, as they locked arms and struggled up then down then up again they resembled two men powering an old manual railway trestle along a stretch of track in the Prairie States of the New World. They were getting nowhere fast though until the old lady pursed her lips and commanded 'heave duck'. Alison managed to swing her across to safe harbor in the basket seat and collapsed panting into the vacant wheelchair. The old lady was struggling to breath at all so Alison patted the pockets of her cardie where she was supposed to store her blue inhaler. Today it was there and she helped her charge gasp down enough of the stuff to cough back a 'bless you duck'. Alison left her sitting there and tried not to let show just how difficult she'd found the whole thing.

The manageress came across her sitting down by the

Councilor Coleman memorial Yucca plant. 'You okay Alison?'

'I don't think I can manage Gertie anymore. Her chest seems terrible and that wheelchair's had it.'

'Yes.' Agreed Mrs. Charles. 'We really need to do a comprehensive risk assessment and get another care plan drawn up, remind me to agenda this for the staff meeting.'

'I just mean I can't lift her safely.'

'Well you're the only one she'll tolerate. Ahmed's too rough and the other two frighten her.'

'So what happens when I'm not here?'

'Well, as I say, we need to discuss this at the staff meeting.'

'We can't leave her in the conservatory till then, she'll...'

'Ah, this looks like Dicky with our new gentleman.' Cut in Mrs. Charles.

'I thought he was called Alan.' Said Alison.

'He is.' Answered Mrs. Charles in a way that put Alison right on both the issues under discussion.

As they looked through the glass from the inside Alison and Mrs. Charles discerned two ghosts shifting slowly into the frame. Then they stopped and began to recede, Alison said. 'He's changed his mind.'

'Well.' Said Mrs. Charles. 'The last time this happened they simply drove round the block a couple of times and had another go. The old chap never looked back second time around.'

ASK ME NOW

'Who was that?' Asked Alison.

'Mr. Collier.'

'Oh, Bobby the footballer.'

'Yes - don't ask to see his medals - hang on there's something happening in the car park.'

The shuffling forms began to fill the frame with a surer sense of purpose this time and the women timed their side of the dance to open the door just as the other two left the gravel to touch down on the smooth red tiles by the entrance.
Mrs. Charles said. 'Hello, you must be Mr. Prince.' He gave her a puzzled if-you-say-so look and asked her to call him Bert.

'We forgot something.' Offered Alan by way of explanation but no further details were brought forward at this point. The delicate business of getting the new admission over the doorstep was handled with practiced aplomb by the manageress who still managed to perturb Bert further when she asked him to call her Teddy. He did, though, take Mrs. Windsor in his stride when she hoved into view and admonished him for not making himself known before crossing the portals. He smiled and told her his name was Bert as she sailed off on her search for the Home Secretary.

'I'd like you to meet two of our other gentlemen Bert.' Said Teddy. 'We can brew some tea and they can tell you a bit about life here. Alison will introduce you.'

They'd reached the office by this point so a smooth separation took place as Teddy and Alan nipped in as the others ambled along to the ladies lounge.

'What's it like?' Asked Bert.

'It's all right.' Said Alison.

As he allowed her to lead him past a room full of people doing nothing Alison was relieved to see that Bob and Harry were still reviewing the television. If they'd gone their separate ways it could have taken some time to round them up again. Best start with Bob. 'Ah, hello. This is the gentleman I was telling you about - Mr. Prince, this is Mr. Rhule and Mr. Rockett.'

'Harry and Bob.' Said Bob confusingly.

Bert didn't speak and seemed to have suddenly lost the thread. She thought it had been going too well. 'I'll pop and put the kettle on.' She said briskly and gave his elbow a gentle brush as she passed him.

'Here, sit you down.' Said Bob, wishing that Harry would find his tongue for once.

Back in the land of sandalwood and social care the two caring profs. were talking about the new gentleman as Teddy perused a comprehensive looking social history. 'Most of this comes from the daughter you said?'

'Yes, she's had a rough time with it all.' He replied.

'Mmm, he's not very old at sixty four. With pre-senile onset it's a bad outlook. Didn't you see her first or something, a two for the price of one deal from old Doc. Watson?'

'God.' Gasped Alan. 'You'll be seeing him in here soon. Sent in a referral for her - you know; anxious and depressed, not responding to Prozac with a brief reference to family stresses. When I contacted her she said she'd rather see me at home, which is generally a bad sign, then when I got there it all

ASK ME NOW

came out. She'd moved in to care for him, the boyfriend had dumped her after six weeks of it and she'd been sitting on it for the best part of eighteen months. It's probably unfair to criticize the GP - I don't think she told him much so by the time the possibility of help appeared she was desperate.'

'As you know we generally like to meet the rellys' as soon as possible. Will she by coming today?' Asked Teddy.

'No. That reminds me, I said I'd give her a ring.'

'How is she then?'

'Better than she was but all this will affect her one way or another. Him liking it here could be as bad as not, if you see what I mean.'

'Not really, no.'

'Well, they're very close, she's an only one and they had her late on. She chucked her job to look after him - what will she do without him?'

'Mmm.' Teddy sounded sceptical. 'What was she doing, before caring for him I mean?'

'She was a potter, her and the boyfriend and another one had some kind of co-operative thing going so maybe that's retrievable. Apparently she knows Claire Todgers though not well.'

'Yes, well - anyway, lets just see how it goes today.'

In the Ladies Lounge the television was off and Bob was asking Bert where he lived. Then, before he could address this question, Harry asked him if he liked acrid milk.

'No I don't care for that.' He replied with some feeling.

'He means Acker Bilk.' Put in Bob. Which puzzled Bert even more.

'You said it was that other fellow.' Protested Harry.

'No.' Said Bob. 'It was you mistaking Johnny Dankworth for Acker Bilk.

Bert suddenly got his bearings and piped up 'Humphrey Lyttleton' with fleeting authority.

'Oh. now your talking.' Affirmed Bob.

'Is he another one?' Queried Harry.

'Yes and he's on the wireless as well.' Said Bob.

This rang a bell with his doubting friend. 'Ah - daft beggar, hasn't got a clue. Acts the giddy goat with Sunita.'

Bob grew testy. 'Oh listen. It's not him who's clueless and it's Samantha, Sunita's in Coronation Street.' It rattled Bob whenever Harrys grasp of their shared enthusiasms seemed to slacken. He'd lost it with his absent-minded mate once and shouted that 'if the sun and moon should doubt they'd immediately go out'. He hadn't had a clue where he'd picked that up from but Harry Rocket had just looked at him, lifted his chin slightly, and said 'appen'.

'My wife's gone to Wetherfield.' Said Bert.

Bob looked at Harry who asked Bert if she liked it there. Before he could reply Alison swept in steering a hostess trolley that caught Berts wandering eye. 'Would you like me to pour now or let it stand a bit?' She asked.

ASK ME NOW

'I think we'll manage.' Said Harry. Bert sat back stiffly and looked anxiously at the television.

Alison felt she should wait discreetly until the tea was poured and busied herself gathering up some stray magazines and a post-graduate level jigsaw puzzle of the Stoke-On-Trent Garden Festival. By the time Alison got the bits back in the box three cooling mugs of County Council blend Assam were as safe as they were going to be and she left them to it.

She came across Alan waiting for the stair lift. A frail looking lady was on her way down and had reached roughly half-way, she was sitting quite calmly hands folded across her lap bearing a look of kindly tolerance. When she reached the bottom he stood back a little and made as if to help her out but she waived him away and beetled off nippily enough.

'Do you know Mrs. Ovenstone?' She asked.

'No but Teddy asked me to keep an eye on her.'

'Isn't Ahmed about?' She asked a bit more pointedly.

'I don't know.'

'Right, well, thanks anyway.' She paused then said. 'You look as if you fancy a go.'

'I went ski-ing with the school once to Scotland and that was enough. Bit of a Godsend here though I should imagine.'

'It is.' Said Alison. 'But it's a great clunking thing, like something in a factory. Look, the teeth are all greasy along the runner. It's about thirty years old.'

As he took a closer look he saw what she meant. It was all

frayed and manky along the inside edges of the carpet and the contraptions functional grey paint was chipped along metal band. However, like Mrs. Ovenstone, it looked likely to last a bit longer..

'How did it go with Mr. Prince Alison?'

'Well I got them introduced and the tea dished out - I think they're still down there. Mr. Rhule's generally pretty good, if there are any difficulties he'll come to find us.'

Alan nodded with one of his serious I-should-imagine faces and observed that they seemed to make the place as human as possible. Alison did know what he meant but was getting a bit tired of his well meant chit-chat, she wondered if this was why Mrs. Charles called him Dicky and if it shouldn't be Divvy. 'Why don't you pop down in about ten minutes, the tea should still be warm.'

Alan thought he'd use up some time by walking in the gardens then returning via through the back door. He could remember a grey steel coloured affair from his last visit leading directly into the kitchens, which had been helpfully propped open with a bag of sugar. It had been a cold day so his glasses had misted over as soon as he'd hit the humid interior. A bellicose cook had waived a pan and asked if she could help him and it had been an uneasy passage to the calmer waters of the corridor beyond. It was a warmer day today though and he felt confident that the panhandler have forgotten him.

Outside the weather had begun to brighten and he found himself in a lesser known area of the grounds where Rose Bay Willow had seeded close to a couple of small headstones. Stained and listing they stood their ground and as he looked more carefully blackened inscriptions gave him some names; Lucky and Robert - two 'grand old lads' who'd pranced and sniffed through better days when the place was new and people just died before they grew too old. A later day Robert had been to pay his respects and Alan looked for somewhere suitable to wipe his shoe. The best he could do was to replace dog-shit with soil but as he rubbed at this with a dock leaf he found that the rims on his rubber sole offered ideal sticking points for the stuff. He got down on one knee to work his fingers ferociously through clean grass.

From the vantage provided by an upstairs window of the building a head and shoulders appeared to watch a younger man lay crimson flowers in the dogs cemetery. As the man outside stood to look with awkward reverence at his feet the other dropped his gaze to the window ledge then disappeared.
'Fuck.' Muttered Alan. Then. 'Shit.' Then. 'Sod it.' He glanced at his watch; all this had taken two minutes. The best course would be to walk about a bit more, watch were he was going so that by the time it was time to go in his shoe should be clean. As he looked over towards the front door it opened letting Alison out. She stood sideways in the porch proffering an arm crooked at the elbow, and then a hand emerged from inside the building. It seemed to stay there frozen against the grey stone for an unusual length of time before anything else happened, but Alison stood her ground and very gradually a small bent woman in a large yellow coat with brown checks inched out into the light. They walked together along the gravel towards a slate coloured bench. As he moved towards them he caught the old lady's reedy pipings, something to do with 'blackamoors' which he assumed had some connection with the coloured lad he'd seen earlier. It all sounded pretty neutral, you didn't come across many reconstructed attitudes in these parts, or much oppressiveness either. Just a blurred world of tethered chaos where words broke free of their moorings and imagination was loosened by uncertain memory. She was trying to sing as he moved away - 'Land Of Hope And Glory'. He did the decent thing and left his shoes in the porch reasoning that nobody would bat an eyelid.

'What's happened to you?' Asked Bert as he rejoined their little group.

'Oh, I went into the garden.' He said.

'I think he means your shoes.' Offered Bob.

Bert looked at him. 'Oh, I ,er there was muck on them.' All ready Alan could sense the older mans attention breaking up and he looked away from him and noticed a portable compact disc player on top of the television. He asked them what they'd been listening to.

'Nothing.' Said Harry Rockett and gave Alan his bland smile.

Bob rubbed his corduroyed thighs with a slightly bogus gusto. 'Nothing yet but you might like this, eh Bert?'

'Can I join you?' Asked Alan.

'Be our guest.' Said Harry, who was nearest to the telly. 'You can switch it on.'

Alan leant across their curmudgeonly companion to rest a finger lightly on the play button. There was a light ping sound then more ordered sound. Beautifully ordered sound; a dancing abstract piano traveling light over pulsing bass and drums and then he knew what was coming next. The antithesis of incapacity, intense rubbery and galvanic, throat-pinched joy forced through a rhythm that made you laugh out loud. Charlie Parker caught, if he wasn't mistaken, by producer Norman Granz in New York around fifty years ago. This lot would have been in their primes then. If Parker hadn't died soon after this record had been made he could have been sitting with them hearing himself playing 'Nows The Time'. He wondered if this was like what might be going on for them now. Their minds fluttering like loose recording tape, catching fleeting snatches of what happened once and getting

ASK ME NOW

it mixed up with something from five seconds ago, their psychic landscapes orchestrated by John Cage.At any rate, Charlie Parker seemed to be bringing them to some kind of shared point in time. The next track was a version of 'I Remember You', which Alan remembered from a Frank Ifield hit. This recital was clearly superior but, he was surprised to find himself conceding, not that much. If Parker had lived he might have tackled 'Waltzing Matillda', maybe Norman Granz had suggested this and hastened the be-bop masters demise.

'What do you reckon then?' Asked Bob.

'Didn't Cliff Richard sing that one?' Asked a puzzled Harry.

'I don't know, probably, but what did you think of that version?'

'Not bad.' Allowed Harry.

'I thought it was great.' Enthused Alan. 'What did you think Bert, Mr. Prince I mean?'

Bert had been looking at Alan's socks throughout but nodding in time to the music, smiling as the thump and ticker of Max Roach's drums came through towards the end of the arrangement. 'Can I go home now?' He replied.

'What about some more hot music?' Asked Alan and looked hopefully at Bob Rhule.

'Hummpff.' Said Harry.
'Good idea.' Said Bob. 'That one he made with Helen Shapero. I'll step and fetch it.'

Alan was becoming confused himself now. At this rate they'd be getting Ronnie Scott meets Alma Cogan, and where did the resourceful Mr. Rhule keep these treasures? What on earth was he doing here at all? Bob returned with his CD of the Lyttleton band and its special guest and they passed a further forty minutes as the radio renaissance mans effortful trumpet accompanied Helen Shapiro's robust contralto through a sprightly set. At the end Bert recrossed his legs and adjusted his posture. Alan, getting a bit desperate by now, decided this was a good sign and tried to catch his eye and test him with a smile. Bert wasn't having any of this but did tap a foot as the last tune kicked off, 'Keeping Out Of Mischief Now'. Bob was obviously enjoying himself, Harry looked anaesthetized and probably didn't mind either way. Alan decide to go and see Teddy. 'Would you just excuse me for a while?' He lingered in the doorway just in case. No one spoke but as he turned to go the lady from the garden appeared before him and let it be known that she wished to get past. He made way as she swept into the room and addressed Bert directly.

'You must be the new gentleman.' She stated.

'Hello.' Said Bert calmly enough.

'Who are you?' She asked, incredibly rudely it seemed to Alan.

Bert composed himself. 'My names Prince, Albert.'
She regarded him coolly for what felt like a long time then hummpfed like Harry. 'Never heard of you.' She said. She then asked him if he'd seen Lord Roberts and dismissed him with an imperious wave when he said no.

Harry reassured him. 'Take no notice, that ones puddled - no harm in her though.'

Alan hung around just beyond the door for a bit then judged it safe to nip off. He hadn't heard Bert Prince say anything else, nor had there been any sign of futher movement. He went in search of Teddy and found her in her office looking over a

ASK ME NOW

drugs chart. 'How's he doing?' She asked without looking up.

'Hard to say. It was a good idea putting him in with those two - Bob Rhule is it?' He seems to be putting him at his ease.'

'Yes, God bless him. Music appreciation is it?'

' Charlie Parker. He seems so much less off it than the rest, how long has he been here?'

'About three years.'

'He could have another fifteen years yet. What's wrong with him?'

'Now you're asking.'

'Well ... what's he on?' Asked Alan nodding to the pile of charts on Teddy's desk.

'Nothing much.' Replied Teddy. 'A homeopathic dose of anti-depressant and some 'Shift-It' for his constipation. When we admitted Bob he was on all sorts, practically catatonic. He'd been wharehoused in sheltered accommodation and started to decompose.'

'What about family?' Asked Alan.

'What about them.?' There's a son who is a musician in America but that's about it, as far as Bob's concerned this is the last chance cafe bleau and he's cute enough to work his ticket accordingly.'

'It's terrible how easily that can happen, especially to men, how frail the foundations can get. If we can't make it stick with Mr. Prince I don't know ...'

'You off to see the daughter then?'

'Yes, I thought I'd go now if that's all right.'

'Leave your phone on.' Advised Teddy.

After hearing from him Briony had unplugged her land line and returned to the kitchen where she'd watched next doors poplars languid swayings as whisky and three nurofens brought about a similar lullaby-of-the-leaves quality in her. By the time Alan rang the bell she was feeling quite composed, if disinclined to rise. She held on to the door a bit like before and nodded in the general direction of the front room. Following directly this time she sat down straightaway in the chair her Father had occupied and gestured with an open hand to the settee. As Alan took his place she smiled, paused, and asked him if he wanted a drink.

'No thanks.' He said. 'I've just had a cup of tea with your Father.'

'Yes.' She said. 'Right, well, he's still there then.'

Alan thought she seemed a bit gone out, and reasoned that she must be exhausted. 'Were you worried he might not be?'

'Well.' She said. 'You know ...'

'I know you've had a rough time of it but I'm pretty sure that if he stays till tea-time we can get him to go again.'

'What if he wants to stay after tea-time?' She asked.

'Lets take it one meal at a time.' He replied.

Briony laughed at this, a bit more fulsomely than it merited he thought, then stopped suddenly to fix him with an appraising look. Alan felt a bit abashed by all this and asked how it had

ASK ME NOW

been for her.

'Horrible.' She said.

She shifted her attention after telling him this. He followed her gaze to find himself looking at a framed photograph on a sideboard. It had to be her parents although he struggled to marry the dignified looking chap in the picture with the hare-brained retiree he'd led away earlier. The woman was familiar from countless anniversary portraits; smiling quietly with a kind of demure defiance. It had been them against the world and, like Mary Tyler-Moore, they'd reached that stage where they might just make it after all. Like every such image it was universal but unreachable. You could sketch out the theme but you couldn't get the picture or know any inside variation on the story. It would be as mysterious as life on Mars or Alzheimer's disease. Alan had clocked up a fair bit of experience, personal and professional, of separation, loss and the ambivalence of dependency so he could essay a rough idea of what Briony might be feeling. Off to the left of the silver frame two elegant pots in a soft brown glaze stood a little awkwardly.

'Are those yours?' He asked as he nodded towards them.

'What? Oh yes - they're waiting to go out.'

'For sale?'

'No, I'm sorting out a lot of stuff - I'm not sure what's happening with all that.'

'You've not been able to do much work recently?'

'No. I just haven't felt like it, you know.'

'Does your Father enjoy listening to music?'

'He used to. Why?'

'Someone put a record on when he got there and it seemed to help him settle, a bit.'

'Just lately the only thing that would settle him was watching for Mum on the telly.'

Alan let the silence grow a little then asked her again what had happened.

'Heart attack, massive - went in one go. He found her flat out on the kitchen floor, told me afterwards that she'd been getting pains round her chest for months. We had a big to-do about that, you know, not saying anything about it, then after about a year he started seeing her on the goggle box. First off it was Fern Britton but now it's Bet Lynch then he gets his delusions mixed up and confuses her with another barmaid off Corrie' who advertises sofas now. I think he thinks that I think it's his fault she died and that I'm wrong because she's just left him. Maybe she threatened to, I could understand her coming to it.'

She pulled ineffectively at an almost empty box of tissues till it came up with the last ones stuck in a clump at its mouth. As she waived the whole arrangement like a floppy cardboard yo-yo Briony swore and wept. The tissues were finally disinterred and she scrunched the container, coloured an aggressive pink, on a bamboo table by her chair. Alan glanced again at the picture frame. Her Mother looked knowing and empathic as if a sliver of soul had been caught in the frozen light and looked out over the sad unravellings of her old front room. He inclined his top half towards the sideboard again which, now he looked at it more closely, was a lightly varnished piece of fifties furniture which chimed in well with the bamboo tables and worn leather settee of a type put together when Linda Barker circled the ether with text

ASK ME NOW

messaging and Tony Blair. Like the people who bought them such sideboards were made to last, he couldn't bear the thought of it set out in the rain at the council tip puckered by rain, the last bits of fluff and scrapings lodged inside escaping to be lost again.He didn't usually consider himself of a spiritual bent but he liked to think that after it was all over we came together again as aspects of soil or particles of plants, making a more useful contribution to the eco-system. Or maybe we all got sucked screaming into Linda Barker land to be respun into whatever terrifying material she makes up her sofas with. Just lately Linda had been bothering him in other ways. It was those adverts; she would wander wraith like through them as an awakened princess with but little understanding of the treasures set out before her. She would caress a chair wonderingly as if such a fabulous thing could never be, pause astounded by brilliant sunlight filtered seductively through the libidinous glass of patio windows then rest gobsmacked on a pure white settee. She would struggle to summon words fit to bear witness to it all. 'I like it.' She would say. 'I think you will.' Briony seemed to be having a Linda Barker moment when words clogged in your mouth like sopped tissue. 'When was that picture taken?' He asked.

'That one? Not that long ago - within the last five years probably. I can remember that cardie.'

'Was it a special occasion?'

'Not really. I was seeing this bloke at the time who was a photographer and I thought it would be nice, you know. It's probably the last one of them together.'

He could see it was well done. They didn't look cross or coy, the lighting was natural and clear from a window to their right. He guessed the daughter was behind the cameraman, both subjects looked back at the lens with poised, slightly quizzical expressions. They were clearly returning something valuable to the lens. Her old Dad looked a handsome fellow with his tie and Greenwoods wind cheater - a fleshier Dennis Norden without the eyebrows.

'It's a good picture, I think.' He said.

'Yes.' She said firmly. 'It is a good picture.' And looked at it a bit longer. 'They'd had their ups and downs you know but they were all right, as far as I know anyway.'

Briony said this in a shrugging sort of way that Alan recognized as a distant cousin of anger. He reckoned on not upsetting her anymore than she was all ready. 'When did you first notice anything might be wrong?'

'With Dad?'

'Yes.'

'Well, it depends on what you mean by wrong. The earliest memory of what I now see was a sign of what later became something being wrong with him was not long after that picture was taken.'

'You said your Mother might have been covering up for him.'

'Well, not covering up so much, not at first anyway.
Maybe you don't immediately think someone's losing it just because they're sometimes not quite themselves. And that's all it was at first. For me I began to wonder if there might be something else happening one May Bank holiday. We went to Southport to play pitch and put, he'd liked his golf, but this was the most he and Mum could manage so I went round with them. About half-way round Dad got the ball and put it back in the hole we'd just played - we thought it was him having a laugh but there was another couple playing that hole by then and when they tried to sort it out he started shouting. It was

ASK ME NOW

awful but Mum seemed to know what was going on and ushered him off. I felt terrible taking the clubs back but the other couple hadn't said anything. When I rejoined them Dad looked a bit winded and Mum said something about people getting hold of the wrong end of the club, I think we had lunch then went down to the beach. That's when I knew really.'

'How long after this was it that you lost your Mum?'

'About two years, or was it more recent? Then it wasn't long before he started shouting at her on telly - and swearing. That's the worst thing; it's just not him. There are times when I look at him but I just can't see him anymore. Isn't that awful?'

'People in your position often say that, it seems to be very unsettling when a bit of the individual they were slips through. He seemed quite settled this morning ...'

'Oh yes, yes he was but then again that's not him - all quiet and docile. I almost wanted him to shout then. What's it like this place ... Peacehaven?'
'Sweethaven. It's pretty good I think. The basic care there is very sound but what really makes it good for me is that the residents are accepted, often to a degree which could look a bit odd.'

'So you'd send your Granny there.' She said then moved on before he could begin bull-shitting in earnest. 'Presumably the people who live there are a bit odd anyway?'

'Well yes, there's a woman there who's gradually drifted into a delusion that she is Queen Victoria. There is a loose connection ...'

'Sounds it.'

'No, I meant with the apparent break from reality. She had married a man called Windsor and people called her Queenie. Also, she ran a local history group at one time and remembers lots of stuff about the nineteenth century. There's really no point now in putting her right.'

'But it is a delusion - doesn't it bother the others?'

Alan felt he'd better play that one with a straight bat. 'Doesn't seem to. Many of the others are lost in their own little worlds anyway.'

'I see.' Said Briony a bit doubtfully. 'I'm not sure, you know, that he's going to like it there - it's all a massive upheaval and shouldn't they be trying to make life more ... tranquil?'

'You mean medication?'
'Well yes - it is classed as a nursing home isn't it, a bit like a hospital?'

He could see they were heading for more formal grounds where he'd have to be less loose with his speculations, more reassuringly professional. 'It's joint funded by health and social services and a number of the residents are on regular drug treatment, to enable as much quality of life as possible.'

'Mmmm.' Mused Briony, then. 'I have to say I've become quite a devotee of tablets since my own peep round the bend. I'll nip and put the kettle on.'

He thought she seemed better, seeing that CPN must have helped. He sat back and looked more closely around the room; if you took out the gauche industrial size television which was tooled in grey steel it could pass as an imaginary set for a fifties radio play. Something set on the Isle Of White, Julian was home for the holidays and the dodgy foreign bachelor was coming round on his bike to give him extra

ASK ME NOW

tuition with his German. His own son had perished during the war and Mummy encouraged a relationship which others on the island thought unwise. Alan dismissed this reverie when Mummy began to resemble Linda Barker then Briony returned with the tea.

'I didn't ask if you took sugar.' She said setting down two mugs. He noticed that she spilled both without seeming to notice. He gallantly flourished a clean tissue but she told him not to worry. He dabbed away regardless and decided this gave him the right to probe further.
'Do you still see the bloke who took the photograph?'

'Why?' She asked evenly.

'Well, I was just wondering who was there for you. You know, it's obviously been a bad time.'

'For my Father - it's not me who's going off their onion.'

There were a number of sallies Alan could make at this and he was very taken with the image hinted at. Your sense of self being peeled away layer by layer till it was all gone, which was how it seemed to go unless nurse pneumonia did the decent thing and carried you off a bit sooner. Common sense told him to slurp his tea and await further orders. After a further ninety or so seconds of quite acceptable silence a lightly scraped pattering announced further life beyond the living room door. It happened again.

'Do you mind dogs?' She asked.

He shook his head and smiled but she was all ready up and heading for the door. 'Come on then droopy drawers.' She sighed.

An ancient yellowish Labrador waddled in and fixed Alan

with a glassy, red-rimmed stare. It must have once been a spring-heeled hunter, keen for walks and petting, now it looked like Ted Heath in old age; pop-eyed and splenetic. It was as well that Charlie couldn't speak; his views on welfarism might have be as challenging as his breath. As if reading Alan's thoughts the dog snorted and lolloped back to his basket.

'He took to you.' She said with a straight face.

He told her about the canine cemetery at Sweethaven and she asked him if he wanted to take the dog too. 'No, no.' He said. 'I was just ...'

'You were asking me about my private life.'

'Well, I was just ...'

'It's all right. You want to know how I'll manage, if I've got an informal carer or something. In terms of blokes the photographer faded away not too long after our little photo session. I do see him sometimes and he was sad to learn of Dads decline but as you'll have picked up from my chilly front the weathers been crap in that particular quarter.'

'You're still seeing Estelle?'

The Community Nurse? Yes she's been a help - what's really not helped was being dumped by my new man who couldn't cope with my old man. Don't be put out, I generally like men, but you have to admit, when it comes to the mucky jobs it's us that get lumbered. It must have been hell for Mum - watching him go like that.'

'You might have had the worst of it.'

'I don't know. I can't help thinking my Mother had more to lose and that it killed her - that he killed her. Anyway, at least

ASK ME NOW

once he really started to slide things began to happen. I'll never forget the relief when the doctor gave me those pills for him. They were more for me, 'to take him off his feet'. Christ, you could block out whole days. I came close to sampling them.'

Alan had a sudden thought. 'Have you still got them here?'

'Yeah, but if I ever get that desperate the railway lines not far. I never wanted to die anyway, just give it some of the old Madame Bovary.'

He was properly out of his depth now, Briony seemed to be floating beyond his orbit. Did this old Madame have a mad Dad.? 'How do you mean?' He asked.

'It's a fairy tale thing - she wanted to slip into continuous slumber and, I suppose awake to find solvency, a constant lover and friendly shopkeepers.'

Alan decided to busk along as best as he could. 'Is that what you need?'

She laughed quite naturally at this and said. 'Well, I'm not sure which would do best. How long has he been there now?'

The bakelite clock on the wooden fire surround said two which meant not far off three hours. 'Mrs. Charles at Sweethaven has your number so she'll ring if there's a problem.'

'Shit.' Shouted Briony as she moved with surprising stealth into the hall. 'I switched the phone off.' She said as she came back more gradually.

Alan tried not to look alarmed as he said. 'Oh well, I've got my mobile on, they can get me if there's a problem. Were there any messages?'

'Briony seemed puzzled. 'Can they do that if it's not on?'

'Yes, usually.'

'God it's hopeless. I got him that phone in just in case and neither of us knows how it works.'

Their impressionistic moment had passed and Briony seemed about to cry again. He registered a firm impression of how useless she felt and tried not to let it overwhelm him. 'I suppose the reason I was fishing around for information is that it seems to me you've been very much on your own with all this. If your Father does stay for an extended period - well, I was assuming you might not want to be on your own.'

'I'd have to stay here for the dog, unless you can book him in too - have a proper clearout.' She began to cough and left the room in search of further tissues.

Then Alan's mobile went off. It's mad chirrup ('The Yellow Rose Of Texas') was muffled by his bag but his reflex apology made him feel daft so that when he answered Teddy Charles asked him if things were going badly. 'Nono.' He said. 'She's pretty upset but it's all right. Why are you calling anyway, is there a problem?'

'No, not really a problem as such.' She said. 'But if you could ask his daughter for a record - I assume he means a compact disc - he wants to play for the lads in the Blue Room.'

'What? Does he want it now?'

'Please.' Confirmed the matron in her best 'well what do you think?' voice.

'Okay, what's it called and I'll ask his daughter?'

ASK ME NOW

He could hear boxy sentences coming in and out of range at the other end as Teddy conferred with, he guessed, Alison. 'It's called 'Out To Lunch' and it's by a chap called Acker, no .... Eric Donkey.'

Alan couldn't take this in at all. 'Do you mean Eric Dolphy?' He asked bluntly.

There was more muffled debate at Teddy's end before she came back with a clearer grasp of what was required. 'Yes that's it - Eric Dolphy, what a lovely name.'

'But how's it going otherwise?' Alan queried in his mildest tones thinking that things couldn't get much more, what was that word he heard Nav use - random.

It didn't seem to ring a bell with Teddy 'Oh fine.' She said. 'They're still listening to records in the lads lounge and someone else has just joined them.'

And now they wanted 1960's free jazz. 'I'll see if Briony can find it and pop back, it's about time I showed my face again - he's alright though?'

'Yes, hasn't said much but he's still here.'

'Fine, see you in a bit then.' He was beginning to feel like Sven Goran Erikson. If Bert was still in the building then they could build from there, if he stayed for his tea they were through to the semi-finals. Anything more would be a bonus. It was the stage following a Michael Owen opener, all very well but they needed that second goal. 'Out To Lunch' though, was somebody having a laugh? It was one of those records he'd heard about but never listened to. It had once been voted number one by the cognoscenti in his hipster's quarterly music magazine and this had put him off straightaway.

After a longer than he'd have thought absence for a hanky Briony returned, still coughing but looking much calmer. 'Sorry about that.' She said, favouring him with a very nice smile in the process.

'It's all right. That was them.'

'Sweetbriar? Is he on his back then - his way back I mean?'

'No, no. They phoned because he wants some music taking over. They've got some kind of hot record club going.'

Briony seemed to take this in her stride and Alan wondered afresh at the strained life of a caring relative. Perhaps you simply got past caring, when he couldn't think of anything else to say he looked at her. She returned another smile in his direction but seemed to be struggling with a similar difficulty. She came to and blinked decisively. 'He wants one of his records, which one?'

'Out To Lunch' by Eric Dolphy. He likes modern jazz then?'

'Yes, poor Mum had a lot to put up with.' Briony made her way directly from sitting to kneeling then moved forwards on all fours to the period sideboard wherein many compact discs were neatly stacked. She began speaking to Alan but addressed the furniture. 'I remember one really bad morning. I'd been required to sit through three hours of tantrums and Cecil Taylor, in the end I gave him one of his tablet number nine take off for the planet oblivion drops and took my mind off it by sorting this lot into alphabetical order. I know they don't know where Dads trouble comes from but listening to all this stuff can't be good for you - aren't most jazz musicians a bit radio rental to begin with? Some of this stuff - I mean, here we are B for Braxton. Jesus only a bloke could like this - Christ his pianist's called Marilyn. 'At this her

ASK ME NOW

shoulders began to move and he cast around for the Kleenex but when she turned round with a CD case in her hand she was laughing and asked him if he thought it was Marilyn from Adam And The Ants. He felt loathe to leave her, grief affected people in many strange and paradoxical ways after all, but he'd already accepted the role of 'cross town record hound. 'Will you be okay?' He asked.

'Oh I think I'll be alright now.' She said with confidence. 'You nip while I have another crack at this cupboard.'

As he turned back at the door he could see that she was still on all fours with her head and shoulders inside what was a surprisingly capacious space. Seen from this angle she reminded him of his mates English Bull Terrier, the dog liked to stand with his head poked behind drawn curtains for long periods of time. 'I'll give you a call.' He said.

'E is for earache.' She replied.

Across the town at Sweethaven Alison closed the office door behind her while Mrs. Charles pushed some numbers on a phone with her thumb while she looked at a letter. In the corridor outside Alison came across her colleague from the morning rota who passed on that Gertie had asked for her again. She also asked for further details of the Italian campaign. Alison made up some business about a heroic resistance unit loosely based on a film she'd seen the previous week, which had depended on plucky British soldiers and went about her tasks with a heavy heart.

The post-lunch crash had upskittled most of the larger group room. Three of its four sides housed snoozing lizards lost in a soothing reptilian slumber. She sometimes wondered if they had dreams where they could run and drink from a cup with one hand and how awful it would be when they woke up and remembered. This part of the day was usually pretty quiet but

Gertie still liked to get about the building when the mood took her.
'Right old girl, let's be 'avin you.' Alison said, rolling her sleeves in mock stevedore mode. The old girl laughed, then coughed, then wheezed and went a bit blue around the mouth and sank back stricken into the cruel bamboo. Her carer remembered then that although Gertie enjoyed a joke you had to pick your moments. 'Sorry, here, sit for a bit then we'll get you up and doing.'

Gertie sat forward till her breathing steadied and deepened then thrust forward her arms defiantly and said. 'Steady as we go.' Alison grounded herself, secured the wheelchair - there'd been an unfortunate incident before involving Gertie, a faulty brake and a left open door - and joined hands with the living.

'After three - ready?'

Gertie nodded and her flickering torque joined forces with Alison's heft. With neither party shifting their footing much a deft delivery was effected. Gertie said 'thankyou duck' and Alison managed a wan smile - her own granny had been a Lincolnshire land girl during the war and spoken fondly of manhandling 'great bags 'o tates' in the plenteous fields. She was minute but nippy, why couldn't Gertie lose some weight?' 'Where to now?' Asked Alison.

'I heard some music before.' Said Gertie. 'What's happening?'

Alan looked in the office as he passed and waived the CD in Teddy's direction, given the thumbs up he proceeded to the blue room, falling in behind Teddy and her charge along the way. 'Has Mr. Prince started a jam session?' He asked.

Gertie seemed disconcerted by this 'What's he say - jam special?'

ASK ME NOW

'No Gert, he's on about the music.' Put in Alison with barely detectable irritation. She felt she was beginning to get Dickies number. Gertie looked doubtfully in Alan's direction and shook her head. When they got there Alison asked Alan to enter first and ensure the door stayed open. His spirits rallied when he came upon a scene enlivened by a calypso from the Humphrey Lyttleton Band featuring Bertie King. The original trio had been augmented by another man in a crimson cardigan called Bimson, he turned to welcome their new member who was already patting the armrest on her wheelchair in time to the music. Bob Rhule indicated a space by Mr. Rocket who looked as if he was almost enjoying himself.

Alan prepared himself to see how Bert was doing. 'Hello Mr. Prince.' He said. The older man looked up smartly enough without saying anything. Alan thought he might be in a different chair now and wondered were else he'd wandered. Maybe they'd simply had lunch and come back, which reminded him. 'I've brought that record you wanted.'

'Ah, let's have a look.' Said Bob and reached across to show it to Harry as well who observed that Freddie Hubbard wasn't Humphrey Whats-his face. 'Don't start that again.' Sighed his mate.

Then Bert said something. 'Harmonically more interesting.'

Well, thought Alan, that was worth waiting for. Harry asked Bob what 'he was at now' while Gertie and Bimson sat waiting respectfully for the treats in store. 'I think he means it's more modern ... eh Bert. Let's have a listen then. Have a seat ... what's he called?' Said Bob to Bert. Alan looked at Bert who tried his hardest but nothing came so Alan sat down and told the group that he was 'looking forward to this'. He'd begun to think that Harry Rocket was more capable than he let on, that it suited them both for Bob to be the only one with enough sense to explain the world and operate compact disc players. He was looking forward to it though, he'd wondered about this musician ever since he'd heard Frank Zappas arrangement of 'The Eric Dolphy Memorial Barbecue' and knew they'd be in for something interesting. Bob did the honours and the music began - or seemed to; there was a shrill piping blurt in the form of a choked fanfare for the brass, then surprised space which seemed to hold a sound that wasn't there, then there was a bizarre parody of march time played by all the instruments and then something incredible happened. The most outlandishly wild and ominously ordered sounds he'd ever heard burst from the speakers beside Berts head - Eric Dolphy was playing a solo on the bass clarinet. Closer reading of the sleeve notes told him the music was nearly forty years old.

He caught Bert looking at him again and found it impossible to divine what was going on behind his watery eyes. It occured to him that the old guy could be all too aware of what was what and be about to denounce him for arranging his humiliation, and after Alan had taken care to facilitate all that choice. But nothing happened again. Alan scanned the notes by the strangely named Bobbi Coolman and came across the phrase Bert had declaimed with such knowledge and authority. It could have been years since he'd last read it but he seemed oblivious to what happened yesterday. Alan hoped he was enjoying this oddly beguiling record, the bass clarinet had blown itself out and the brassy panache of the horn man who wasn't Humph. had given way to a quieter passage for chimes, percussion and softly plopping bass. In relation to the fantastic racket which had preceded it this felt lovely and Alan wanted it to last. The next piece had a similar feel; Eric the bold was still wielding 'the big pipe' as Coolman had it but the overall affect of the music seemed profoundly moving - slow and passionate but very direct and reachable for all its abstraction. The overall effect was suggestive of a freakish threnody. He checked the cover, it was called 'Something Sweet Something Tender' and Alan felt sad to also learn that

ASK ME NOW

Dolphy had died soon after recording it. As he looked about the room he could see that Bimson and Gertie had been touched by the sounds, he began to wonder again about free jazz and cognitive dissonance. If Bert were to stay they might be able to transfer his music library over here bit by bit. Briony could get on her bike each week, the process a rite of passage, healing and redemptive as Father and Daughter grew together apart, and music therapy took off at Sweethaven.

'How much longer does it go on for?' Rasped Harry.

'Oh, there's more yet.' Assured Bob.
'Right.' Said Harry decisively. 'Time for a hit and miss.' And shuffled towards the corridor. As he got as far as the door Alan noticed that Bert was signaling his intention to follow by waiving a hand in Harry's general direction and making as if to launch himself from his chair. He was clearly having trouble escaping the sun boiled upholstery so Alan looked for the care worker who'd delivered Gertie but she'd gone. What did they find to do all day? Bert got himself up unaided by twisting sideways and prizing himself out via the chair arm. He stood panting like the old labrador up from his basket and ready for the off. Harry had been aware of these developments as he hovered discreetly beyond the doorway.

'You too?' He said. Bert answered by waiving an imperious finger which indicated that should Harry care to lead he would follow. An understanding thus established the two men took their leave.

Alan calculated that, given his struggle with the armchair, Bert would be in no shape to escape and settled back for more 'skewed swing and weighty philosophizing' from Eric Dolphy and his Feetwarmers. The selection now playing was a swifter moving piece with more marimba and some bird like flute. 'Lovely whistle on this bit.' Observed Gertie.

The man called Bimson nodded and added. 'Sounds just like that express used to rattle past the end of Surtees Street.' And Alan felt good about all this; for all the cobblers on record sleeves the common listener got there anyway, and this had to be to Eric Dolphys credit. Sweethavens too, in most places this lot would be more likely to be flattened by Kylie Mynogue - they should be so lucky. The band then dished up some more of the skew whiff stuff so Alan decided to see where Bert was.

As he turned into the long main corridor he saw Teddy in the distance bidding a joshing farewell to two men by the door. They were carrying out an unusual amount of clear plastic and brown tape. He couldn't be sure over the sounds of an altercation in the kitchen, but he thought he heard Linda Barkers name being bandied about by Teddy and the men, then Bert appeared just in front of him from a side door bearing a small mounted illustration of a small boy peeing into a bowl. He was followed by Harry Rocket who left his new friend looking around fretfully as he headed back towards the music room. Bert looked blankly at Alan then turned purposefully on his heel to head for the open door. As he got there Teddy came back in smiling to herself, pulled it shut and Bert stopped to look to his left. He then let out a gargled cry of seeming recognition and made a sudden totter into a room in front of him.

Teddy said. 'Oh - Mr. Prince.' Then seemed to think better of it and turned to Alan. 'It's alright, we've just had a new settee delivered - courtesy of the friends of Sweethaven - and I haven't quite decided where to put it yet.'

'Ah.' Said Alan.

'Yes, anyway.' Said Teddy. 'Someone has to sit in it first.'

When they looked in to see how he liked it he was not alone. Mrs. Windsor was seated in Queenly splendour and looked to

ASK ME NOW

be granting Bert permission to join her. His demeanor greatly surprised his social worker; he was standing in a winded fold with hands on knees as he gasped for breath. The old lady began to console him and pat the red leather beside her. She then asked him if he knew Lord Salisbury and as Bert puzzled over which Freddie Hubbard album he'd played on she said not to mind and that he would do. As he settled himself beside her she patted his hand and told him tea would be ready soon.

'She's right about that.' Said Teddy. 'Shall I set him a place?'

Mike Pearson

CLOSE TO YOU

And now we go over to Ambridge where Shula's been shagging the Vicar again.

'Nmnngh gag thoop, eh?'

'I thought I'd turn it on to drown out your snoring.'

'Sorry, here, I'll sit up – have you got another pillow?' Much lifting and effortful shifting as the guest makes himself comfortable. 'It's worse at this time; I think I get unusually persistent colds. I'm generally better by September.'

'Oh well, if I feel like inviting you back I might as well wait until then.'

Alan was getting to know Cindy a little better and enjoyed her mordant wit but there was something not quite right in this, something chiming dully at the back of his mind. Something to do with Shula Hebden. 'What's happening on The Archers, Shula was saying … something when I woke up.'

'I dunno, she was in a tizz over something the Vicar had said – her lardy cakes were flat again I think.'

For Alan an everyday story of country folk meant family Sundays, Adam the Sunday Express gardener next to the advert for Sandeman port, the taste of treacle on Yorkshire pudding. Disturbing his Dad getting his leg over (why didn't he continue on his way over mummy, who looked as if she was asleep, on the journey he was surely making to the wardrobe?) The Pinky And Perky show then Dr. Finlays Casebook then bedtime then oblivion. Alan didn't want to think about his Father after that carry on with Bert and Briony Prince, everyone holding their breath in case he should take it in to his head to run away. He hadn't of course which simply confirmed he really was three sheets to the wind. But was he happy? The business with the sofa of memory and the old Queen coming together to make sense to him. Was that right?

'Do you think History happens quickly Cindy?'

'You what?' Sighed Cindy as she struggled with her bottom drawer.

'Well, you try to arrange your life to handle what you think might happen but the stuff comes at you sideways, then it's done and you have to make sense of it, and sometimes you can't.'

'Yes, well, maybe. Has something happened to Tony Archer?'

'Possibly, but I was just thinking generally.'

Cindy found the top she was after and stood up. 'Alan, you have a lie in if you want, I said I'd see Claire for lunch.'

'Yeah could do, I couldn't get back off again this morning. I can't seem to get going at the moment. It must be old age accelerating on the blind side.'

'What's brought this on? Is it a sex and death thing or something?'

He propped himself up and considered telling her what was on his mind. 'I think it's that bloke I admitted to Sweethaven last week. It was a bit of a soft sell job, but then it usually is, I got enough of a glimpse of what he might have been like before his marbles went. He liked jazz and his daughter told me some things.'

'What kind of things?'

'Not much really, just about him and her and her mum who'd died. There was a picture, I just felt an impression, then he was there in front of me all knocked off and lost to himself. Do they know it's coming or when it's there?'

Cindy sat carefully into her antique wicker chair in just her knickers. 'Maybe there's something built in to blind us so that we don't know till we get there and then keep forgetting. Doesn't despair rely on a memory? Does a dog recognise death? Perhaps it's best not to know.'

'Yes, perhaps.' Mused Alan and lay back. She pulled on a green top; her thick black bob bounced up and out and she shook her head as she stood to get into a pair of khaki cargo pants. He tried to picture her with brittle bones and liver spots but as she leaned over to kiss him goodbye he sensed the firm swing of uncapped breasts and wondered if he'd nap just yet.

Alan eventually resurfaced at noon feeling bad all over. His face ached at vague and scattered sites behind the eyes and a stab of neuralgia sliced across his left cheek. There was a nagging feeling of unease at the back of his mind; a faint version of the jitters he'd noticed before at odd times. It usually scuttled off but seemed to hang around even as he ignored it. His knee was playing him up too but he made it to the bathroom in time remembering to open the window before doing anything else. It wasn't that he believed women shat in lavender bags or anything, it was just that they didn't make such a palaver of it and Cindy's bathroom seemed to reflect this; you came in, did what you had to do and the whole thing was as comfortable and utilitarian as it needed to be. Then there was the male fondness for farts and farting, he was in an ongoing state of giving this up but like a soft-centred recidivist he was regularly letting off one last-one. Then there was the denial – delusion more like – that other people didn't notice or if they did that they didn't mind. Perhaps if he picked his nose more he might fart less, it beung well known that blokes couldn't multi-task. Sexual encounters could bring out the reflective side in Alan; being naked in her bathroom while she was out made him more conscious of himself as all the tellingly personal bits of her pressed home an odd sort of intimacy – the soft green towels, her choice of soap, a straw hat hung on the wall. How did he look in her eyes?

Back in the bedroom he pulled on yesterdays clothes, lay back down and fiddled with himself absently. This was another common pursuit he'd been giving up for as long as he could remember, each time would be the last, the transitory pleasure not worth the farcical shame and more lasting mess. He couldn't reconcile whether men were basically dogs or apes, their lives one long scratch and sniff experience, helpless self-pleasurers waiting for mummy to smear dirty hands with salving ointments. Tommy Smith, the psycho-therapist at work, had spoken of these things one lunch-time setting out with persuasive know-how the male fondness for part-object relating which was in its turn related to the male fear of intimacy. Alan hadn't been sure he'd got much of what Smithy had been on about and thinking about it now he hadn't struggled to grasp the bits of Cindy he'd been only to happy to relate to recently. It was bound to be more complex than that, most things were. He put his hands in his pockets and thought in a very focussed way of the psychotherapist as a whole object. He was plug ugly and fond of blue shirts with white collars and this did the trick for a while. Then he caught sight of Cindy's bangle on the bedside table. He'd read somewhere that the most beautiful part of a naked woman was her face and he knew this to be true, last night had included quite a bit of the social workers Karma Sutra and one or two side orders he hadn't bargained for but what he'd really liked, what had really sealed it together for them was how she looked, especially how she'd looked at him. If you forgot about yourself and disregarded the detail sex really could be wonderful, so was this love? His body seemed to concur and though the Frankenstein image of Tommy Smith loitered in the background the monkey in Alan won the day and he succumbed. As he cast around afterwards for some suitable wiping material the door banged.

'Hi.' Trilled Cindy. 'Fancy some exercise?'

Fuck, thought Alan. If only you'd been ninety seconds earlier. 'Yeah.' He called back. 'Won't be a minute.' He spavined his way across to the bathroom with one hand holding up his trousers and the other cupped slimily below his paunch. As he closed the door with his backside he had to wonder if it had been worth it. He hoped Cindy hadn't meant sex when she'd said exercise, he'd have to put her off somehow.

'You all right in there?' She called up.

'Yeah, well no actually. I think that curry's done for me – just give us a minute.'

'Oh dear. Fresh air's what you need, it's lovely out.'

Alan thought he was getting enough as it was reflecting with a sinking heart how soon daily deceit wormed its way into these affairs. He had another clear up, flushed away the evidence of his sin and gave himself further comfort with the notion that if this Cindy business worked out he might be able to stop wanking and be happy. He skipped down the stairs keen now to set eyes on her again.

'Alan.' She said with some gravity. 'I think last night might have been a mistake.'

Shit. 'Well, I, er – yeah.'

'You do sound bad, anyway I should have followed my instincts.'

'Yes, yes. I suppose so.'

ASK ME NOW

'Alan sit down you do look pale. Yes, anyway we should really have gone to 'Green Acres', nobody comes off second best there.'

'What?'

'That Indian – a bad idea. Look at you, come on you can walk it off.'

'Right … what's Green Acres?' And now he did feel properly poorly. Cindy seemed a very modern girl and treated everything with an equivalent weight of seriousness so that where you went for your tea was intuited on a similar plane as who you went to bed with.

'Its that new vegetarian place on Portland Street – part of the Green Judgement set up. Claire told me about it.'

Right thought Alan, should have known. 'I thought you were seeing her for lunch.'

'I was but her mobile went soon after we got to the pub, someone had overdosed at The Lindens – so, do you fancy going out this afternoon? We could go up to the Moors, I'll drive if you're off it.'

He felt a total wanker now; if women were from Venus then men must be from Macclesfield and had he really imagined she'd want to jump straight back into bed with him? She'd left him alone and he could hear her muffled movement as she passed across from bedroom to bathroom. He was able to identify the strappy slap of sandal on lino then a headache scrape of window sash raising by no more he reckoned than six inches. There was a pause; flushing cistern and running tap then the gathering creak of antique stairs before Cindy presented herself before him. He thought she looked lovely with her green fisherman's jersey and just washed flush, as he stood up she came forward to embrace him without saying anything. For all last nights honking and bonking it seemed to him the most intimate thing they'd shared. They remained like this for almost a minute before Alan felt he should say something. 'Are you putting any socks on?'

Cindy pulled away looking a bit put out. 'You what?'

'Your socks – you haven't got any on. Aren't we off for a walk?'

'Oh.' She said matter of factly, disengaging from his curry-flecked fleece. 'There's a pair in the hall by my walking boots.'

'Right.' Said Alan. 'It does look nice out.'

As they sat in his Punto he gave Cindy a run through of the controls while she adjusted the seat and patted the mirror. 'It's a bit like that Fiat I used to have.' She said. 'Except the indicator's on the other side.' After more twiddling and similar comment she got the ignition going and reversed out. He watched her working the pedals in her socks and the stretched line of her neck from behind where her hair fell back as she twisted to see behind her. It was true, he thought, that you always felt more vulnerable as a passenger, more aware of the hard clash between unforgiving surfaces and softer packaging. He looked again at her firm strong feet pumping the controls, a driver had too much to think about plus the illusion of control to feel frightened. She effortlessly elided the stiff clutch with the accelerator and moved them into the Sunday lunchtime traffic on Haslington Road.

'Do you ever get fed up of driving Cind.?'

'How do you mean?'

'Well just every day, you know – up and down the road, stuck in traffic. Getting in and out all the time.'

'How else are you supposed to get anywhere? It's like housework, it simply needs doing, besides, it means you can get out on a Sunday when you want to. Al.'

'Oh yeah, yeah I know really. It's just that faff on on Thursday then having to get to that tribunal at Rampton the day after.'

'That sounded like a bad one – the admission, what happened?'

Alan gave this some thought, trying to knock together a narrative that didn't make him look too daft. 'Well the chap had calmed down quite a bit by the time Dr. Wallace and the GP had done their bit so it was decided that an ambulance wasn't necessary. I would drive him over to the ward with his Father coming along to make it all right.' Cindy was looking ahead frowning slightly so he continued quickly. 'And I think that's good practice whenever you can swing it, as well as good use of resources …'

'But that's what they're there for.' Protested Cindy.

'Yes but its a bit heavy end for the old service user – and they can take ages to turn up.'

'Tell them it's an emergency.'

'What and have them turn up with their sirens wailing?'

Cindy changed down to let a lorry past. 'So what happened then?'

'Well, it was half-six by the time we got going and it was bumper to bumper on the by-pass and he was getting agitated again so I took us round by the County Ground but there was a game on ... so we got stuck there and his old man asked me how long I'd been qualified. I should have called the ambulance really.'

He hoped the note of contrition would stop Cindy probing further. In the end, which had taken a further forty minutes, he'd had to call them out anyway to ensure safe passage for a by-then dangerously deluded patient. It had all been glossed over when they finally got to the ward and Alan had been accorded hero status by the nurse in charge who'd probably heard the unedited version by now. 'Oh well.' Nurse Norris had said. 'These things happen.'

Two cars that had pulled up untidily ahead of them had diverted Cindy's attention. As they drew closer he could see a huddled group looking horribly vulnerable and exposed as they stood around their vehicles. As far as he could tell no one was badly hurt and the cars wore only slight crumples but he experienced an angry kind of shock that was like spotting the top shelf of the newsagents.

'You've done that before haven't you she said.'

'Done what before?'

'Risked it without an ambulance.'

'You don't always need to and it's often better not ... '

'Oh, sure but you'd probably have done better with one the other night to begin with, then there was that time with the man in the camper van. He was hypo-manic wasn't he? Could have done anything.'

'But he didn't.'

'But you couldn't have known that. Estelle couldn't believe

ASK ME NOW

you'd taken such a risk.'

'She would. It's all right for pissing CPN's they don't have to take on stuff like that, God help us if they ever give them powers under the act.'

'Alan, my point is that you don't have to do stuff like that. It's the Inspector Frost approach to statutory social work – a male approach if you don't mind me saying so.'

She took them past Gibsons auto wreckers and out towards more open country. Alan tussled with a familiar goblin within; of course he didn't mind her saying so, why should he? She'd said it anyway; at least he didn't turn up late for dates in a greasy old trilby. 'You mean feeling we have to sort out an immediate answer to something?'

'No, not that – a situation like that clearly needs sorting out, it's more ... the caped crusader bit. Do you think Catwoman would have done it like that?'

He quelled an unkind caveat about it depending what was on telly that night and conceded that, no he supposed she wouldn't have.

'Estelle said that old chaps daughter was very impressed by you – you know that chap you took to Sweethaven.'

Cindy was very fair minded he thought. 'Briony Prince, she's a right character do you know old, well he's not that old really, her Father turned out to be a jazz fan? Piles of CD's stashed away in an old sideboard.'

'Did anyone else like it?'

'Don't think so, not the daughter anyway but it turned out that another chap at Sweethaven did.'

Cindy thought about this. 'I really liked that one you had on yesterday, it seemed much friendlier than most of the stuff you usually have on.'

'Monk.'

'Yes, I liked that – it sounded as if they were having fun.'

So where were they going? The Moors then back home, then where? Back to bed, to see her Mother? Would she want that window fixing or a lift to the shops?

'How're we doing for petrol Alan?'

'Should be all right, I filled up on the way back from Rampton.' He saw her look anyway and noticed with a heavy heart that he was all ready half empty again. Had she looked before she'd asked? He seemed to spend so much time with women wondering what they were really asking him or if what he'd just said was what they wanted to hear. His last proper girlfriend had explained that so much of it came down to a fundamental gender split in ways of communicating and brandished a surprisingly slim volume on the subject by some Canadian woman by way of reinforcement. From this he'd learned that men asked questions from a position of testing or establishing dominance while women wished to clarify things or request information. This led to confusion and deep-rooted mutual incomprehension. She'd been a football player who'd had trials for Bedlington Terriers and rubbed home her point by playfully winding him. But he liked women; he'd always liked them and in his more reflective moments considered it a small miracle that they bothered with men at all. If he was a woman he wouldn't. All this Cindy stuff had caught him off balance; he'd known she liked him and he'd always fancied her but why hadn't he made his move before now? He had wondered at one time about her and Claire Todgers but Graham had put him right on that one when he told him that

ASK ME NOW

'Cinders, was 'doin' a bit' with a smooth junior doctor they'd had on placement once. He wondered how best to seek clarification on these points.

'We're not far now Al, where do you fancy stopping?'

'Isn't there a National Trust place round here somewhere?'

'Probably – yes up ahead a couple of miles.'

'Good, right, we'll be able to get a cup of tea before we start.' He said.

He felt her smile at this and the rest of the short drive passed in companionable quiet, as if they were practicing for the kind of trip they might make in twenty years time with some tea all ready made up, a blanket and a dysthymic west highland terrier who wasn't that fussed about his walkies anyway. They passed some bored looking sheep idling in a field, and then he saw the moors climbing ahead of them and some brown signs indicating the visitors' centre. Cindy seemed to know the way and rattled them slowly over a cattle grid into a wider road dotted with ramblers and similar souls who wandered about as if motorists didn't exist. They seemed to him a smug set of passive-aggressive types with their excruciatingly reasonable behaviour and scruffyposh country wear. He reminded himself that the middle classes had their rights too and managed a few fierce 'good afternoons' to people he'd never met before as they scrunched their way across the gravel. He suggested they walked first and had their tea later, in case the weather changed.

'That's a good idea.' Cindy said. 'I'll just check to see what time the café shuts.'

To reach the main walk taking them upwards to the wilder parts they had to pass through a wooden gate opened by a complicated metal clasp fixture. It took Alan a couple of goes to work the thing while an annoyingly sociable couple waited on the other side passing suitable remarks about the complexity of the mechanism and the wildness of the weather. Cindy laughed quite naturally and nattered politely while he fiddled. As they passed on their ways he asked her if she'd known the couple.

'No.' She said. 'Why.'

'Just, you seemed to recognise each other.'

Cindy looked at him sideways and said she was simply being friendly. 'Do you think formal introductions would have been more in order?'

'No of course not, it's just it's sometimes a bit bogus, you know – but it's easier to do it than not to – even if it is a bit dishonest.'

'I think we had a conversation a bit like this before, you've got this idealised notion of authenticity or something. There's a connection with Brenda Blethyn isn't there?'

'Oh yeah I know, I sometimes get a bit Will Selfish about all those feel good films.'

'You said they were pornographic in their way.'

Alan winced. That sounded about right. 'I suppose they are pretty much fantasy. I mean, you don't look to films for much else.' They had found a comfortable pace and all ready the bits of Slaithwaite below were looking like croutons scattered about an untamed tablecloth.

'Well.' Observed Cindy. 'I think films are like anything that tries to dramatise what happens in the world; some of it gets close to our experience and some of it doesn't. People might not believe in 'Billy Elliott' but it's something to aim for – a world where it could happen. Incidentally I think there is a dancer who started out from a place not too far from the kid in the film.'

'Maybe he had a Julie Walters dance teacher.'

'Maybe he did.'

They came to a big flat rock by the path and sat down without speaking. She leaned against him as he used his arm as a support for them both. She undid one of his jacket buttons to put her hand against his chest. 'I can feel your heart pumping.'

'There's hope for me yet then.' He said.

'Alan, you seem to get cross about these things. How do you feel people should be portrayed?'

'I suppose a bit more warts and all. It seems to me that the more the sunnyside is pushed the more you can't help wondering about the other stuff. Isn't sentimentality the superstructure for brutality or something ?'

' Is it? But would we want to see that?'

He held her a bit more firmly and she pushed a bit further in, he felt himself beginning to respond. They stayed like this for a while and he began to pick out detail on a larger stretch of land which, if he'd got his bearings right, should lead across to Huddersfield. 'That's Saddleworth Moor over there isn't it?'

Cindy sat up to see. 'Yes, I think it is.'

He squinted to try and see more but at that moment another

walker drifted past, they exchanged painless enough 'hellos' then as the other moved off he had the effect of wiping the view clear so that Alan could see better. There was something there he didn't like; there were no dots of life moving and the place carried a dull greyish flatness. It looked a place you wouldn't want to go. Another couple, with a chid – a girl he estimated, no more than twelve, came back down towards them. He didn't venture a greeting this time, as they were pre-occupied with something funny the girl was saying. The man squeezed the girl closer, her small head tucked behind his shoulder, and she laughed again. Alan looked back across to the landscape in front of them and his breath shortened. Cindy felt this happen and asked him what the matter was.

'It's Saddleworth isn't it over there. Saddleworth Moor.'

'Yeah.' Answered Cindy.

'Where they think that kid's still buried.'

'Somewhere over there, he could be anywhere.'

'Didn't they let him out once – he was going to show them where to dig?'

Cindy stayed where she was, talking into Alan's tailored donkey jacket. 'They didn't find anything. All it stirred up was more slow torture for the families and the umpteenth hoo-haa in the papers.'

Alan now felt bad about his twitch of arousal and felt he should sit apart from her. He remembered a photograph he'd seen of Brady and Hyndley frolicking in a field like lovers do; they were laughing at whoever had the camera and she was trying to get away from him. He looked handsome with his thick bushy hair and a poplin shirt; she had on a cheap patterned dress. They could have been anybody. The image had shocked him because it suggested things that were sealed

ASK ME NOW

off by the two police mug-shots which everyone knew; she gormless and guilty with her awful bee-hive; him whey-faced and pasty looking with a mouth that seemed to say cruel. The frolic in a field picture was slightly unfocussed but it showed them alive and potent, normal. This was what bothered him – Brady was usually described as 'her lover', was this how it started? He was Cindy's lover – where might this go? What sort of muck festered at the back of our minds? Was it only a question of time before the tape recorder and the shallow grave? He'd recently bought an old bri-nylon shirt from Save The Children.

'What are you thinking about.'? She asked him.
'Them. The Moors murderers, do you think anybody goes up there now?'

'Yeah I should think so, people forget then there are the curious.'

'They could be walking over that poor kid.'

'Who knows what we're sitting on here.' She said.

Alan straightened up but held on to her hand. 'I was thinking about the newspaper pictures, that's all I can think about really not, you know, not what they did. Sitting here looking across, it just seems mad. Or maybe it really is evil – the Ripper came from just over there. They tried to say he was a paranoid schizo. Didn't they?'

'Did they, I'm just glad they caught him – eventually.'

'Christ, do you remember his mug shot – his beard and that bubble perm?'

'I do actually, I remember people being intrigued that he was good looking.'

Alan looked into the distance again. 'The child they never found, do you remember his picture?'

'No. I thought they did find him when they dug that time.'

'No, they didn't find anything. Brady was just taking the piss probably.'
'What about his picture?' Asked Cindy, looking directly at him this time. 'Have you seen it recently?'

'He's about ten with a knitted balaclava and National Health specs. He's laughing, must have been his Mum took the picture.' He kept on looking at the distance and pictured old Thames Trader vans and boxy sixties saloons, their head lights raking the murk, a bad man digging his way into the collective unconscious.

'It really bothers you.' She said quietly.

'Yes. Doesn't it you?'

'Yes, but perhaps in a different way.'

'How do you mean?' He asked.

Cindy thought for a bit while she blew her nose with a soft churfing noise, which involved releasing his hand and sitting up quite formally. 'Well, I suppose that you feel it more personally …'

'Because I'm a man?' He said flatly.

'Well, I don't know – maybe. I'm not getting at you personally, besides he wasn't on his own was he?'

'No but it was him really wasn't it – Brady, Sutcliffe, Fred West, Donald Neilson. Never trust a man with bollocks eh?'

ASK ME NOW

'I think that's a big mistake myself but the difficulty is that some men are like that and it's hard to tell.'

'Well yes, okay but what if we are all more or less capable of going that way, or if we're not but everyone thinks so anyway?'

'By everyone you mean women?'

Alan gave of the air of a man struggling with an inner conflict and said. 'Yes.'

'Well.' She said. 'I can understand that but I'm glad you're a man Alan and do you really think I'd be here with you now otherwise?'

He managed to not notice the subtle strains of a yes-well-run-along-and-wash-hands-for-dinner-now edge to Cindy's patient peroration and felt free to ventilate more of his inner fires. 'I don't know whether it's a kind of generalised gender guilt or what but I get so pissed off and scratchy about the way it seems to go. You know, like we're all potential monsters or something – I feel that what they did was just unimaginably awful, I mean how much further can you go – I mean … fuckin' ell.' He hesitated but Cindy seemed content to let him have his say. 'When she finally snuffed it there was a few of these what's-it-all-mean? Doodahs on the radio, although the one I'm thinking of might have been on the box, anyway they'd got old Dea McKenzie on and she was pushing the line that women like Myra Hyndley – I think she actually called her Myra – were indeed hapless foot soldiers recruited on account of their vulnerability by these men who could spot a helpless victim when they saw one. I couldn't help wondering if it wasn't the other way round.'

He looked carefully at Cindy who said. 'I'm not sure where

we're going with this – I suppose with these deadly partnerships you have to wonder if either one of them would have done it without the other and perhaps that's how it works with couples anyway; the peculiar chemistry making a marriage work for fifty years or fester into a pair of sadistic monsters. Without her Ian Brady might have been just another low grade shitbag but that doesn't make it her fault.'

'It doesn't make her a victim either.'

'No. No it doesn't, it's just more complicated than that and, if you press me, I'd have to say that without him I believe she'd have had a fairly familiar flat, passive and unhappy life.'

'Sometimes inaction can be power, it wasn't her who shopped him.'

'Wasn't it?' She said. 'You seem to know more about it. I can't help noticing that for all the interest these awful crimes generate it's the women everybody talks about, whether they're vixens or victims. I could never understand why she wanted to get out of prison, she wouldn't have lasted five minutes, the newspapers would have run her to ground inside twenty four hours.' Cindy took a breath and blew her nose again. 'If you really want to know what I think, I would bet she was a powerless, needy and probably abused individual … but that doesn't mean he was all there either.' She put her hand back on his leg and said. 'Do you think we've come far enough?'

'Eh, oh yes – what time does the café close?'

'Four thirty, its now a quarter to.' Said Cindy.

Alan looked back across Saddleworth Moor for the boy with the balaclava and wanted to hold both of Cindy's hands, help her up with maybe a kiss at the end of it but let her rise unaided. The walked back to the shop and Alan's heels began

ASK ME NOW

to rub on the uneven ground. 'I could do with a cup of tea.' He observed lamely.

'How's your belly?' She asked him.

'Bearing up, how's yours?'

'Mmmm – I think my periods due.'

Alan felt favoured by this discourse; it returned him to the surprising nature of intimacy – how shared moments uniting details of latent diahorea with budding menstrual blood could bring together a woman and a man. He was certain Cindy wouldn't share this with just anyone, well maybe Claire Todgers. God only knew what passed between those two over the Special Brew and candyfloss. 'Sounds like there was a bit of a crisis at The Lindens.'

'Yes, that reminds me I must phone Claire. Have you got your mobile Alan?'

'In the car.'

On the way back Alan advised a man struggling with the gate who told him it was 'needlessly arcane'. He smiled at this and made a note to remember it for Graham. The aggressive shale gave way to smoother slabs then Cindy went to get the teas in while he fetched the phone. They parted by a building resembling a Swiss chalet that put him in mind of a model one they'd had at home. It had lived on a Welsh dresser next to the Greek urn from the Bishop Auckland branch of Woolies and when you lifted the lid it played a madly syncopated strain from Strauss. He'd seen it quite recently during a visit to his mothers where it had been transplanted to a remote window ledge. He'd lifted the lid to a silence, no one had wound it up or else the spring had gone. Home really was so sad. He opened the passenger door and was touched when he saw the drivers seat pulled forward; he decided to offer to drive them back. The phone was in the glove compartment, as he fished it out he selected a cassette copy of 'Monk Live In Europe' to put on later.

Once past the dark wood doors of the visitor centre Alpine charm gave way to a briskly functional entrance area with an information point. The gift shop to his left had just closed so there would be no stylishly embossed biros to take back. Through some swing doors ahead of him Alan saw Cindy sidle carefully away from a till with a brown tray. She couldn't see him and as he watched her glide carefully across to a corner table he felt an exquisite tang of something deeply troubling. He could hardly bear to bring it to the front of his thoughts; it was a cold, fleeting but powerful impulse to rush through and push her over. It was barely an image or a worked out idea, just a cold bad possibility that came from nowhere. It was the last thing on his mind. He really didn't want it squirting out with Cindy. As he neared the table she was inverting a saucer over one of the cups. 'I didn't get us any cakes because of your ... you know.'

'Oh, yeah – here there's still a fair bit left in the battery.'

She took a little while to acquaint herself with his mobile then phoned her friend. Alan sipped for a bit then took himself off for a tactful piss. He returned after about four minutes and sat back down with a discarded Mail On Sunday, Cindy pursed her lips at him to indicate complicated doings at the other end and said 'right, about ten if I can' before returning his phone with a sigh. 'Trouble at Willow Gables?' He ventured.

'Yes. I'm going to try to get over tomorrow to see her. Could you cover duty for me till lunch?'

'Sure.' Nothing ever happened on Mondays. 'What's happened anyway?'

ASK ME NOW

'One of the residents took a serious overdose, they're over at the General now – it's touch and go.'

Alan wondered if it might be the woman he'd got in the other week and asked if it was anyone they knew. 'No the chap concerned came from Puddingdale but he has a family connection over this way and hopes to be re-housed locally.'

Alan found this odd. 'But someone from the team should know him – Claire wouldn't take someone without a key-worker. Dr. Wallace must have agreed to be RMO?'

Cindy gave him her tired look and told him that the respective consultants had shared a phone call, a fax had materialised and a transfer agreed. Cindy didn't know for certain if anyone from Northfield had ever clapped eyes on the individual in question, let alone set about the process of engagement.

'Claire must be pretty fed up.' He said.

Cindy sniffed and nodded. He felt he should make some kind of contact across the table so he stretched to shape a hand round her bent elbow. She smiled, he said. 'It's like at work, watching the trolleys trundle across to the morgue – the only end of life being there all the time only you don't see it.'

'I'm not with you Alan.'

'Well, someone must have found this poor guy ...'

'Couple of kids, down by the cow parsley – he was actually very lucky.'

'But they weren't and that's my point. It's like us up there suddenly realising where we were then having to face it.'

Mike Pearson

'Sometimes it's best not to.' She said.

'Sometimes you can't help it.' He replied.

Cindy put down her cup and mirrored Alan's hold on her arm with hers. 'It seems to really bother you.'

'Doesn't it you?'
She looked directly at him. 'Only if I think about it.'

'You make it sound like there's a choice.' He said.

There was a lot of finished-for-today noise coming from the kitchen as plates were clattered and cutlery spangled from dishwashers. A young woman appeared from behind a swing door to survey the room, they were the only punters left. Cindy smiled in her direction and said 'nearly done' so he stood to faff with his buttons as Cindy helpfully stacked their pots for the girl.. As they walked out into the car park he overheard voices from the other side of a small opened window letting out warmer air; 'might as well go self-service' someone said in wounded tones.

He offered to drive and she made herself comfortable as he slipped in his cassette. By the time they'd reached the A640 to Milnrow Cindy was snoozing along to a freakish lullaby set forth by Thelonious Monk and his merry men. It was called 'Ugly Beauty' and its heartbeat implied a balanced stagger across great distances, it seemed so right in itself that the band just had to play it as written to project the affect. This was a live version though and the sax player took a solo sustaining the mood miraculously over several choruses of blue rinsed invention then Monks tinkly piano took charge, with what he'd read somewhere was 'much spidery chromaticism', to bring them back to the theme. There was the tumbling sea sound of distant applause from some discerning Italians then they took off on a more conventional swinger called 'Well You Needn't' which offered space for all the men to have their say. The drummer got a solo on this one, flutterbumping like the clappers causing Alan to clap the steering wheel in time till he realised that, well he shouldn't. At that moment he felt happier than he had for ages, in the film of his life he would be (a happy) Timothy Spall and Cindy would be … Kate Winslett? Kirsty Wark? Diedre off Coro.?

'Ernmmm.'

'What say ducky?'

'You what? Where are we anyway?'

'Just coming round the 'Dale. Home soon.'

The by-pass took them past the round lights of Ridsdale spotting out the line of the conurbation. He liked it like this; dim lit with vague shapes appearing then subsiding sketching out lines that never became clear. Monks music was the perfect soundtrack for this subterranean half-world, very occasionally human shapes would move in and out of corporation yellow, vehicles would whiz by on their way somewhere. The line of traffic slowed to a halt allowing him to look across Cindy toward the back of some sort of factory unit, the tape had come to an end and without the feeling of movement Ridsdale seemed much less allusive. All he could really see through the mucky wire fencing were a dirty white fuel tank, yards of shut up workshop and random piles of metal draining the light from a security lamp. It still seemed better to him than it did in the daylight.

'What are you watching?' Asked Cindy.

'Oh, just what's out there.'
She looked, winding down the window. 'What, what's out there?'

'Yeah, I like it in the half light.'

She coughed as she wound the window back up. 'It reminds me of 'Erasurehead' I think David whatsit must have come round here for inspiration.'

'Oh right.' Said Alan. 'The squelching chicken and the rotten baby – some folks imaginations.'

'Yes, well Alan, believe it or not I'm hungry.'

'Shall we stop at that chinky at the end of your road?'

She struggled with this for a moment. 'Just get some chips – I'll heat up some pasta sauce.'

He began to feel uncertain of his way again, like a boy with his mummy. He'd known Cindy would never say chinky but he hadn't since he was fifteen and feeling up lasses behind the youth club. He remembered the girls; they all seemed to wear that perplexed and puzzled 'well-if-you-really-want-to' look that sometimes played around bigger girls faces, like Cindy's. He'd had one of his big-boy-now chats with Tommy Smith about this and learned that it was another aspect of object relations theory. He'd recalled that the rough kids at the club had evolved an entire lexicon for girls parts which drew on their parallel passion for motor mechanics; adjusting her plugs, giving the cylinder head a seeing to could denote any kind of sexual activity short of a full service. It had been widely believed that Howard Green had really shagged Linda Ford and words had fallen short of celebrating the lovers tryst until someone had pointed out that Fords were always real goers. Greenie had gallantly bottled this kid and for all anybody knew might still be committed to the lovely Linda. He wondered what kind of school Cindy had been to. All girls he hoped. An old man shuffled past pulling a faded poodle then a group of youths pitched up on a street corner making a bad noise as they tried to sound older. Ordinarily his

ASK ME NOW

sympathies would be more or less with them, he knew where they were coming from, that there was little real harm in them but just at that moment he wanted to shout them down, humiliate them, take the trouble away.

'Little boys.' Remarked Cindy evenly enough.

The take away was lit up in blue with a full-length red curtain in the window, Cindy stayed in the car as he went to place their order. A bored Chinese kid behind an inclined plywood counter wrote it down and held out his hand for the money without comment. Alan waited on an incredibly comfortable hardboard sofa to watch the end of Corro' and wondered vaguely if Tracey would slap Karen for adjusting Steve's points in the previous episode then the chips came through in a neat brown bag with handles. The kid met Alan's eye this time and said 'there yare mate' without a trace of the Orient. He noticed then that the place was called 'Kung Food' and wondered how many people had been. He smiled then and was rewarded with a seasoned 'see ya mate'.

They tootled back to Cindy's little house before their chips could cool and were soon tucking in by the gas fire in her front room. 'Ah, just a minute.' She said and put her plate of gooey red fries to one side. Before he could empty his mouth to ask anything she pressed a button on her new looking music centre. It gave out a high-speed whir, clicked to a stop then began to play automatically. The Archers theme began its clog dance from Hades out of the tiny but resonant speakers.

'How did you ...?'

'It's this gadget. I can set the tape to record for as long as I want to while I'm out then stop as soon as I've got what I want. Alan couldn't be bothered to hear any further details so nodded as interestedly as he could and remarked judiciously on the deliciousness of the supper. Cindy nodded with her mouth full and they settled into a companionable huddle as the early evenings broadcast from the land of lardy cakes and set-aside manure unfolded. It transpired that Neil Carters cat had gone missing and Pat Archer had neglected to cancel the papers prior to a fortnight at Sheringham. Also, Caroline and her new partner were looking to the future. Alan felt moved to comment. 'She doesn't want to come on all precious and ambivalent just yet.'

'What do you mean?'

'Well.' He said dismissively. 'She's always been like this, makes Shula seem astringent but underneath she's very calculating.'

Cindy thought for a bit looking evenly at the curtain pole. 'You don't always like women very much do you.'

He felt his chest go a bit tight but she wasn't looking at him as she felt around the side of her chair for a tissue. She soon gave up and wiped her fingers on her jeans. He affected an air of settled reflection, quite up to the challenge she'd set. 'Well, I wouldn't say I dislike women … I mean I like you, but that's not what you mean, is it?'

'No.' She said after a pause. 'You've still got loads left, aren't you hungry?'

'Oh, here, have some.'

She munched on with her faraway face and seemed happy enough with the way things were going so he piped up.' Do I come across as one of those men who fear you but dress it up as something else?'

Cindy sucked her teeth till a satisfying sthpop sound slapped softly from her mouth as an impacted particle of chip shot

ASK ME NOW

back down with the rest. He experienced a sudden unwelcome memory of his mother eating bacon when he was a child; how she'd pull the fatty bits from his plate and gobble them up, sometimes in her dressing gown. He knew now why his father took his through to the back room. His brother would prattle while mummy ate the fatty bacon, he didn't like them much. Not then. 'No.' She said. 'Not like I think Graham might do.'

'Well that's something.'

'It's just that you do seem to carry a bit of a chip, you know what I mean?'

Not as much as some of the women I take tea with he thought. 'Here, have a few more.' He said instead.

'You sure?'

'Yeah, my appetites gone - I don't think I've properly got over last nights yet.' And what about tonight? It was work tomorrow and nothing had been decided, signposted or otherwise settled on. Cindy seemed oblivious to the whole thing and began stacking plates, piling papers and generally getting things tidy. She left the room with sundry items for the bin bag balanced on the plates. What did she want him to do?

While he pondered a short recital came through from the kitchen; the sleek cushioned shimmer of a bin bag taking in papers cued in the sound of a tap then the tight muffled click of an electric kettle. He liked to listen to free chamber music and imagine outlandish domestic doings but it didn't seem to work the other way round. It wasn't The Wireless Workshop Group in there and the sounds were too closely tied to whatever else might happen. If one way to understand people was to listen to the silences between them where were he and she heading? The kettle clacked off and he picked up china being arranged, Alan thought he'd fish out that Lester Young record he'd lent her with 'Tea For Two' on it then thought better of it. Instead he picked through her neatly racked collection; Lester was there but so too was 'The Carpenters Greatest Hits'. He considered Karen Carpenters moony aspect and her goofy brother with his footballers feather cut from 1974 then flicked forward through a predictable trawl of classical stuff, a fair bit of opera, the soundtrack from 'Twin Peaks', Talking Heads (cool), The Eagles (oh dear) but nothing to disarm a discerning hipster such as he.

She came back in with a wobbly wicker tray and motioned for him to put something on. He toyed with 'Twin Peaks' but it made him think about the moors murderers again so he slipped out the box for 'The Four Seasons' but there was no disc within and the line of CD's fell forward partially leaving Karen Carpenters importuning maw at the head of the queue. It would have been like kicking a kitten not to choose her.

'I didn't know you liked The Carpenters.'

'Why should you?' Fair enough.

'Your 'Four Seasons' is missing.'

'Oh it's probably in the player.'

Of course. He stretched finger and thumb to get it out and replaced it with a plink in it's jewel case. As he closed it an artist's impression of Vivaldi appeared, he was poring over manuscript paper like Tom Hulse did in 'Amadeus'. It didn't seem to suit the music that always seemed to him finely tooled charm and languorous poise, but then most Mozart belied the midnight oil. He chose not to share these thoughts with Cindy. On the day the angels …. Waa aah aahhh close to you. Had Burt Bacharach really written all that?

'Crap isn't it.' Observed Cindy.

ASK ME NOW

'I dunno.' He hedged. 'Lots of people like it.'
'You don't like it though do you?'

'No, not really, don't you either?'

'I wouldn't say I liked it, I've just got it.'

'Why?'

'Present from my mum.'

'Shall I…?'

'No leave it on for a bit.'

As they listened Alan was aware of Cindy connecting with the music in some way. She came over and parked herself by his foot, leaning against his chair. He rested a hand on her shoulder and she gave off a quiet rueful sigh. 'They used to play this when I was a kid – Sunday mornings before their friends from down the road called round for coffee. I could sing it in a squeaky voice and my mother got me to do it along with the record once when they were all there. I think once was probably enough but she remembered and got this for me a couple of Christmases ago.'

All this brought out the librarian in him. 'There's that poem somewhere about home being so sad. Music in piano stools, vases placed where they were when you left years before. Sometimes it's incredibly irritating or a bit frightening, suddenly clapping eyes on chipped door frame you caused when you were ten then sensing for a mini-second your whole life since then siphoning out and away from you like it all never happened.'
'I should bring this up next time you're chatting to Tommy Smith Alan.'

'I think I know what he might say – failure to separate. I'm confusing severance with true separation. Issues aplenty.'

'Mmmm' She said. 'I'm beginning to see why those feel good films wind you up.'

They sat on through the balance of the toothsome twosomes greatest hits – what a lot they'd had – and he learned that this was the first time she'd listened all the way. But how was he doing? He rubbed her shoulder and she yawned then smiled, then said. 'Right, time you were off.'

Right. Okay, fine. Then it seemed to him that he was suited and booted before he could say Anne Robinson and she was embracing him quite ardently on the other side of her doorstep. 'I've had such a lovely day Alan.' She said and kissed his bald head.

For some reason he caught a dim memory of a tea advert and wondered if he should ask for a second cup. She smiled and added. 'You're in at work tomorrow aren't you?'

As he nodded she began to close the door. 'See then then.'

ASK ME NOW

IS VIC THERE?

Alan was sitting in Val Meatings office trying to stop trying to make sense of his Sunday with Cindy. He gradually took his mind of it via a disgruntled dog which leered at him from his managers computer screen. The beast looked more like a clapped out ram rescued from a bucolic Northern high street of 1901. He felt it was a good picture though, the photographer expressed a feeling for the subject, also, the image implied a whiff of wet dog. He could sense the horse muck matted about the mouth, the toxic breath and sopping paw. Val had brought him into work once but an anonymous team member had agended health and safety at the next day's sector meeting. Cal hadn't been sighted since. This could explain the hangdog screen saver.

She entered the room backwards finishing a conversation with Dr. Wallace about anakastic personality disorder. Did her dog have one? She turned in to face him, backed the door shut and spattered a pile of files onto her desk in a way meant to convey that this was the most fitting thing you could do with them. The effect floundered because the files were unevenly weighted for such a roustabout and several fell on the floor where she left them.

'It's all right Alan, I've got your supervision notes here. Thank goodness they're soon to be a thing of the past.'

'Files you mean?'

'Yes, roll out the paperless workstation. I can't wait.'

'Do you think it's realistic, I mean what happens when the systems go down?'

'Well, the Health Trust are taking the lead on this one and they've ring fenced a budget for a state of the art job. I ran into Tommy Pollard at BINSS last week.'

'Eh, are they selling computers now – I know we're taking on private finance these days but I can't see House of Fr ...'

'No Alan. Best Investment In Nursing and Social Services. You must master your acronyms if you're serious about management.'

He laughed at this. 'I'm okay with the daft ones like Personal Initiative Support Team or that one Graham brought back from Harry Kirk House. Something to do with brief interventions.'

Val wasn't seeing the funny side. 'I'm sure it must all seem very risible to you but what's the alternative? We need effective ways to communicate and share information especially now that we're finally working in tandem with that lot.'

Alan took this as an invitation to be serious too. 'Are we going to be getting training from Health? You must remember what a fiasco it was last time when our lot installed the old system; stuff vanished, printers cracked up and someone logged the department onto a chat line which siphoned off thousands.'

'Yes, I remember it well. Tommy tells me this one has firewall security.'

'What is it?' He asked doubtfully. 'Have you heard of it?'

'It's the Nationwide Information Technology System ... and what happens when it spots a problem is ...'

'Val, they can't be serious, you know what they'll say when it crashes.'

ASK ME NOW

'Well, this system doesn't crash ... apparently.'

'So we'll all be getting nits.'

Val looked wistfully at her dog. 'Yes, hmmm. I see what you mean; anyway we'll all have to learn to love it because by next year everything will be on line. There'll be documents scanned in pro-formas ready, the lot. It has to be better than this pile of cardboard and paper clips – papers fluttering to the four winds. Confidentiality is a joke.'

'What about the medics?' He asked with a friendly frown. 'Dr. Wallace often writes straight into the notes as she's seeing her patients. I can't see them learning to love nits.'

'Tommy's meeting the doctors next week; anyway, lets go through your caseload. How's Mr. Clayton doing, he's back home isn't he?'

'He's been out on leave for the past week, Lyn's seeing him in out-patients today and she'll probably discharge him then.'

'Good. You'll follow him up for a while then close it?'

'Yeah err, I'll go out to see him and find out how they want to play it.'

'Okay but when the Rehab. and Recovery team are up and doing we'll need to be handing cases like this over to them. What about pointing them in Mind's direction?'

'I'll see what the Claytons say.'

'Well sort something out, there's quite a backlog building up at the referral meetings.'

He managed to fence and parry for a further forty minutes

before they'd both had enough. At one point he thought he heard a trace of Cindy's laughter and had listened with more interest to his manager to distract him. She'd noticed this and asked him if he wanted some tea before going on to explain that having a more supervisory role would 'dovetail nicely' with his commitment to taking students. As they drew to a close she said. 'Alan, I really think this is a good time to re-position yourself with all the changes taking place at management level. I'll leave you to reflect on this and we'll talk again next time.'

Alan reflected that he'd best show willing and said. 'Right, okay. Shall we set a date now?'

'I'd better get back to you about that. What are you up to this morning anyway Alan?'
'I'm visiting the Claytons at eleven.'

'Do you think you'll be able to close it?'

'I'm not sure – have to see.'

'Well bear in mind what we've agreed – ah, that sounds like Dr. Wallace, I'd better nip.'

Left to his own devices Alan moved hopefully across to his office. There was plenty of paper there but no other people though Cindy's desk showed signs of recent use. Freshly slopped coffee browned the edge of a pink memo, a white envelope disclosed a blue memory. He thought he caught a faint echo of her bathroom smell then Graham came in and asked him if 'Woodbine Winnie' was about.

'I haven't seen her, is Cindy in?'

'She was, maybe Fagash has nabbed her – apparently there's an assessment in the offing and I could do with not doing it

ASK ME NOW

Alan's angst over Cindy caused him to chide his slippery workmate. 'For fucks sake Graham, it's got to be your turn. When was the last time you …?

'Dickie old mate chill, eh. I only meant my car isn't going properly and anyway, there was a queue at the Gents.'
'A queue? You can generally have forty winks in there. Anyway, what's wrong with your car?'

'Oh, I don't know. It wont start and it was sort of coughing yesterday.'

'Well.' Mused Alan. 'It's either caught a cold or become allergic to carbon monoxide – I should change the plugs.'

Graham looked scornfully across the office. 'I think your plugs want seeing to this morning. Isn't that O.T. down the corridor a dab hand with cars – sorted out Cindy's cylinder that time?'

This was said with a straight face but their abrasive badinage was stirring complex reflections and his thoughts began to drift. Graham was sticking with the business at hand. 'Gypsy Larry, lives in a caravan down Badgers Drift.'

'Oh him.' Remembered Alan. 'Last time I was out with Romany his own car conked out.'

'Plugs?' Queried Graham.

'No, but something like – clutch cable, that was it.'

'Ah, social workers.' Trilled Dr. Wallace as she swept into their blokey domain. Suddenly the room seemed edgy with Dutch Tobacco and her subtly challenging vivacity. These men – these social workers – were malleable shapes, slack cables for her knowing boots.

Emboldened by what he saw as Grahams besting over the spark plugs Alan said. 'Presumably you only want one of us.'

'Oh yes, it's another Police Station job. We can go in my car.'

Alan then remembered that urgent phone call and busied himself with it as Graham lumbered off in his awful blue car coat. The clock on the wall told him to look lively. If he left in five minutes he could reach the Claytons on time. If he left now he would be able to not see Cindy and therefore avoid seeming bothersome, clingy and generally preoccupied with where things were going in their relationship. Something he sensed would prove a bit of a turn off for her. After a further fifteen minutes of faff and dither she still hadn't appeared. After ten more in road works by the bypass he reached his eleven o'clock appointment as 'You and Yours' came on the car radio.

He's late. I wonder if it's harder for him than me. They all seem so anxious to please, make you better, nurses, community workers, socialist porkers. This one seemed right enough, let me drive all the way over to the bin – right round the bend. They think you won't remember, that it won't matter when you're better. If you play along with it maybe they won't remember what you did and said, the water works, the shouting. Then there's the stuff you don't let on.

Alan turned round in the road parking behind the camper van, hoping it had been somewhere more interesting since last time. There was another van just ahead with a big picture of Steve Owen from 'Eastenders' on the side. Someone else was having a new sofa delivered. He concluded that Linda Barker must have fallen off hers.

Betty's fussing in the kitchen. She won't join us unless I ask her to. My main carer entitled to services in her own right. If I'm such a pissing burden why did they bother sending me

ASK ME NOW

back? Why did she have me back? Some days I don't feel much better then there's others when it's a bit different – a bit of the time. I'll find myself looking through the kitchen window, cock of the walk in the new trousers she brought me to come home in, brown of course.

Best show willing. It would be a poor look out if she has to answer. Same as last time. Steady as you go – yes-fine thanks, milk but no sugar isn't it? Sit you down, Betty's brewed, now you're talking. I don't remember too much about it all to be honest, first two weeks were a bit of a blur. I think I slept a lot, must have been the drugs. Err, red ones. No more like little chips then some at night to help you sleep. I don't need them now.

No I meant just the ones to help me sleep.

About six-o'clock most mornings, sometimes a bit later. I try to get straight up though, it doesn't go too well if I just lie there, not after the first couple of minutes anyway. It's strange really, when I first come to I feel all right and that there's nothing much wrong, I ought to be able to keep that going then it all goes bad again and my stomach turns over and then I have to get up and it's horrible.

Yes, a bit round teatime then we can watch telly together and by bedtime it's not too bad. I think I'll wake up next day and hold on to the mood but it never seems to work like that. I got better last time, didn't I?

Dr. Wallace was on about that. Long-term she says, perhaps for the rest of my life. They never bothered me before, blood tests weren't too bad except one time they gave me this daft lass at the Doctors – made a right mess of my arm. Still I made a decent job of that myself didn't I?

I'm sorry? – no, it's all right. I'll just get that tea, maybe a biscuit, if you like.

Help yourself to a fig roll, I might join you.

I don't know, possibly. These cords could be getting a bit tighter. I've been looking at that pamphlet thing; early morning wobbles, weight loss, persecutory anxiety – Dr. Wallace told me I'd got a full house of symptoms, you know, bingo you've gone bonkers.

Well yes I suppose trying to be funny is a good sign but none of that stuff in the book tells you about the mad stuff does it? I don't mind being called that, I really was mad, it's just, you know – why does it happen? I know you can't tell me, Dr. Wallace couldn't really, and maybe I was just too far-gone at the time to take it in. She talked about - stress variability is it?

Oh is that it? Vulnerability model, like something you get in a kit at Christmas? The stress comes from trying to put the thing together. This group support thing – I remember something like that from before, can't say it was much good but I stuck it out till the end then they let me go. We're an ungrateful lot aren't we?

Yes of course I'll give it a go, as long as it's not at that hospital.

Oh right, where you and Dr. Wallace work, where I go to see her. One of those H-Block affairs. I'll drive myself this time.

Well, that's that then. He's a funny one though, sits and looks at you; I think I prefer the prattlers. You don't have to tell them too much. Couple of the nurses on the ward were like him – tell them something just to get shot, then they'd come back for more. Sometimes you really don't remember things and I think that's best – if I try hard enough it might go away, like a good shit. Flush it all off and away with the rest of it. Is

ASK ME NOW

that what this group is like? All of us, men and women, sitting round in a circle on individual toilets with our trousers down enabling one and all to bear witness with our arses, have them inspected, wipe each other down, then when we've done that … where's Betty? I've got to stop this; she's the only one who knows – think of something nice. The way it felt when next doors dog brought you his ball in the back garden and Mr. Murtagh said 'hello' then you realised he'd sent him through on purpose. Rags left you his little jobby as well but that didn't bother you then. Betty cleaned it up. Good she's gone out, who'd want to hear this, off again with his self-pitying gobshite twattybollocks – why can't I be a good boy and just get on? Papped me pants again mummy. Mr. Murtagh's a nice chap, bet he doesn't think about opening his mouth to say hello and his tongue shooting out like a lizard with a furry white dog turd on the end. Bet he wouldn't send old Rags round if he knew what went on. I told Dr. Wallace one or two things; she just sat there nodding. Too busy with sloppy tea and medical notes to comb her hair, she must get to hear some things in her job. I couldn't make her out, always the same. I decided that I could tell her anything and she'd just sit there – nearly did one day. The one about the baby and the boiling hot bath water, the pensioners day trip to Sodomy-On-Sea in kind Mr. Clayton's nice new camper van. And there's more.

I'm not a bad person, why should I think these things? One day I thought my head would explode. I can understand these people taking all these drugs, on a bad day I once asked for more. I'd take them forever; never stop again, if they would just lay me out for a couple of weeks. A nurse told me why they couldn't – as if I didn't know. He also told me that in the old days they would dope people up for ages in a long sleep. They had to keep an eye on them of course, turn them, take them to the toilet, get stuff into them. There'd be a right how-de-do if they did that now. I wouldn't have minded. Apparently it never did much good but nursing was less stressful. I got a bit interested; in the real old days they'd whirl you round in a big chair till you stopped mythering, or breathing. Now it's little white pills to put in your mouth like mothers milk.

Where's Betty taken herself off to? Shops I should think, she could hardly have invited me along what with Mr. Duright here. Thought it best to pop unannounced, nothing if not tactful my Elizabeth, the demure Miss Dickson who turned out to be nothing like. That's all gone now of course, they tell you with a straight face that anti-depressants can cause sexual dysfunction. Well, not as much as depression they don't. Funny thing this morning though, woke up with my hand on the old fellow pissproud and half-mast, and where there's life there's … what? Think about Mr. Murtagh and his little doggy, his kindly smile, the dog's blind faith, the way I felt. Like nothing mattered for a moment. Feel like seeing me again then?

Alan's ignition turned over four times untill the engine fired then chugged fitfully for the length of the street before hitting a rhythm. He pushed on the radio to distract himself and caught the off-station muffle of The World At One where plans for a new Mental Health Act were being debated. He de-tuned to Radio Ridsdale where the Spotty Wilson show was hosting a phone-in around issues raised by proposed changes to the refuse collection system. Several sectionable callers had their say then the radio refuse man wrapped things up with an emollient summary about such being life before moving on to this weeks 'Spot Spotty' competition. Keen Spotty watchers had apparently spied their man as far a field as Warrington and, in one case, on top of Old Smokey – he cut this one short, perhaps sensing smut in the air. This week's winner had correctly identified him at – where else? – Spotfields where he had been seen suffering with the rest of them as 'Dale had been toyed with by Hartlepool. The plucky North-Easterners had gone top of the division on goal difference as a ring rusty Ridsdale counted their bruises after

ASK ME NOW

a 5-1 pasting. Alan hoped the new mental health act would come in soon.

There was a red light at the last set of road works before base. He looked out of his window, he couldn't see Spotty anywhere but began to enjoy the light as it dappled from the canal against a warehouse wall then a woman walked past. Her hair could have been bobbed and as her bare legs moved in and out of the shade he thought he recognised her ankles. This made him feel anxious and when the guy behind him parped briefly to let him know the light had changed he wound down the window to yell 'fuck off'. It was at this point that he knew for sure he was in love.

Back at H.Q. Val Meating met Alan in the car park and squired him back to his work station chatting forcefully of the new degree course at Trafford University (formerly Wetherfield Poly.) The course literature referred to 'train and transform at Trafford', which Alan thought was asking for trouble but he kept his counsel because he'd worked out what was happening – she wanted him to take a student.

'How did it go at the Claytons?' She asked.

I dunno.' He parried.

'What do you mean, is he on the mend or not – hasn't Dr. Wallace discharged him yet?'

'From hospital, but I think she'll be seeing him in out-patients for a while yet.'

She became disobliging at this. 'Yes I know all that, but is there a role for you?'

'There might be.'

'Alan, I really feel we need to be more pragmatic about what cases we're keeping open and what we think we're trying to do with them. I expect you to have given this some thought by the time we have our next supervision session.'

Alan decided to be more helpful. 'The new course sounds interesting.'

'Yes.' She said taking Cindy's vacant chair. 'They're very excited at TAT – I think we need to be in at the beginning on this one. The department has a firm commitment to offering student placements and we've struggled to make our quotas for the past three years. When did you finish your practice teaching course?'

'I got the certificate in June last year.'

'But you haven't taken anyone since?'

'No ... they're looking for a placement then?'

Val pushed three-quarters of a Twix bar into her mouth. 'September ... five months ... final placement.' Which, baring a name, was all he needed to know.

'Right, well, as long as we can provide a desk that shouldn't be too much of a problem.'

'Excellent, and, Alan, think about Mr. Clayton and any other cases you can close. You'll need space for a student.' She then did the decent thing and lingered long enough to let them both feel there were other things she might value his views on then set off for the afternoons divisional management meeting. Rather you than me he thought before sitting back to think about Bill Clayton.

He knew the poor sod wasn't as well as he reckoned to be. You didn't need to be very much better to get off the ward

ASK ME NOW

these days; Bill had figured this out and worked his passage accordingly. Alan couldn't blame him but all the signs were there to tell any halfway decent worker that Bill Clayton was just the sort of subtle high-risk type to quietly slope off one fine day and top himself. He'd do it too, no messing about with aspirins in the lounge while the wife's away. The question Alan struggled with was why hadn't he? He was pretty sure they'd avoided something untoward when they'd admitted him and he'd seemed pleased when Alan had seen him on the ward, maybe there was a role for him. To do what though? Listen, advise, help and support, exasperate, irritate and advocate? Take responsibility for keeping alive? You could be the Wayne Rooney of community mental health work but if Bill Coleman chose to kill himself on your watch he would. He hadn't been able to believe his ears one day when Dr. Wallace had solemnly abjured some poor lad in outpatients to promise her he wouldn't do it again. Perhaps that was as good as anything you could do with them, as far as he knew the youth in question was still whizzing about in one piece. A less trenchant medic. would have diagnosed a borderline personality disorder and referred him for 'individual work', and that was where the taking of responsibility began.

Alan knew that as social workers went he wasn't a bad one, on his better days not bad at all. He also knew that over the years, with some modest training and occasional clinical supervision from Tommy Smith, he had become perfectly capable of delivering supportive counselling, and that there were times when it appeared to work. But he wasn't a therapist and too often that's what people thought they were getting or what you were giving, and things that weren't really there never really worked. This was no doubt what Val Meating was getting at but he wasn't one of those workers – more common among the nurse-trained workers in his view – who seemed to need their clients more than they needed them. He knew it couldn't be his job to save Bill Clayton – Bill must know that, his wife certainly did; her watery tolerance and perfectly polite reluctance to digress from the strictly business-like told him this. Maybe Bill just needed someone to talk to, people often did. Someone other than their nearest and dearest or the bloke down the pub. Someone you could tell things to and it didn't matter, not as much as it would to the others and in a way it made you matter, a bit, for a while, and they, Bill and the others, where entitled to expect you to know your stuff and not talk like a twit. And that's where a different kind of responsibility began.

He was distracted from further thought by the phone on Grahams desk, which sounded as though it might go on forever unless answered. Becky told him it was Dr. Lokum Effendi and made the connection without pausing. 'Izgram.' Said the phone.

Alan hesitated then cottoned on. 'No, it's Alan Duright here, Graham's out at the moment.'

'Ardik, you tell him this …'

'I can pass on a message or let you have his mobile number if you like …'
'Grrr … nobloodygood – you tell him this.'

' …?'

'Ewetheredik …?'

'Still here, what should I tell him?'

'Thank you … tardik.' Click.

'Is he having a laugh?' Alan asked the phone which then rang again. He snatched it up.

'Is Vic there?'

ASK ME NOW

'No… it's Dick not Vic – and, anyway it's Alan.'

'Are you having a laugh?' Asked an unfamiliar voice.

'No, sorry – whom am I speaking to?'

'It's Dave Bamber here from Trafford Uni. I'm Vic's tutor; I'm ringing to sort out our pre-placement meeting. Vic should be with you by now, anyway if you're Alan Duright it's you I'm after.'

Alan asked if there'd been some misunderstanding and Dave Bamber fell silent very briefly before referring to 'Val' and if she'd talked to him about 'the placement'.

Oh yeah.' Said Alan. 'In September.'

'No, starts Monday. Didn't she explain?'

'Not that bit.'

'Right, well, sorry about this but it's all got a bit complicated – we're having to rejig things on the course, tweak a few fine details. You know how these things take on a life of their own. Val really should have given you the full SP on this'

Alan had to admire Bambers pitch; deftly indicating where responsibilities lay, smoothly aligning himself with Alan – just another pair of hard-pressed public servants doing what they could with scant support from management and treacherous organisational quick sands waiting to pull them under. It did the trick. 'You say this placement starts on Monday today's …'

'Thursday afternoon as we speak. We'll have to get something organised for tomorrow, I can come at any time so when Vic turns up just set a time then phone me. They'll get a message to me if I'm not there.'

'But I don't know anything about this Vic. What's he look like, he could be wandering about the place now for all I know.'

'Yeah, sorry mate it's all been a bit rushed. Actually he's very easy to spot; think Cornish Mick Hucknall before the hair cut. He's called Curno and he's very keen to do a mental Health placement.'

'Yes, can't wait to get here.'

'Yeah, sorry mate … anyway, lets get something sorted out for tomorrow. We're really very grateful for this Di .. Alan.'

You devious so-and-so thought Alan, stitching me up like a kipper. He should have known there was something fishy afoot when she'd waited for him in the car park. Trying not to get carried away with more images of sprats mackerels and marlin spikes he went off in search of a Simply Red look-a-likee. He wasn't sitting around in reception, no messages waited in his tray. Alan decided that a determined walkabout would focus his thinking and clarify his perceptions. There was something about facilitating learning outcomes which brought out the berk in him. It also came to him that he hadn't thought about Cindy for about twenty minutes. He knew that she fancied Mick Hucknall and tried to remember if she also liked pasties or cream teas.

There was no sign of 'Vic' or anyone like him in the building but, if he was a smoker, he could be outside. He soon came across Dr. Wallace in the small transparent bus shelter affair where the dirty smokers went for their fixes. Someone had helpfully stuck a skull and cross-bones by the industrial sized ashtray. It didn't put anyone off. She was re-igniting a half smoked dog end and as he glimpsed her she looked very tired

ASK ME NOW

and alone but as she caught sight of him she laughed and said. 'Anything to get out of the Trust Management Group.'

'Has anybody else been round here?' He asked her.

'I haven't seen anyone – who are you after?'

'A man called Vic. He's got long ginger hair.'

'Nope. Who is he anyway?'

'A social work student, he's coming on placement.'

'Oh really – presumably he's interested in psychiatric work. What's his experience in the field?'

'I don't know, I haven't met him yet.'

She looked at him for three long seconds and said. 'If you haven't met him how can you take him on? He might be totally unsuitable to work with patients – you'll be responsible for him Alan. I'd never take an SHO on the nod – does Val know about this?'

'I'm not sure ... yes I mean.'

'Alan I think you probably need to sort this out, is he just wandering about the place or something? Somebody needs to take responsibility.'

'It's not that, I think what's happened is ...'

What happened next was that the doctor's dog end described a contemptuous arc on its path towards a blameless rhododendron and Alan passed on to a seldom-visited area behind the clinic rooms. He didn't think he would find Vic there but he badly needed some time. Student placements weren't usually arranged after Raymond Chandler but he was beginning to think bad thoughts about the slippery tongued Bamber – but there was no way Ina would dab him in it. His mood began to lift as he toyed with the notion of a social workers course taught from the mean streets of pre-war Los Angeles; risk assessment with Moose Molloy, counselling skills with The Thin Man, Harry The Horse could tutor the unwary in the mysteries of transferable skills. Everyone would be required to smoke heavily and drive unreliable cars to remote, dangerous areas of town. Perhaps Vic was already sleeping with the fishes?

Behind him a high window opened suddenly and a falling voice said 'two weeks time'; the depot clinic was in full swing. Alan sloped off adjusting an imaginary hat, it was all he could do to stop himself muttering 'farewell my lovely' to Ruby from rehab. When they passed in reception. His eyes raked the room but there was no one there.

'Are there any messages for me Becky?'

'No I don't think so – no, nothing.'

He checked his waterproof Timex. Only an hour to go and he still hadn't made that call, and he couldn't get that broad out of his head either. 'Is Cindy in do you know Becky?'

'No ... not having much luck today Alan.'

'Eh, oh no – not really. Listen, if a tall chap with lots of red hair called Vic should turn up it's me he needs to see, he might seem a bit confused but don't worry.'

'Right.' Said Becky. 'I'll let you know. Is he a patient of Dr. Wallace's.'

'No, no he's actually a social work student, supposed to be coming here on placement on Monday.'

ASK ME NOW

'Right.' Said Becky, more quietly this time and looked keenly down at her tool bar.

'Yes, well, I'll be at my desk.' He said and moved off with a sudden tightening of his stomach. He was sure he'd upset Becky in some way and thought he'd better come up with something lightly bantering to make her laugh. Nothing came so he went through to his office feeling worse, all his playful musings around Moose Molloy had fallen away and he just felt very silly, and something else. Something taking shape at the back of his head, on the borderlines of affect. Something damp and dirty. There was no sign of his manager or anybody else so he pressed on the tape recorder by his desk. The therapeutic sounds of Stan Tracey using a piano keyboard to hammer down some loose floorboards helped reign in his senses and lend astringency to his thoughts. What had seemed discordant soon became harmony, of a sort.

It was looking less likley that Vic would show and this made things a bit easier. He decided to assert some control over events and phoned Dave Bamber who asked him to please leave a message after the tone, as 'your call is important to us'.

'As your student hasn't appeared I think we should meet here at twelve tomorrow – you'd better contact him.' This made Alan feel better.

Almost as soon as he'd put down the phone it rang and he felt anxious again. Becky explained there 'was someone on the other end asking for him'.

'Hello, Alan Duright here, who am I speaking to.' He always felt a prat saying that but he hoped it would set out a suitable tone with his elusive trainee.

'Ooh, I'm not too late am I.'? Queried a less commanding voice from the other end. An older voice, a Harry voice, or a Bob voice. Or a Bill.?

'Oh hello Mr. Clayton, how's it going.'?

'Oh, all right thank you. It's not too late is it?'

'I don't think so. Too late for what??

'To call you, don't you finish at five?'

'No, of course it's not too late – anyway, how can I help?'

Bill Clayton gave this some thought before he replied. 'Can we get together again soon. If it's not too late?'

'Yes of course, I've got some time tomorrow – I could call in the morning. Would ten be all right?'

'Just hang on a minute.'

Alan heard vague tapping sounds, something like the diminishing swish of an enormous curtain then the sure but faint murmurings of human speech. There was then a sudden loud scrape and Bill said. 'Yes that will be all right.'
There wasn't much time to reflect on this because the phone went again and as Becky connected him he said directly. 'Is Vic there?'

'No, it's me, Cindy. Who's Vic.?'

'I don't know.' He said.

'Right, well I'm phoning to say I won't be back in the office tonight and to ask you if you wanted to come round for a cup of tea. Say if you don't.'

ASK ME NOW

'No, yes, that will be fine. Vic is a student who's coming on Monday, apparently.'

'For the morning or all day, have you got something lined up?'

'For three months actually.'

'You never said anything. Where's he going to sit?'

'In here somewhere.'

'Well don't stick him next to me. I'm still trying to forget the horrific halitotoid from Huddersfield we got last year.'

'Cindy the department has a commitment to taking students and as a professional group …'

'Yes, well as long as they send them housetrained. That one could have transferred his skills to stripping paint if he'd failed his course. Anyway, does your professional commitment extend to taking them before you've met them now?'

'I'll tell you about that later.'

'Okay, come straight over if you want.'

Alan felt much better and decided he'd just been tired earlier. It was time for some purposeful paper pushing and another crack at that stubborn stain on his desk. He might have to share it with this Vic if he ever materialised. Val Meatings meeting must be finished by now he thought, if he hung around he could nab her on her return and avoid pitching up at Cindy's too soon. It could also help him formulate a plausible assessment of the whole caper when she started asking all the obvious questions.

The building began to empty, faces appeared in doorways to say 'see yous' but not to linger. Alan felt relieved by the time most of them had gone and turned over his tape. This time Stan The Man was to be heard weaving a dream of strange beauty for solo piano with many a nod to Bartok and Les Dawson along the way. The piece was called 'Bi-Bitonal' and caught the moment perfectly for him. He fished out Bill Claytons file, looked at the notes he'd jotted after this mornings visit and became aware of movement across the corridor and a door closing quietly. After about five minutes the door opened letting out light and Val Meating who slipped smoothly away from the range of his peripheral vision. He was sure she'd seen him. 'Is that you Val?'

'Oh, Alan – you still here?'
'Yes, can I have a word?'

'Of course Alan, has something happened?'

He felt his dander twitch at this; her well-practiced concern, the whole how-can-we-sort-this-out bit that told him she knew what the crack was. 'That student we discussed this morning, for a possible placement later this year?'

'Yes that's right.' She said.

'Not on Monday.'

'On Monday?'

'Yeah ... Dave Bamber from TAT was on this afternoon looking for Vic.' Alan twiddled his fingers at this point. 'Who wasn't here anyway, but is clearly expected to be starting his three month placement with us on Monday. I've agreed to a pre-placement meeting here tomorrow.'

'Where?' Asked Val. 'What time?'

ASK ME NOW

'Here at twelve.'

'Right I'll be there, this needs sorting out.'

'I know but where did Bamber get my name from and …'

'Alan I really need to head off, there's a MIND committee tonight I ought to get along to. We'll talk tomorrow.'
'And that's all she said?'

'Yep, then she was gone. I'd had enough by then anyway.'

They were standing in Cindy's kitchen waiting for the tea to mash. She'd kissed him companionably on arrival but there was a clear that's-it-for-now feeling in the air as the leaned against the waist high work surface. He considered the mystery of whatever process had hastened him over the doorstep last time only to bid him return today and reasoned that she wouldn't have popped the kettle on unless she really wanted him.

'You really are a berk sometimes Alan.'

This set him at his ease. 'Yeah I know, I should have told Dave Bamber it wasn't on.'

'Well, either him or Val or both of them are stringing you along – and this guy never appeared?'

'Nope.'

Cindy busied herself with the tea and frowned with her bottom lip pushed forward over her top one. He thought how odd it was that once you'd had sex with someone watching could feel more intimate than touching them. How we were all different but the same. She was looking in a cupboard now. 'I'm sure I've met this Bamber bloke, do you want something to eat?'

'But not this Vic?'

After a listless rummage she waived a tin of sardines. 'On toast?'

'Yeah, that'd be nice.'

He sat at the old pine table and scanned the Indie; Wimbledon had signed a new player and the others had signalled his acceptance by burning his tailored leather tracksuit. Was this a prank too far for the Crazy Gang? Not a bit of it; Mazza was happy to make light of their lovable ways but served notice that there'd be other things he might make light of in his own good time. The manager took heart from this quoting that 'the new 'un' would fit in well and strengthen the team spirit, a combustible mixture by the sound of it. Elsewhere David Batty had been sick in the showers again and Trevor Brooking, 'no stranger to conformity', had become embroiled in controversy with Sky Sports. All this seemed shocking to Alan, such goings on would never happen down the 'Dale – tailored tracksuits? In leather?' Billy Cocklehurst was felt to be a big time Charlie with his personalised number plate (don't ask) but that was about it. Football was still the people's game up here, if Cindy would come to a match with him ... best take things slowly, sex first, Spotfields later. She dished up in due course supplementing the promised fare with grated carrot and curried beans. He was touched. 'You said you might have come across Dave Bamber before.'

'Yes I think he was that one that went to court in his trainers then got his manager into trouble by going to the papers about it. You know the class of cobblers; authoritarian institutions, fatuous value systems – state oppression if I remember it right, a complete tosser. I hate that kind of thing, they're invariably shit workers too. Yes, it's coming back to me now,

ASK ME NOW

his manager was Linda Weller in the old child-care intake team, Claire knows her, what they did when he left, they got hold of his trainers somehow – I think he kept them at work – and burned them round the back of Oakhill. It must be the same bloke – just the type to go into teaching.'

'If you burn a mans shoes maybe it means you don't want him to leave you. There's something in the paper today about some footballers burning a team mates leather track suit, do you think that could be something similar?'

'Maybe the other players are all vegan and took exception.'

He knew she was having a laugh and began to enjoy himself, but what did it all mean? Everyone holds dreams and darker currents, occasionally they break the surface but mostly they don't. What makes the difference, were dreams just for those who sleep? Something told him to keep this kind of stuff to himself for now, people didn't talk like characters in a play.

'I want to construct spaces for people to find themselves in.' Said Cindy.

Careful. Take your time. 'Pardon?' He eventually managed.

'Here, halfway down. Christiana Belletriste a green architect challenges traditional notions. She's just won a commission to design a new housing project in Oldham, what do you think she means?'

'Perhaps she felt a bit lost when she found herself in Oldham. I bet she's not from round here.'

Cindy perused her Indie'. 'No, graduated from the Sorbonne – Swiss by the sounds of it, you doing anything tonight?'

'No.' Answered Alan. 'Nothing special ... how about you?'

'I usually stay in on Thursdays, winding down the week you know, also, it's good telly – Eastenders then there's a thing on Four about depression which looks good.'

Ordinarily the evenings programme as just set out would hold limited appeal for him but the deeper currents began to stir; she was asking him to stay the night, or part of it anyway. 'Sounds interesting.' He said.

'Good, you go through and put the fire on while I clear up.'

He switched on the main light in Cindys parlour and showed a masterful hand with her rickety gas fire. Unfortunately he couldn't get the telly to work so he sat down on the two-seater settee and hoped he hadn't damaged it in some way. He was about to have another look at it when she came in. 'Oh, is the box playing up again?' Without waiting for any further comment she nipped down behind the set and tinkered knowledgably with the cables, plugging in at the same time what proved to be a small lamp by the CD player. 'There.' She said switching the television on and the main light off. As she sat down beside him Ian Beale pitched up on screen shouting at a tearful woman that she should expect 'nuffink' from him.

'Devious little twat.' Observed Cindy.

The next half-hour passed in a similar vein as she showed an informed grasp of the plots and a blue stockinged insight into what it was all about. 'This whole thing with Den and his family is 'King Lear' crossed with 'Twelfth Night'.

'How do you mean?' He asked, trying to retrieve anything he knew about either play.

'Den's kids have been to Spain where they got lost but were reunited in Walford after many trails and tribulations and initial failure to recognise one another. Then Den gives up his empire of dodgy enterprises expecting them all to get on and run things for him. It all goes wrong of course and they end up hating him, I think one of them will bump him off in the end.'

Alan was very impressed. 'Where does Ian Beale fit into the picture, he looks pretty star crossed to me?'

'Oh Ian runs the café.'

Something rang a distant bell for him. 'Wasn't he married to someone called Cindy at some point?' She laughed at this and curled her feet beneath his thigh. 'Someone else rang me up this afternoon.'

'Mmm, who was that?' She asked absently as the credits came up.

'Mr. Clayton – the man with the camper van.'

'Is this unusual, doesn't he use the phone or something?'

'Well I'd only seen him at lunchtime and I was really surprised to hear from him again at all. I don't think he's as well as he reckons to be but we had a fairly routine natter about looking ahead, managing the jitters and all that. I just got the impression he was politely saying thank you very much now you can fuck off, then he phones up all nicely nicely and asks if we can get together again soon. I'm seeing him in the morning.'

'You must have done something right. Did it surprise you when I phoned?'

'A bit, but I'm glad you did.'

They sat on in easy silence and watched the Channel Four thing on depression; he thought it wasn't bad for a pre eleven slot. It had secondary gains too; suitably sombre music from Jan Garbarek, all keening cries over sparse pianos, and a provocative plea from Dorothy Rowe around the notion that all we need is love. He thought the old girl might be beginning to lose it a bit but it certainly more inspiring than bio psychosocial interventions. Happily shortfalls in the services were glossed over and the conclusion that depression was a common aspect of the human condition had both viewers nodding sage assent.

'Ooof.' Said Cindy as she pulled her feet from beneath Alan's leg. The manoeuvre caused her to move towards him then off and away like something underwater breaking free from a rock, then there was fleeting difficulty as cramp made her fall back and steady herself against his shoulder. He hazarded a free arm of his own about her waist and she softened briefly before proposing more tea and heading for the kitchen. So, he thought, where's it going, how'm I doing? Could he take her as he found her? Would that work both ways? If she'd been two minutes earlier on Sunday she'd have found a total wanker and washed her hands of him, there were times when he really didn't like himself very much. But not tonight, not so far.

'I've got some of that stuff you and Graham like – singsong whatsit.'

'Lapsang Souchong, yeah, great.'

She came back with biscuits and mashing pot, it all felt so homely he wished he'd worn his cardigan. How would Cindy cope with that? She took up her former position and let her hand rest on his green corduroys. All this and biscuits too, it was better than sex then a passing cloud drifted onto the telly. It all started innocuously enough; a bog standard advert for British Gas featuring a trainee class of gormless youths who

ASK ME NOW

were being instructed by a fading dominatrix played by Brenda Blethyn. He thought he could be hallucinating and closed his eyes. This shouldn't be happening, it ought to be Linda Barker or at least Sarah Lancashire but no, there she was when he opened them again acting the giddy goat with an adenoidal moron. 'Isn't that your favourite thesp.?' Asked Cindy.

'Yes, Mike Leigh must have got the gas contract but lets not spoil the evening with talk of high culture, is there anything else on?'

'Have a look.' She said handing him the Guardian guide as she reached for the teapot. The wet smokey smell drifted across, it made him think about being young and worrying about girls, so plus ca change, he reflected, and all that. He found the correct page, pick of the day was the Channel Four thing they'd just watched and elsewhere there was a Taggart he'd all ready seen, pro-celebrity dominoes on Five with Neil Morrissey. Doin' The Old Man Up with Lotty and Totty or Julie Walters in a heart-warming drama about women who cook too much. Just his cup of tea.

'There's that thing where those too posh bints sort out your husbands wardrobe.'

'I usually enjoy that; I want them to do Graham. They'd have a field day – I bet he's got a set of cardies.'

'Do you fancy watching it?'

She sipped her tea and blew across her cup. 'Nah, I fancy an early night; I'm getting period pains. Do you want to stay over again?'

Alan tapped his foot to make sure the rug beneath his feet wasn't moving and stuffed a whole biscuit into his mouth to buy some time. As invitations to a lady's favour went this was unprecedented, as far as he could tell. He could hardly say no, not that he wanted to, but he felt that he was beginning to understand Cindy in a deeper way. When somebody offered you his or her dreams you should tread carefully.

'Of course – maybe if we think about Vic and the mystery of the missing placement we'll work it all out in our sleep.'

'Do you think it really is a mystery Alan?'

'Well it's all a right mystery to me.'

'You don't think you've just been done over for a mug?'

'I don't know. What do you mean, who by?'

'I think that's the mystery. I agree it doesn't sound like Val Meating.'

'The smooth talker from TAT goes to the top of my list.' Said Alan.

Cindy offered a dubious 'mmm' then pointed out that the more of this sort of thing the team tolerated the more they'd get. 'I mean, how long did you spend this afternoon traipsing round after someone you'd never met?'

Hang on, he thought, we're not married yet. 'It's hardly my fault, I was only trying to be helpful.'

'There speaks a proper social worker.' Scoffed Cindy.

'Look Cindy what was I supposed to have done. What would you …?'

'I wouldn't have accepted responsibility for it so quickly. I know what it's like when you answer the phone in an empty office but you can always play daft. Graham wouldn't have got himself lumbered like that.'

'Yeah well, he doesn't take students anymore, not since that case of mistaken identity and the elected member.'

'Yes.' Laughed Cindy. 'He's blacklisted at TAT which takes some doing but at least he doesn't get himself caught up in capers like this. Did the CPS ever get the full SP on all that?'

'No it all got hushed up but there's an informal injunction keeping Graham from within a mile of City Hall, Councillor Coleman'll clock him one if he ever sees him again.' He then set up a familiar refrain ' None of this is my fault you know.'

'No, I know but your name's stuck to it now. Like marmalade to a blanket, there's no getting it off – have you sorted out an induction week?'

'Christ, I haven't had time.'

'Well it's you they'll moan to if the student is sitting around all next week reading books. I'll have a word with Claire, she'll take him for a couple of days, then they're usually back in College one day, health and safety should take up a morning and one of the CPN's might offer something. It'll be Friday before you know it and you can bring up study time then. Could you run me a bath while I sort out down here?'

Fair enough. talk of the fair Claire generally made him smarten his ideas up but coming out unfavourably in any comparative study with Graham was more than he deserved. Anyway, Cindy's astringency had clarified a few perceptions and signalled ways forward. He had a crack at the bathroom while downstairs the ordered clatter of washing up and siding away gave form to his thoughts. It was all of a piece with women; patterns, logic, common sense, was that why we needed each other? He trailed a hand in the deepening waters and remembered Bill and Betty Clayton, about how much she'd have had to put up with, how irrelevant a carers assessment might seem to her. Maybe it was her who had got Bill to phone him today. Cindy appeared in a lime and yellow kimono with her hair gathered severely in a black plastic helmet. 'I'd leave the water in for you after only, you know.'

'Yeah, sure.'

'There's a new toothbrush up there anyway. I'll give you a call.'

There was enough steam about the place to make Cindy look like Tokyo Rose returning from Pearl Harbour in a mist, enjoying the image he made himself comfortable on the bed and noticed that she was re-reading 'Middlemarch'. He leafed through to find her place marked with a postcard from Porthmadoc. It showed a prelapsarian British jazz musician winding up his hurdy gurdy for some bored locals. The image reminded him of the last time he'd seen Keith Tippett down the Arts Centre, he avoided noticing who'd sent it and opened the book further on. He found a bit he particularly liked where it all begins to unravel for Squire Bulstrode, his old mucker from 'Nicks London days' reappears by a tree in a field and threatens to expose him to the good folk of Tipton. This was familiar to him from the Beebs production where the Raffles character had been played by Fred Elliot off Coro'. To Alan most aspects of culture was rinsed in a world of lather. He skimmed on; Mary and the geese, dark doings on the town council, Ladislau in his breeches then Dorotheas sad steps. Which always seemed to him to be genuinely moving, and a world away from Dot Cotton. Cindy came through and told him there should be plenty of hot water in the tank.

Stripped down before the sink Alan thought himself homely plump. Cindy didn't seem to mind and once he'd sounded her out successfully with a couple of quips about his baldness he

ASK ME NOW

hadn't really looked back on that score. After ten minutes he returned to the bedroom smelling of roses. She was curled into the middle of the bed with her head facing his pillow. He wanted to get straight in to hold her and felt relieved that they were keeping sex out of the bedroom; it was another digestive biscuit moment. Alan slid carefully in as Cindy lifted her head to settle on his chest and settle an arm across his belly. He began to stroke her hair, working his fingers through to her scalp, she mmmed a bit so he continued. When her breathing began to deepen he picked up 'Middlemarch' with his free hand and read as the book fell open. Mr. Brook was being cruelly mocked by a bunch of surly farmhands who were unimpressed by his ad-hoc election speech. He had to retire after a bit more rough handling from the crowd and the affair became a notorious fiasco, the result it seemed of the wretched fellow agreeing to speak at the last minute then making a hash of it. Brooke came out of it badly, looking like a well-meaning booby. It was generally agreed that he should have said no in the first place or at least found out a bit more about what he was committing himself to.

Alan put down the book and tried to empty his mind of conscious thought.

Mike Pearson

ASK ME NOW

THE WINDMILLS OF YOUR MIND

'Cindy won't be in today, not very well.'

Becky registered this without comment so Alan went through. There were two security pads between the reception area and his office but nothing between the desk Becky used and the public, this could be a bold statement of anti-oppressive practice or an oversight on the part of the joint steering group charged with supervising health and safety. Becky would sometimes raise the issue after a visit from Marjorie Razorblade but nothing ever changed except Marjorie's medication. Graham was all ready at his desk running down the bullet points of an internal memo. 'Anything interesting?' Asked Alan.

'Yeah actually. It's the outline guidance for electronic case notes. I think it could be good news – we'll all have to go minimalist.'

Alan smiled at this. 'Should be fun, Cindy's sick by the way – Beck's just told me, asked if I'd sort out her diary.'

'Eh? Oh, right. I thought you might be ill anyway.'

'No, just a bit held up.'

'Ah.' Said Graham. 'Ina's been looking for you.'

'Is she about?'

'No, had to nip apparently.'
Alan busied himself with the coffee arrangements as Graham took a phone call that he hoped would divert his mates train of thought. When he'd finished he asked him where their manager might be.

'I don't know but she was in a right old tizz about something.' Graham was unable to tell him anything else because Nav came in looking for Cindy who had been expected 'at that CPA meeting for Mrs. Bremner'.

'Off sick mate. Apparently.' Said Graham as Alan scanned the car park.

'Right, great.' Sighed Nav. 'What are we supposed to do now?'

Alan reckoned that Graham would be looking in his direction so he affected a sudden interest in something that seemed to be unfolding outside, although all he could really see was a tiny Yorkshire Terrier defecating what looked like half of its body mass over by the bushes. Haunches aquiver, it looked up at an old man in a bomber jacket who mouthed something and slouched off. 'Look.' He said. 'You can't keep dumping on Primary Care every time there's a problem. The world doesn't stop if Cindy's not here.'

''But this is your problem Alan.' Protested Nav quietly. 'Cindy is the key worker in this case.'

Graham had returned to his bullet points so Alan felt obliged. 'I'll have a look through her stuff.'

'Won't it be locked away?' Asked Nav.
'We share a drawer, it's easier.'

'It's a very friendly arrangement.' Put in Graham. 'Lets him use his key.'

The bastard, thought Alan, he wouldn't dare push it if Nav weren't here. Fortunately their colleague was more mindful of the roasting Dr. Wallace would be warming up for him if the review went tits up. 'Great.' He said. 'See if there's anything in there.' A green pro-forma headed 'CPA Review' was found

ASK ME NOW

but it only covered the complexities of a Mr. Boylans case.

'Keep looking Dick, I bet they're in order.' Urged Nav.

Next up was a plain sheet of A4 with 'notes for Dottie's review' and a stream of consciousness text. 'What's this lady's first name Nav?'

'I think it might be Dorothy.'

'Well this will have to do.'

'But what if it isn't? I'll look a right one.'

'Look.' Said Alan. 'This isn't your responsibility – just explain the circumstances, confirm what details you've got with Dr. Wallace and do your best. Can't do no more eh?'

Nav pondered Alan's team talk then said, without much conviction. 'Dorothy Bremner, or could be Doris.'

'Or Billie.' Offered Graham as Nav moved off down the corridor. 'He's never not right that lad.'

Alan began to sort Cindy's diary. After a couple of phone calls and an e-mail to Claire Todgers her day had been re-framed so he turned to his own appointments. 'Do you know anything about this student we're taking Gray?'

'Ina said something about it earlier but she was in such a flap I couldn't make any sense - all a bit rushed apparently. What's happening?'

'Well, apparently, someone's coming over from TAT this lunchtime to meet us, then it'll start on Monday. He's called Vic.'

'You're kidding. You can't set up a placement like that, it's not fair on the student – tell 'em get stuffed. What sort of Herberts do they take us for? No wonder Ina's made herself scarce.' More bluff common sense from Graham in a similar vein persuaded Alan to set off early for his appointment with Bill Clayton.

The journey over to Coleridge Crescent featured enough road works, punch ups and top of the range powered wheel chairs to make time for the first side of 'A Love Supreme'. Alan wondered, not for the first time, if he really liked this stuff as much as he let on. It seemed to him that Burt Bacharach evinced a surer grasp of the spiritual pulse than John Coltrane ever had. He switched tapes before arriving and as Sonny Rollins began to play 'How Are Things In Glochamorra'? He started to feel better and remembered why he loved jazz. The Claytons front lawn looked ominously tidy but Bill answered the door promptly enough, bidding him sit down in the back room while he mashed the tea. Alan was relieved about this given the painful memories he associated with the other room. He took up one of two comfortable looking recliners either side of a wooden fire surround. One of the perks of a social workers life was the privileged access to other people's homes, a licensed look at their most intimate arrangements; how they positioned their soft furnishings, where they stacked their brown envelopes. Bill and Betty's pile was tucked discreetly behind an empty vase at the far end of the mantle piece. The end closer to Alan displayed an ashtray from the 1991 RSPCA dinner dance. It made him think of Cindys face when she was naked, that these were the things that mattered, the small quiet things in amongst all the louder stuff.

'You don't have sugar do you?' Said Bill as he came through with the tray.

'No, just milk.'

'Right, there you go.' Bill sat in the other chair and tried to

ASK ME NOW

sip his tea though it was obviously too hot. Alan looked away as Bill put down the cup and waggled his scalded fingers. He was struggling to come up with something to say and Alan knew his role was to help this along.

'How are things in Gloc … I mean how are things going … you rang me yesterday?'

'Yes, I hope I didn't drag you away from anything important.'
'No, no I'm glad you phoned …'

'Yes well, I wanted to ask you something.' Alan proffered a quiet smile and Bill furrowed his forehead and said 'Am I going mad?'

'I don't think so, no. How do you mean?'

'I don't know, it's just … is the tea all right?'

Alan sipped a bit, it was still too hot but he said 'fine' then. 'What do you mean by going mad?'

'Crackers.' Replied Bill. 'Doo lally tap.' Fair enough thought Alan and asked him as gently as he could if he sometimes feared that his thoughts were spinning out of control. Bill pondered this and fiddled with his ear lobe. 'I don't know – my heads not right I know that much.'

Alan decided to deploy a bio-psychosocial intervention, draw on the teachings of the stress vulnerability model. 'How has it been since you came home from hospital?'

'Bit up and down.'

'Do you feel you're getting any better?'

'Since they let me out you mean? I reckon they'd got fed up

with me you know.'

'Of course they didn't. You were discharged when you were well enough to come home.'

Bill thought about this as he tested the side of his cup with a finger. 'I didn't want to come home, not then, but I didn't want to stay in there another minute. Now I sometimes wonder if I've started to go down bank since I came back here. Doesn't that sound a bit mad to you?'

Alan had recognised some familiar strains. 'I think it can be a difficult time in between life on the ward and getting used to being at home again. Particularly as there'll be more time alone and that can be a bit tricky to begin with, you know, things seem much quieter all of a sudden. In the hospital there's always somebody there.'

'But I didn't like it in there. I think it made me worse – there was a lad in there tried to hang himself. Only nineteen, drugs or some such.'

'What makes you think you're going mad?'

Bill sighed and sipped his tea. 'Oh I dunno.' He focussed on a pile of videocassettes beneath the telly; Antiques Roadshow thought Alan or Wednesdays Corrie. After a desultory rummage Bill sat up straight and clapped both knees. 'I've told Betty some of this and she reckons I should tell you.' Alan waited then Bill began. 'I keep thinking I'm going to think something really bad.'

'Something really bad?'

'Yes, something awful – I get frightened and sometimes it gets worse. I don't want it, to think these things. They're the last things I want but I can't stop, that's why I think I'm bonkers.'

ASK ME NOW

'Could you give me an example?'
'Well it's like – I never do anything – it's just ideas, pictures, odd ideas in my mind. Possibilities if you know what I mean – things that could happen. Horrible things. Why would I have to see a psychiatrist if I'm not cracked?'

'Did you confide in Dr. Wallace with these frightening thoughts?'

'A bit. She said something about persecutory rum something and that it would fade with time, didn't seem to put her off but then nothing seems to – stuff she must hear about.' He looked to Alan with fear in his face, the hoped for fading hadn't happened yet. This was something Alan knew a bit about.

'Was it persecutory rumination she mentioned? Thoughts that get stuck in your mind going round like a circle in a circle.'

'Or a wheel within a wheel.' Added Bill helpfully. 'Well it's all very well hoping it's going to fade but she left me feeling it was something I do to myself – self-persecutory, that's it. Why should I persecute myself, what have I done that' so wrong? I want to get better.'

Alan sensed his therapy-lite nerves stirring to conceptualise an internal world of persecutory anxiety threatening the insecure citadel of bad objects generating the manic windmill of anger turned inwards to mill a cold harvest of neurotic (major) depression. But he quelled all that and tried to make Bill feel a bit better. 'They're just thoughts Mr. Clayton. We all know you haven't done anything – the only person they hurt is yourself. I've come across this kind of thing before and it can often be the worst part of serious depression. It's a good thing to tell someone.'

'Other people get it then?'

'Yeah, the thoughts that trouble them the most seem to be about disgusting things they'd never do in a million years. Sometimes it's just a cold, fleeting idea about something that could never happen but it's enough just for it to come into your mind for the awful feelings to follow. It's awful but it is a normal part of many peoples depression. And it does go – I can see myself that you're on the mend.'

Mr. Clayton nodded slightly but his focus seemed to be turned a long way inside himself. Alan often felt that your mind was located inside your face – somewhere behind the eyes, or just inside the bridge of your nose. Definitely at some point from the neck up. He was most aware of his own as a series of facial impressions, often inside his mouth or around his cheekbones. Other people seemed more centred in their bodies; trustful of their feelings – putting their best foot forward, divining gut reactions. Bill seemed an introverted type like himself and too much withdrawal could take you too far out. Cut off from reality. A bit mad, but Bill didn't seem too keen on madness as a concept. 'So, if I told you something you wouldn't hold up your hands then beetle off back home?'

'No of course not. Do you want to tell me something?'

Bill filled up at this and looked away. 'Not really – you and Dr. Wallace say it's normal and not to worry – I do listen to what you say but you don't know what it's like … why does it come and does it really go away?' The poor guy was in turmoil, it was written all over his face and Alan wondered if he should be there. Bill began to weep so Alan passed him a man-sized box of tissues.

They sat on without speaking for a full three minutes. In a neighbouring garden someone was demolishing something; there was a hurried command to 'shift the cat' followed quickly by a hurried swish and cushioned crash. Bill seemed

ASK ME NOW

oblivious to this but his breathing had deepened and the commotion from outside served to point up a more settled affect in the room. A dog yapped. 'That'll be Rags from next door, canny little dog.' Said Bill, then he carried on crying.

'What are you thinking about Mr. Clayton?' Asked Alan as gently as he could.

'I wouldn't hurt him – I'd never do anything like that, how could anyone … ?'

'How do you mean Mr. Clayton?'

'With a dog.'

'Of course you wouldn't want to hurt the dog – you worked for the RSPCA.'

'Came across some things there I can tell you. Nothing like this though.'

'There's something about this that's really bothering you at the moment isn't there.'

It wasn't the most piercing insight Alan had ever come out with but it seemed to help things forward. Bill looked directly at him and said. 'It was something I read in the newspaper; it was some literary chap in a book. He used to pleasure his Alsatian bitch – that's what it said. I don't want to read that in The Telegraph … then, later I was looking through the front windows and next door was taking their dog out. He'd been chatting to me that morning and the dog had been there then, and I was seeing them going out and I thought about what I'd read about that other man and his dog and I thought, well it just seemed to come to me. It was terrible – I didn't mean to think it. Then I just went cold all over, I didn't know what to think'

'But nobody was affected except you though were they?'

'No I don't think so. Well, no.'

Alan smiled with genuine sympathy. He didn't think there was anything he could have said anyway.

'There's been other things too, horrible stuff, shit and sex and things. I'm not like that but it comes into my mind. Why does it come?'

Sounds of further demolition came over the garden fence, and a further yelp followed by. 'Fuck that stupid animal'.

'I've never heard Mr. Murtaugh swear like that before.' Said Bill.
'He seems to have a right job on next door.' Said Alan.

'Eh? Oh I blame myself for starting him off when I took it into my head to be a lumberjack. I think his wife's promised him a new shed if he gets topside of their back. I ought to offer a hands turn really.'

Alan had learned how easy it was to underestimate depression, Bill Clayton had all ready begun to slacken off into the quotidian, the man next door, his house and garden, no more stuff from the dark side for now. Alan's job, his task, was to keep them in the here and now, get him to consider the preposterous notion that it could be all right to be not all right. Someone else had said that fear is in your head/so forget your head and you'll be free. Wonderful as it was this would not wash with Bill, what Alan had to do was help him find some hope. 'You said that you took it into your head to be a lumberjack and that it was your fault.'

'Well who else's fault was it? There's too much of that now – blaming all and sundry for the things you do. People should

ASK ME NOW

take responsibility not go on the telly ... who's that fellow with the sun tan, grins like an ape?'

'But you were poorly, very poorly. That wasn't your fault and, even though you're on the mend, the horrible ideas you get are part of the depressive illness. As you improve they'll fade. I think you mean Killroy.'

Bill nodded evenly and appeared to be focussing on Alan's shiny shoes. 'Would he be part of a horrible illness do you think?'

'Oh he's just a clown.' This was strong stuff from the social worker and he made an effort not to lapse any further into the brittle mateness he knew to be a regular pratfall in the getting-to-know-you stage. The delusive appeal of the getting-to-hope-you-like-me impulse had messed up many an intervention, Bill didn't have to like Alan, just take him seriously. 'I've heard people say before that they felt as if they were going out of their minds, that their thoughts were in chaos and how terrifying it is.'

'Yes but you tell me that isn't going mad – it is like losing your mind a little.'

'But you said it is like losing your mind. It's the as if bit that makes the difference, it might feel like losing it but you didn't. When someone's properly mad – psychotic – they're lost in something that isn't real. They're convinced the television's talking about them or God's chosen them for a secret mission. Depression's different.' Alan knew he was glossing over quite a bit here because, at it's worst, Bill's experience could have taken him as far as the outer ring of psychosis. The main thing was to get him through the next couple of months. He wondered how Mrs. Clayton was coping. He also wondered how much Bill wanted to remember from his earlier breakdown. If some well meaning wise acre had told him then that he'd get better they'd have been right, but then he'd got ill again so that was best left alone for now. He pressed on with what probably fell within a cognitive view. 'The way you stand back from it just enough to say what it's like keeps you from losing it. It's very frightening but it's the illness not you.'

'It might be better if I went all the way round the bend then, maybe it wouldn't bother me so much.'

'Does it help to know you're not on your own with it?'

'What the making yourself feel terrible business, the stuff you say isn't mad?'

Alan looked a bit harder beyond the television. There were a number of books on a shelf in a corner. He could make out the spine of Great Expectations and a P.D. James leaning against some hardbacks stacked the wrong way. 'What are you reading at the moment?' He asked nodding to the books. He toyed with the idea of introducing Mr. Dick; the image of a man sending his troubled thoughts into the sky trailing from a kite on a hill at Betsy Trotwood's cottage was one of the most elegiac images he knew.

'Nothing much.' Said Bill. 'I can't seem to concentrate for more than two minutes then when I do it's some filth in the Telegraph. It used to be a decent paper, now it's full of pictures of Liz Hurley in a bikini and dirty books. That poor Alsatian, in my day we'd have gone for a prosecution.'

Stifling his curiosity about the Telegraph Alan tried to move them on a bit. 'I was thinking about a book we've got at work I could lend you. It covers a lot of the things you seem to have been struggling with – tells of other folk who've had it and how it happens. It shows you you're not on your own, that you're normal.' Bill seemed not to be listening and he couldn't blame him. You phone your mental health worker

ASK ME NOW

and he turns out to be a travelling librarian.

'Well.' Said Bill. 'Maybe it all helps ... you say other folk get this?'

Before Alan could dispense call up wisdom the front door opened followed by the unmistakeable bustle of a woman back from the shops. Bill sat a little straighter and watched the door. After the accelerating rustle of full plastic bags on cushioned kitchen floor diminished Bills significant other appeared. 'Does he want a biscuit?' She asked without looking at Alan.

'Err no, its all right, I'll need to get off soon.' Alan said watching Bill who watched his wife disappear again. Then the back door banged and a would-you-credit-it type of exchange began then trailed away into the garden.

Bill seemed oblivious to whatever it was that was going on but had taken in something of Alan's counsel. 'And you say this book you've got might help me?'

'Yes I think it will, you can borrow it as long as you like.'

'What's it called?'

''The Successful Self' by Dorothy Rowe, she's a psychologist – she's really good. Titles a bit off putting, I think.'

'What, you mean 'Madness Made Simple' might pull them in?' Offered Bill deadpan. 'Well, bring it along, when do you want to come again?'

Alan fished out his diary but before any further arrangements could be made the back door re-opened and a snatch of conversation about 'neighbours' and 'mending fences' drifted through. Then Betty Clayton stood in the doorframe nodding

Mike Pearson

nicely, this time in Alan's direction as another friendly, but flustered figure made himself known behind her. He too gave a sociable, slightly deferential gesture towards Alan in the manner of someone in a classic sit-com of 1968 greeting the Vicar. Bill could be Eric Sykes, Betty Hattie Jacques and the man from next door would have to be Derek Guyler. In fact the man – the mysterious Mr. Murtaugh – gave off something of Derek Guylers' amiable menace. He was tall and gangly with an incongruous baseball cap and Alan remembered what had been said to the dog. 'I say Bill.' He said. 'Would you give me a hand with this shed, only it won't fall right?'

'I'm afraid it's caught the fence Bill.' Put in Betty.

'Well I'd best be off.' Said Alan as Bill left his chair and peeled off his cardie. He felt this signified a willingness to help rather than the prelude to a fight with Mr. Murtaugh and, having set a date for the next week, he let himself out.

On the way back to Northfield Alan tried to focus on the next task in hand, the student placement. He persuaded himself that he couldn't really kick up too much fuss about this. Even when they'd had months of preparation time, with opportunities to introduce, set in place and generally get their fingers out nobody ever gave much thought to the thing till the last minute. So this Vic affair wasn't that different really therefore the view that he was being had for a Wally wasn't an issue, as such. The taking of a student was a right palaver though, especially the first couple of weeks, all the mentoring and explaining, all the questions. What was social work? What do you do? What does this mean? What happens now? How should he know. Then there were the competencies, the verification of which should be underpinned by values, the theory which had to be integrated with effective practice, the inequalities to be identified and challenged while difference was acknowledged, and separately but at all times must anti-oppressive practice be burnished and honed under the seasoned guidance of an experienced practitioner. But he enjoyed taking students, he'd never met one yet who wasn't sceptical about the bollocks even as they effectively integrated them with the cobblers to pass their courses. They tended to be older now and had done something else occupationally, to be generally made of sterner stuff than his generation of red-bricked layabouts with their half-hearted commitment to the revolution and a keener interest in the pub and relationships (copping off as was). They'd all hated Thatcher but he could see that she'd made them grow up and that social work education was better now. He would sometimes dust down his old copy of 'Radical Social Work' and not know whether to laugh or cry, he still fancied the woman on the cover, the bloke had his foot on the desk. He was wearing sandals. Anyway Cindy had given him some good advice and there were plenty of willing colleagues to 'give the student some time'. It would all get sorted.

He parked up by the consultants rust bucket and couldn't help noticing a cobweb strung out from the passengers side. Her sills wanted looking at too. In reception Becky was explaining something complicated to one of the outpatients. He was struck again by her patience and unforced empathy, had she ever considered a career in social care? This particular punter seemed quite pale and disturbed so Alan wondered if this was a mental health act a brewing. She came to the end of her part and said. 'Ah, here he is now.'

The man – a rough cross between Wild Bill Hicock and Angus Deyton in detox – looked up and wheezed 'Right.' He then looked down again so Becky smiled and left them to it.

Horrified but trying not to be Alan said. 'You must be Vic.'

The other laughed mirthlessly and said. 'Vic won't be joining us, at least not in the form you've been led to expect.'

Badly ruffled by this Alan asked him whom he was talking to

in the briskest tone he could muster. 'My name's Bamber. Dave Bamber .' The man replied.

Alan thought he should have guessed but what on Earth was going on and who, where, or what was Vic? Then Val Meating appeared to say she was terribly sorry and it was all her fault. Would they like to come through so she could sort it all out?

'Ah.' Said Bamber.

'Oh.' Said Alan.

She led them through the security doors to her office. It was a typical Friday afternoon; no one about and the offices baking with a week's central heating and clogged with anticipated release. It was like an August afternoon in Rome; everyone else has already left and the space that used to sizzle and buzz seems flat and melancholy, the only intimations of life an empty crisp packet twitching in the street. Even the Tiber has stopped moving. Alan reckoned he needed a holiday.

'Come in chaps.' He and the time locked lecturer took their seats and waited. The phone rang and Val asked Becky to take a message and not put any further calls through for the next half hour. 'Well really I should try to explain what's happened – basically 'Vic.' (waggling her index fingers in parenthesis) wont and never will be joining us. It's all my fault, I've really got things arse about face on this one, so apologies all round, It's a proper lash up and no mistake.'

Bamber was content to hold his tongue so Alan asked the obvious question. 'So who is Vic. And where is he?'

'Virtual Information Collapse.' She said baldly. 'And he came by these here parts last week. It's like I was saying about those little old acronyms.'

ASK ME NOW

Alan was seeing a new side of Val; loose lipped and flippant, though she needed to decide between the breezy top sergeant with a swagger stick or Wilbur Cobb from The Ren And Stimpy Show. 'Well.' Said Bamber. 'If that's that I'll saddle up and say adios.' And before either one of them could say Blazing Saddles he'd reached the corridor.

Then the phone rang. 'Becky I said I was in a meeting … oh all right. Alan hang on I think this could come to something. Yes, fine … put him on.' By the time Alan reached reception Bamber had made good his departure. A right set of cowboys thought Alan, and no mistake. He went back to see how Val was getting on. 'Well no.' She was saying to the phone. 'This wasn't … I don't think … but I don't think that's possible … ' At this point she flashed Alan a stricken look and bid him return to his seat with flapping hand gestures. Bound to be a Mental Health Act assessment he thought as what was a very one sided telephone conversation unrolled. Val was just about able to put in the odd 'hang about', 'yes buts' and 'couldn't possibly's but eventually wrestled the initiative 'on this one' with an odd précis concerning roll out times, power points and staff being no-where near ready for 'on-lining'. She then put her phone down and turned to him. 'This is what it's all been about.' She said.

'Right.' Said Alan. Was that him then?'

'No Alan, I've all ready explained – he or she is a virus which has somehow mutated out of an inherent incompatibility between our computer system and health's. It's caused no end of trouble and that was Tommy Pollard telling me at one thirty on a Friday afternoon that everything stops at midnight so they can sort out a major operation by Monday morning. Oh and, as they're paying, we're expected to fund our own training – of course there'll be nobody available in Department S this afternoon.'

Alan was beginning to get his head round it all. 'But if Vic is a virtual fantasy why did Dave Bamber turn up all ready to discuss the placement?'

'I don't know. He took himself off pretty smartly though didn't he?'

'I'll have a word with him; he could have been anyone for all we know. It's great though isn't it when health and social services get together the produce a love child computer virus called Vic. Do you think if they warm to it they could conceive one called Bob? Imagine the fun they could generate, reminds me of that one where Ulri …'

'Alan shut up. It's galling enough to think how much post-modern mayhem this has caused all ready. Didn't you spend most of your afternoon looking for him the other day?'

Somewhat stung by this Alan asked her why she'd gone along with it so readily. 'Well, oh it's been a busy week what with one thing and another, when you're under pressure you want to believe what people tell you. Life gets awfully complicated when you start questioning everything, it sounded right so I decided it was.' She paused to sigh. 'Isn't that terrible? They always say that when you get into management you should stop being a social worker; you have to be tough-minded not ruminative, decisive not creative. You have to stand firm and anticipate conflict. Christ, if one of you had been so soppy with someone who promised not to jump off the roof or stop bashing the kids … '

'Mmm – we all want the world to turn as it should and nearly all the time it does. I can't understand what Dave Bamber was playing at though; he must have come along prepared to blag his way through it making it up as he went along. What a nerve, no wonder he showed us a clean pair of plimsolls when it all went tits up.'

'What a charming expression Alan. Well I'm sure we'll hear

ASK ME NOW

about it eventually – there's Annette Kirton on that course.'

'Eh?' Alan was having some difficulty with this. Would it be parted to disclose the risky doings of Dave Bamber?

'Netty Kirton, an old mate of mine from the Chatterbox Club. Brilliant group worker, she teaches at TAT now, I'll have a word with her, I gather he's got previous.'

Alan thought about what she'd just told him. Several issues came to mind. 'What was the Chatterbox Club?' He asked.

She laughed at this. 'God, that was years ago. We'd both just qualified – Cindy reminds me of Netty a bit – and we were all up at the old General then. There was this old Chinese consultant up there called Dr Foo but everyone called him Funny Pong because ... well anyway he was a nice chap and would take an interest in the community and what social workers and community nurses got up to. Every now and again the cultural divide would prove too great for a patient and he would ask them if they would like to chat to a socialist worker, and some did. He used to say that chatting was good for you, and who were we to disagree so Netty and I decided to run a modest group therapy group type thing. We got one of the psychologists to supervise us and it grew from there. I'm not sure how much good it did but most of them came back each week and we enjoyed it. Netty had a real flair for it, I wonder if she's able to teach much of that at TAT?'

Alan sensed Val unwinding as she talked and thought that she might miss all that. 'Did people really call him Funny Pong?'

'Yes but not to his face, and we all liked him. It was a few years ago now. There was an African Doctor there too called Chittapo – everyone called him Noggs, even the other doctors, even some of the patients. No one seemed to bother.'

'That reminds me.' Said Alan. 'Dr. Effendi phoned me and I really struggled – he wanted Graham for something – all I could catch was 'thank you'. I mean if English isn't your first language it can be a real problem for the older patients.'

'Or for the hard of understanding – Alan, we're supposed to be living in a multi-cultural society now aren't we?'

'Are we?'

She thought about this. 'I don't know really. I don't know that we can sometimes but it's very difficult to think aloud on this at the moment. Netty's told me some horror stories from TAT, Dave Bamber would be less likely to get into trouble over this afternoons caper than if he practiced oppressively – and you can do that in your sleep. Especially in your sleep.'

'It can be a right old minefield. Cindy told me some stuff about that Cultural Awareness course she went on last year, sounded like brief cases at dawn.'

'How are you and Cindy getting on?'

'Oh fine. We managed to get the window sorted out by my desk so we can open it now.'

Val looked at him doubtfully and said. 'Right, well, I suppose I ought to do something purposeful before Monday comes around. Have a good weekend.'

'You too.' Said Alan.

He went off to tidy his desk, thought better of fiddling with his computer for half an hour and went off in search of Graham with Dr. Effendis' message. His partner was nowhere to be found so he left a note with reception rather than risk trusting it to the information black hole that was Grahams desk. He noticed a flustered young man of Eastern ethnicity

ASK ME NOW

trying to make himself understood to Becky. The general drift was that he'd been badly delayed in traffic and hoped he might still have his meeting with Mrs. Meating 'to make plans for Vic'.

'Val's still in.' He said to Becky, then 'She's been expecting you.' To the man he sincerely hoped was not Mr. Foo.

Mike Pearson

FILL YOUR HEART

On Saturday morning Alan came to alone and tried to hold the fleeting stay of grace separating oblivion from memory. Once it had all started to start up again he had a go at inverting the process by retrieving a dream but all he could snatch back were a few stray images; a kimono, and Val Meating intoning 'Happy Talk' in a monotone to a blank computer screen. Ordinarily it would have seemed funny but all he could feel was a dull after ache of things leaving him behind.

This troubled him but he hadn't woken too early and wanted some toast so it wasn't forced to be the old grey mutt demanding an extended run round the block. He'd been all right for ages anyway, and then he remembered he was in love. In love with Cindy Watson who put the wind up Graham and half the other blokes at Northfield. Lovely Cindy with her hair in a bob, an encyclopaedic knowledge of the Mental Health Act and unsuspected reserves of carnal know-how. How on Earth had this happened?

Alan made some tea and toast, the activity helping disperse some of the chill flatness he'd woken to. He took his breakfast back to bed and selected some music, settling on 'Miles Davis And The Modern Jazz Giants', a troubled quintet recorded by the legendary Rudy Van Gelder on Christmas Eve 1954 and now an undisputed classic. Legend had it that Miles had been at his meanest on the day and been fantastically rude to everyone, and hadn't Thelonious Monk clocked him one for his troubles? No one really knew and he thought it was likely to have been greatly talked up after the event; anyway the music was glorious stuff. Some said that jazz was night music but Alan could generally listen to it at anytime. Saturday morning in bed was especially good. Propped by an old Habitat cushion he sipped his Russian Caravan like the last Romanov in Ridsdale while the sounds unwound in his bed-sitting room and Milt Jackson's milk bottle vibes chimed as Miles and Monk clunked and spat. He

ASK ME NOW

knew the recording so well though it was never quite the same, but this morning, like the first familiar hint of a cold coming on, the music was out of reach and wrong. The idea was there in theory but he wasn't really getting it, instead there was an old odd strain he'd forgotten, till it came back. The edge of a sadness, of losing touch. He felt the sketch of a heartbreaking image of a child on a station watching helplessly a train full of his classmates pulling away into the light, laughing families crowding the hot compartments leaving the dark platform. But he'd arrived too late, there was no choice but to turn round with Mummy, go back home to be a good boy again and forget all about uncertain journeys into the light. He didn't know where the image came from but it carried a weight of exquisite sadness, and fear – the child was beyond comfort, destined for disappointment, and another thing.

He ate some toast and tried again with the music; they were onto 'Bemsha Swing' and he knew what was coming next – Monks amazing solo, obtuse tappings and shuffleplonk rhythym. One of his favourite bits of music, ever. He got it but ... the feelings were like they should be but disturbing in their slight remoteness. Like a known face seen through a dirty window. He pressed the music off and made himself get up. John Peel was on the radio asking someone who's Father had suffered a stroke if the old man had liked Captain Beefheart, Alan decided to go out.

After a good twenty minutes of cleaning up, reordering his CD's and choosing an outfit he found himself out on the street wondering what to do next. He thought he'd go back in and phone Cindy – after he'd been up to Londis for some bits and bats. So he returned to the flat to see what he needed then came straight back out and headed for the shops. He lived in a shabby-genteel part of the town where much of the housing stock had been put up in terraces somewhere between the old Queens death and the Great War. Many streets were named after soldiers or campaigns and he was intrigued by the notion of smaller private events and conflict happening inside each beautifully built house. All the familial strife and trench warfare that Natal Street had framed, the reconciliation's and unifications negotiated along Gordon Road.

Also, he had learned that they'd been constructed during a golden age of craftsmanship when the standards reached in carpentry and brickwork had brushed perfection when there had been the time and money to do the job properly. Even now with half of them hacked into multi-occupancy or plastered in cladding the houses kept their dignity; they'd seen an awful lot come and go, nothing much could bother them now. He got to the top of Surtees Street then turned down Cartmell Terrace. The houses here were smaller and less tampered with, from his vantage at the bottom of the row he saw the facing parallel lines as inclined cliffs with lots of lives packed into small cells. He reckoned as many as two hundred people living off the street hidden away in there at this time on a Saturday morning, it seemed wrong; how on Earth did they live, what did they do? How could they all be happy together?

After Alan had walked up and down one side of the street three times he came to a stand still at a house painted purple. A man in a turban emerged and asked him if he was all right. 'You seem a bit lost mate.' He said in a mildly concerned way.

'Umm, no, no it's okay.' Alan said as he moved away. When he got back to Surtees Street he realised he was crying.

He walked home feeling slightly better and set about changing his bed. The gentle exertion, folding, straightening, the smell of fresh things helped him on a bit further so he made a list of similar such tasks and divided the day ahead up into rough sections on the basis that by six o'clock he'd be crisper too. The trick was to keep moving. He knew depression was recurrent; there wasn't much he didn't know about it one way and another. He also knew himself to be intelligent, have a creative streak, to be goodish at his job, not unattractive to other people. Something he'd done with Bill Clayton had seemed to strike a chord, or maybe the older man had simply spotted a fellow delicate.

He ought to be feeling alright but felt like a stupid boy now, grinning inanely over some great shame. The sound of Lena Martell singing 'One Day At A Time (Sweet Jesus)' was going round in his head so he put on his favourite Stan Tracey record. It was called 'Hello Old Adversary' and on the cover Stan looked lost in a transport of deep blue rumination. Alan very nearly laughed. He composed himself as he usually would to listen, he could tell how good the piano sounded but the overall effect was to show him how far from his norm he really was. Wise counsel from the days of doublets and hose advised that he should be not solitary or idle and of course there was always Prozac. Really, there was very little reason for people to be depressed these days. Particularly for him, now that he'd clicked with Cindy. He thought he'd phone her again but didn't. For some reason this seemed to be the hardest thing. Trying to read the Indie only made him feel more agitated and he began to hope that Steve from downstairs wouldn't ask him if he fancied a pint and an afternoon at Spotfields. Only the very undepressed could watch the 'Dale. He knew he ought to, Steve was virtually a friend, they'd shared one or two serious talks down the pub where each had confided candidly of weighty notions and the ways of men, and Alan had made him his tea once. Cindy would doubtless encourage this course of action, women in general being more naturally inclined to the communal. He was pretty sure she talked to Claire Todgers about him but he wouldn't dream of mentioning her to Steve, did Steve have a girlfriend? He wasn't sure – he knew he worked on the Echo, liked rap music and Irving Welsh and, that was about it. Well, blokes took their time over connections; nobody wanted to come on like Brenda bleeding heart Blethyn did they? If there was a knock he'd pretend to be out.

The disc clicked off but he didn't know if he wanted to hear the other side or switch the radio back on. He thought he could hear muffled shuffles behind the door, then the phone chirruped. If he answered it the furtive shuffler would know he was in. He felt paralysed, his mind banged like an iron maiden, his belly boiled like a mad pan – he wanted to shout and evaporate simultaneously. The phone stopped and the visitor shuffled off. None of this was right.

At such times the radio was the best bet. On 'Any Question' a wiseacre from Westminster was blandly informing the audience that the governments recent proposal regarding something or other represented the most sensible initiative set forward by anyone at anytime ever. Then some helpful soul asked a question about the green paper on the mental health bill – weren't there many people, dangerous people, out there in the community who we should be locating and treating? There was no getting away from it. Then the phone went again. He picked it up and cleared his throat, his tongue felt like a dead weight so he was glad that the voice at the other end was the lady of mystery with news that he had a message. He pressed the right buttons and Cindy came. 'Hi, it's just me. Wondered if you fancied getting together today – let me know. Bye.'

Talk about any questions, this one could take up the afternoon. He had enough sense to ring her back directly but when she answered he thought it was her taped response. It was only when she asked who it was in a sharper tone that he said something. 'Oh, it's me … Alan … I got your call, earlier I mean.'

'Right, well thank goodness for that. I thought I'd got a weirdo on for a moment – you sound out of breath. Are you all right?'

ASK ME NOW

'Eh?'

'You sound a bit wheezy.'

'Eh? Oh yeah.' He said without elaborating.

'Anyway, I'm feeling a bit better today and I wondered if you fancied getting out for a bit. Maybe up to the moors again – we could have a drink on the way back. Perhaps you could use some fresh air.'

What would have been expected here, he thought? He summoned up a hidden slice of normalisation. 'Yeah … yeah, that'd be nice.'

'Are you coming round then?'

'Yes … umm what time is it?'

'Alan are you all right?'

'I, slept in … sorry, a walk would be good.'

'That's a yes then. It's half-one, I'll see you in a bit.'

'Yes. I'll come right over.' Alan noticed himself feeling brighter and took a look at his freshly folded bed. He thought about lying there with her and Middlemarch. He would be all right. On the way out he knocked on Steves door to say hello but there was no answer so he drove to Londis to buy a plant and pay the papers. On the way back to the car he met the man with the turban and smiled firmly at him. His new friend muttered a wary 'all right mate' as they passed which immediately flattened his mood. He recalled what Cindy had said about a weirdo and decided to make more of an effort to be himself.

The route to Cindys took him past the football ground but it was impossible to tell that there was a match due to be played. Whenever he went along with Steve it seemed a small miracle that anybody turned up at all but by kick-off there would be two thousand of them all practicing their personal brands of cognitive re-framing; convincing themselves that something bad was somehow good or that it was so bad it was good in another way. Also, given the conditions the players had to contend with – which were never properly delineated – they did well to put on a show at all. They'd like to see 'that swarthy little cheat' Maradona ply his trade in the English lower leagues, he'd have to leave his fancy foreign ephemera in the dressing room with his Matalan suit and muck in like the rest. The fact that he'd left the entire English defence for dead on a wet night at Wembley when he was seventeen didn't count, let alone making merry with the likes of Peter Reid at the World Cup. Had it been Graham or him who'd dubbed him 'a dago twat'? He wished he hadn't remembered that. Maybe he could coin a joke about the plant being an Argentine Climber,'Maradona Duplicita', she might laugh – or think him a precious berk. When he got there he left it in the car.

She smiled at the door and ran her hand down his upper arm companionably. 'Come in Alan, do you think this weather'll hold?'

He looked back; wispy streaks pointed to more substantial lumps of grey mashed potato in a sky that was still basically blue. 'I dunno.' He said.

'Oh well.' She said. 'Lets go anyway. You still up for it?'

'Yeah – blowin' the blues away. Fresh air.'

'What?'

ASK ME NOW

'Horace Silver.'

'Oh, right.' Said Cindy in a slightly tired voice.

He stood in the kitchen while she went upstairs. All ready bits of the place were becoming parts of his life; a plate he'd eaten from lay flat on the draining board, he'd enjoyed her Modigliani poster from a different angle as they'd sat down to supper. When she'd opened her door the curtains had asked him what the matter was. Things would pick up when they were out. He heard the rush of water then the headache scrape of window sash.

'Right all set. Do you mind driving?'

'No, course not.'

As they left the house he found himself puzzling over a phrase that had replaced Lena Martell at the front of his troubled mind. Something about an iron street and windy curtain, or was it the other way round? Why did it matter? Before he could bother himself further Cindy clapped eyes on the plant. 'That looks nice, is it coming with us?'
'Eh?' Alan was properly puzzled now. 'Oh, no, I brought that for you.'

'That's sweet, shall I pop it in the house now?'

'Yes, oh yes. I must have forgotten.'

Cindy favoured him with a kiss and a gentle frown as she popped. He could see her from the car at the kitchen sink. She had her head down and was running water as she plucked deftly at his careless offering. He reflected that he'd have made a hopeless bowerbird leaving his gaudy bawbees all over the forest floor. Unable to locate a mate he would end his days alone wearing the bowerbird equivalent of a Littlewoods cardigan.

'That'll do well in the yard, they can climb up anything can't they?' Said Cindy as she clunkclicked herself in.

'I don't know to be honest; I just liked the look of it in Londis. What is it?'

'It's a hardy Latin vine type thing – quite aggressive to less virile blooms, I can't help thinking it's their own fault for being soft enough to let them.'

Alan looked ahead in some alarm and started the car. 'Have I imagined this or is there a plant called 'Sluggish Peter?'

Cindy thought about this. 'You're not thinking of Saltpetre are you?'

'Probably.' He said with relief. 'Where do you fancy going - same place as before?'

'God, I feel so much better today.' She said. 'Sounds like I missed a strange day at work, did you manage to get things sorted?'

'Oh, I think so.' He said managing an authentic chuckle before recounting a version that hinted at his part in the proceedings as trusting then firmly critical rather than as a hapless twerp. Cindy left it at that.

'That Dave Bamber is a slippery beggar – just cleared off without a word?'

'Yes. I think he must be the academic version of that vine.'

She laughed at this and stroked his thigh. 'You all right with it?'

ASK ME NOW

'Yeah, it's just – well nobody feels comfortable trying to work out what's happening when you've only heard half the tale. I think we all like to feel we know what's happening.'

'Hmmm.' She said thoughtfully. 'Well when we get this wizzo computer system up and running we can find out what's what.'

Alan laughed again and wondered why he'd worried, everything passes he thought, even Ridsdale's midfield. 'Do you mind if we have local sport on for the latest scores?'

'No, shall I tune in?'

'Please.'

He enjoyed her unfussy facility, how she'd fluffed out that plant and was now twiddling his car radio with her simple poise. He thought this was a woman thing, men having to make such a production of everything by contrast. Women seemed to just get on with it and make it work as best they could, whether it was a car radio or reforming the trade unions. Sure enough she found the live broadcast 'from around the region'; Bury were nil-nil away at Lincoln, Stockport were struggling at Scunthorpe and at Spotfields ...

'Why did they call it Spotfields?' She asked.

'I think it was supposed to have been Sportfields but they couldn't find their r's.'

She gave a demure chortle and he missed most of the bulletin apart from 'Dale 'having it all to do now'. 'Oh well.' He said. 'I think we can manage without the live commentary – get the result later.'

They fell into an easy silence. This was something else he

liked about her, he'd come to a conclusion about one aspect of the man-woman stuff; people were wrong about the talking issue. It was usually men who couldn't shut up and as for not expressing their feelings where did that come from? A bit more taciturnity in that quarter wouldn't go amiss. A car pulled out to overtake and he felt smug as he slowed to let it pass.

'What's this tape like?' She asked as she clipped it back in and pressed play.

'What?'

'The tape you mentioned earlier – 'Blowing Bubbles About' or something.'

At this point the music came on, quite loudly. It was a particularly stormy passage from John Coltranes' 'Ascension' recital, all blaring brass and flaming reeds underpinned by the customary pots and pans. Cindy pulled a face and remarked that she'd sooner have the blues back if this was the alternative. 'Oh this isn't Horace.' He assured her.

'Well, can we hear from him then?'

'Hear from Horace?'

'Yes. The one you were playing on the way over to my house – the one you were telling me about.'

'I think I might have got that wrong, we're nearly there anyway. This bit's a bit smoother – did I tell you about the music appreciation class at Sweethaven, that Teddy Charles is a character ... '

'Alan, what are you on about?' She said with some irritation.

'Don't shout at me Cindy.' He responded in his patient, long

ASK ME NOW

suffering voice.

'I'm not shouting at you – Alan what's the matter?'

'I don't know.' He replied after a telling pause. The rest of their journey didn't take long but the mood in the little fiat had turned from smooth sailing to choppier waters.. By the time they were facing each other in the car park Alan felt as bad as he had all day.

Cindy came towards him. 'Alan, what is it?'

'I don't know. I don't feel too clever.'

'Oh Alan, you should have said something sooner.' She gave him a tight smile and a hug. He marvelled at her normality. How did people do it? He felt anxious for the car park man as he fielded questions from an overwrought motorist – how could he do that job? It would defeat him.

'I'm sorry Cind. I feel awful.'

'It's all right, I thought you seemed a bit off when you came.'

'How do you mean?' He asked with obvious concern.

'Just a bit vague – not your normal self.'

'Do you think I'm depressed?'

'Do you feel depressed?'

'I don't know. More scared really – I'm all right for a while then it just goes and everything falls away.' He pondered as she stood back to see him. 'It's happened before.'

'Come on.' She said. Lets start walking then you can tell me if you want to.'

'Are you sure you want to … '

'Alan, for fucks sake what do you think of me? We're big people now so spare me that otherwise I will shout at you.'

He had enough sense to take that as meant and held his tongue as they took off between a straggled group of four wheeled drives and some smaller vehicles. Last time they'd come it had been a bit dull and he'd not wanted to go far but today was different; blowy and mutable. A sudden whoosh caught Cindy from behind, forcing her hair forward over her face to make a perfect parting just south east of her right ear. She turned to face the wind and him moving her head with a subtle adroitness that he found suddenly beautiful. She laughed at the weather and said. 'Come on, I feel a Kate Bush moment waiting for us up there.'

They linked arms and bent into the wind with their heads down. He noticed the rough slabs peter out to less certain stuff as they hit the track. There was no one else in sight and he marvelled again at Cindy's sense of purpose as she led him to the point they'd come to last time. He remembered the moors murderers and felt that that was probably the first time he'd been aware of the monkey poking his shoulder. When they past 'that'seat he wouldn't look across to Saddleworth. Cindy didn't stop either and he was content to follow her lead as the path took them along a ridge then to a dip where there were rocks and some spikey looking evergreens. 'So, what's been happening?' She asked, not unkindly.

'I don't know – I mean I do … it's just, I feel so stupid.'

Cindy waited for more as they reached the little copse He noticed one of the trees was festooned with used condoms and felt a bit sick. A pair of big stones formed a rough settee near the tree and the sudden conflation of careless love with Linda

ASK ME NOW

Barker put him in a curious mood. He sat down the better to contemplate the sadness of his life, Cindy joined him and regarded the condom tree. 'It must be awful when you've got nowhere to go, do you think Heathcliff and Cathy had to make do with this?'

Alan smiled at this. 'I thought they never got round to making do at all, besides he'd have had to travel to Leeds for one of those reusable sheaths made from sheep's bladder, they'd have been better off not bothering. Cindy I think I'm going bonkers.'

She moved closer and he felt the warmth from her leg. 'What do you mean by bonkers?'

'That my minds not right. I don't know what I'm going to think next, I'm watching myself all the time and I don't like what I'm seeing – I keep feeling terrible. I think I must be depressed ….. I can't believe it's happening again. I'm not bad some of the time but it won't go away. I'm sorry.'

'Don't apologise, you say it's happening again?'

'Yes, let's face it I ought to know. I just thought it might go away, I mean, you do it's no good stalling at the first fence.'

She put her hand on his knee and placed his over it. 'How long do you reckon it's been like this?'

'I think the first time I felt something was the last time we were up here. That Sunday, do you remember? It had been a really nice day and we sat on that seat back near the centre. I remember this clearly; a fleeting echo of a bad thing. I knew what it was but it went away. I decided I was just tired, which I was but that might have been another straw in the wind too.'

'I remember the day.' She said. 'It was a nice day but I didn't notice anything in you … except I noticed you were going on a bit about Myra Hindley and what they did. I'd never heard you talk like that before, almost as if you were taking some kind of responsibility. I know all that stuff happens but we don't have to think about it.'

'Well that's just it, I can't stop, sometimes. It's one side of me roasting the other, that's why it's bonkers.' He said then the wind found it's way in to lift one of the condoms away from its branch and deposit the thing with a faint plop on an adjacent stone. A thin trickle of watery spunk seeped over it's bloated pink collar which seemed to be offering itself up to him with it's gummy carp lips. The soggy toggy would bother him all day. She gave him another nice hug. 'I've felt pretty ropey today Cindy. I suppose I'll have to go to the Docs.'
'Right.' She said. 'When can you make an appointment?'

'Not until Monday I should think.'

'Which practice are you with now?'

'Eh? Oh, the Rio Grande lot, down South Way.'

'Ah, they've moved haven't they. You don't see old Dr. Pointon do you?'

'Old Dissa? No I usually see Dr. Rose – I like her she's made a fair few referrals to the team, seems very interested in mental health generally.'

'Well make sure she doesn't refer you.'

'It's not a laughing matter Cindy.'

'I'm not laughing.' She said as they disengaged. 'I think they're switched on to some sort of key pad system like they have when you want to book seats at the flicks.'

ASK ME NOW

'What, you can make an appointment like that?'

'I think so, lets have a go.' She said fishing around inside her jacket for her works mobile.

'Do you know their number?' He asked wonderingly.

'I've got them all keyed in, here you are.'

'No, you do it.'
Cindy accepted this without comment and deftly tapped and listened as the wind pulled her hair about. He couldn't credit it that this drop dead Nefertiti of the keypad liked him and could do the things she did. 'Right.' She said and switched off the phone. 'Monday ten to five.'

'You can do it just like that?'

'Yes, it's good not to have to talk.'

'Thanks Cindy.'

'Shall we go on or would you prefer to go back now Alan?'

Oh Christ, he thought. He'd learned that at times like these the best policy was to act on an 'as if' basis; make up the answer you think you'd normally want and sometimes you did. 'I'm not sure.' He said and began to feel a perverse attachment to their little bower and distress that they would leave it. Cindy made their decision by walking on ahead; as he looked back at the bushes quivering in the wind he began to fill up. They were soon climbing again and he could see the beginnings of West Yorkshire and Bronte country proper. He asked Cindy if she'd had her Kate Bush moment yet.

'Not yet.' She laughed. 'We could always play hide and seek out here, play out some epic of elemental space and separation, calling to each other across great divides. When you're better maybe.'

'Well it's good to know you've got faith.'

'Of course you will, come on Alan, you know as well as I do how common depression is, and how treatable.'

'What about the bonkers material?'

'What about it? They're just thoughts in your head – the only person you're hurting is yourself. As you say.'

'Is this how you talk to people at work?'

'I'm not at work now Alan. Would you prefer it if I started wittering on about persecutory anxiety or obsessional whatsits and other gubbins I only half understand?'

'Of course not but that's what a lot of it is isn't it?

'Well yes, I dare say it is and if having a brain in your head and a persuasive grasp of psychobabble was the remedy you'd be able to sit at home with the Jazz Misanthropes for company and think yourself better. Do you think that's going to do the trick?'

He thought about this as he looked back to where they'd come from. The path up from the copse of copulation had disappeared from view and they might have to find a new way back. He found this comforting and it made him wish to stay where they were for as long as possible. The wind had got itself up to the point where even his minimalistic mullet was atousle. Her hair was all over the place and she was laughing at something he couldn't catch. He moved closer to her and the held each other in defiance of the withering height.

'Christ.' She shouted. 'Dare we go on?'

ASK ME NOW

'Is there another sheltered bit further on?'

''Lets find out.'

As she reached out to pull her hair back from the wind Cindy felt her knuckles graze the bedroom wall. She fell awake to a receding trace of a great puzzle; an impossible mathematical calculation or a race with no finish. She tried to fall back but it wouldn't come so she lay and thought about the day to come, and Alan. They'd agreed to spend Sunday apart while she visited her Mother and he spent some time with a friend who he could tell what was happening. She was due to see him at teatime after his doctors' appointment. An uncomfortable echo of her dream found its way through and she felt overwhelmed again. Experience told her to lie still, let her thoughts come and go – then the radio came on automatically and a broadcaster shouted at a politician which drove her to the bathroom where she eventually lay like a Betjeman business girl to lap her loneliness in heat.

Before setting off she tuned into the local station where Nina Desousa was able to give a helpful rundown of road works, diversions and likely trouble spots. This meant she could chart a smooth passage to Northfield where she was almost the first in.

'Feeling better?' Asked Becky, who had seemed to be on her own.

'Yes thanks, Alan won't be in today – I saw him on Saturday and he wasn't too bright, he phoned last night and asked me to let you know.'

'Right.' Said Becky as she tapped at her keyboard.

Cindy's thoughts as she reviewed the day ahead were a

strange brew of concern for Alan and a jarring feeling that this was more than she'd bargained for. She didn't like feeling mean or mixed up and this complicated her feelings about him further. If she was going to be any help she'd need to dish out the old tough stuff; sign post limits, allocate responsibilities and all that, not become 'over involved' – a phrase she loathed. There was something else kindling away under all this, a bad thought she had covered over till it drifted into an idea; that in some way she might be part of Alan's dark night of the soul. That she could be disrupting his equilibrium in ways she couldn't understand. He'd seemed so happy during their salad days and one of the things she'd come to like about him before they clicked was a seeming solidity along with the quirkiness and lop sided sexuality. He liked making her laugh as well and perhaps this should have alerted her. Basically the last thing she needed right now was a complex production with a significant other, not now that her Mother was leaning north by north-west. Naturally as the daughter, and the one in the caring trade, something her brother had been quite carping about, until now, she was expected to know what to do and make it happen. Fix her up with Teddy Charles had been her only plan as she'd returned from the rough and ready affair that had been Sunday's lunch; quiche with custard, roast pork put in the fridge to cool. Pee on the carpet, worse in the bath. At that rate the problem would take care of itself soon enough.

At least with Alan she did want to be close to him. With her Mother it was more like calling occupants of interplanetary craft, something she couldn't think about. She phoned Claire Todgers. 'Oh Hi, yes it's me. Yeah fine – listen can I come round at Lunchtime; I could do with a natter. Yes, and Alan – I'll get up for one … see you then. Bye.'

Val Meating paused en route to her room as Cindy put down the phone. 'Mornin' Cindy, feeling better?'

'Yes thanks – bit of a virus then my period came.'

ASK ME NOW

''Well it won't be that with dear Dickie. Becky says he's bad today, possibly reactive stress from our bizarre Friday. Remind me to tell you about that – oh, and don't touch the computers.'

'Why not, what's happening. I need to get at my e-mails.?'

'Oh, the usual IT cock up but there's someone coming over this morning to sort it out, I think he's Chinese, they know all about computers don't they?' She then executed her smooth trundle, a rarely seen but greatly admired phenomenon. Basically a seemingly effortless movement across, and sometimes along, corridors as if powered by tiny casters while continuing a diminuendo conversation. Done well, as it was today, little movement should be apparent from above the knees. This one was as persuasive as French mime, as breathtaking as a Michael Jackson moonwalk. Cindy couldn't help laughing and wondered if she would ever be able to ask her how to do it.

Graham was on a days leave so she had the office to herself, which suited her. She glanced at Alan's' desk. The tape player was there and still plugged in so she pressed play. The aural nightmare that emerged suggested a quantity of furniture being tipped down some stairs in the warehouse at the end of the world followed by a choir of course grained blurtings at full volume. She switched it off directly and unplugged the player. She knew that not all jazz was awful, that even some of it could be quite pleasant and that not much of it sounded like that – though quite a lot of the stuff Alan seemed to like did – it just seemed to be the kind of music you really needed to like a lot if you were to enjoy any of it. And she just didn't, to the extent that it seemed incredible that anyone did, but they did and they often seemed to be blokes like Alan. So there must be something to it – like depression? She wandered to the kitchen to make coffee and encountered Dr. Wallace.

'Cindy, I'm glad I've caught you, have you got much on this morning?'

'Errm, I've an appointment at One but I think I'm pretty free till then … yes, nothing too pressing. Why, is something happening?'

'Possibly. Do you remember Mrs.Brestbohn from Aqueduct Street?'

'No, I think I'd remember the name.'
Dr. Wallace nodded and smiled briefly. 'She married a Dutch chap who left her with three kids, the whole lot of them are a right set but they generally rattle along well enough. I think it was before your time when we had to section her – she's been all right with some long arm support from one of the CPN's from Assertive Outreach, I know that doesn't make sense, but he's on a course this week and something seems to have cracked off on Saturday night. Can you have a look?'

'Yes of course.'

'Good, have a word with the med. Secs. – I think there's a fax flying about somewhere and I'll catch up with you later.'

Linda the med. Sec. Eventually found the fax on Dr. Wallace's desk beneath an out of date MOT for her Fiesta and last months British Journal Of Psychiatry. Cindy scanned the index and one of the papers caught her eye. It was titled 'Masked Male Depression: A New Formulation' and she made a mental note to nip back later. Linda handed her the details. 'Here – Brestbohn. Here's the word o' de lord.'

'Eh?' Said Cindy.

'Connected to the neck bone.' Said Linda and waggled her palms helpfully.

ASK ME NOW

Cindy decided racism didn't count when you were as black as Linda and enjoyed watching her beautiful pink tongue wagging instead. 'Right, yes. The word of the out of hours duty team, sounds like a proper how-de-do.'
Hoping she hadn't caused offence with the last bit Cindy moved decisively back to her office re-reading the fax as she went. The gist of it was that the Police had been alerted by a long suffering neighbour sometime round midnight due to more than the usual amount of noise filtering through the adjoining wall. Sounds suggestive of falling masonry. The put upon neighbour later reported vague shapes moving about the front garden. The even more put upon Police duly diluted the worst of the commotion before handing over to the emergency social workers, who turned out to be the vague shapes in the garden. Were they 'on duty' there all the time on a just-in-case basis wondered Cindy and waiting for back up? The implication was that the Brestbohns were mad but not that bad and probably safe to know so long as you were forewarned. There were no mentions of damage to persons or property but great play was made with a 'baseline formulation' that more than one borderline personality was at work in a manner 'not otherwise specified'. Mrs B. was living in parlous circumstances; a single parent to a dependent family group with special needs. In other words she was crackers and they'd made her that way, or was it the other way round?

She had a quick look at the medical file where it transpired that the GP had kept the consultant up to speed for some years. Julie Brestbohn had managed off medication for some time and the only real cause for concern had been a number of complaints about the 'unorthodox' pattern of life the family practiced which the Housing Department had passed on to the team. Dr. Wallace's' main service to them had been an ingenious series of measures to stall any further action and 'review the situation' in a manner which seemed to keep everyone happy and no-one called upon to do anything. Filled with a fresh dose of admiration for her colleague Cindy set off.

People were often surprised at the varied social strata the 'Ridsdale lot' got to work across, the spread of race, class, sex and soft furnishings. Though there were times when they went down familiar lean streets redolent of a certain stereotype of a social workers lot and the Brestbohn family seat was situated on one. Summer Street formed the main artery along a typical post-war council estate gone wrong; all the properties had decent sized gardens but some had scruffy looking cars in them, there were trees though one or two were decorated with bike parts and some of the homes were numbered, in large painted figures on the brick work by the door. The places that didn't catch attention like that looked neat and well cared for with lovely planted out borders and little men on sticks who caught the wind and danced. They were often nurtured by older couples with small but obese dogs on leads. During the holidays the streets would be full of kids straggling round together in a way you didn't see any where else, well looking kids in bright clothes and even in the rough looking house fronts people sat around drinking from mugs and rolling fags. It enraged her whenever she heard other people putting them down yet given the choice she wouldn't move here and she knew enough to know that the bad bits could be pretty bad; the casual brutality of the boys and young men, the hysterical machismo and disdain for anything remotely feminine – even from some of the women. She wound down her window as a girl of about, she guessed, thirteen approached pushing a buggy with a baby in it. 'I'm looking for number five.' She announced. 'I can't seem to find it – there are two number sevens.'

The girl simply turned and pointed behind her in a way that suggested she knew who Cindy was and what she was about then tottered off. Cindy could see a chubby fist jiggling about from the side of the buggy; from the back she glimpsed fresh

ASK ME NOW

nappies. Another girl appeared to kneel down laughing softly at the baby. Cindy got out of the car and walked over to the house. It was on a corner and enjoyed more land around it than most of the others with a virile Lime casting gently mutating patterns onto the building. In the long grass several metallic shapes also caught the light and a corroded car engine rested beneath the front bay at a point where the smarter houses sported tubs of flowers. The only immediate sign of life came from the house next door where an old man in a denim jacket and Stetson stared at her from his window.

She pushed the letterbox carefully but there was not an answering yap, muffled scrape of occupancy or brassy rebuke. She listened harder and heard a mysterious creaking sound and distant laboured breathing. It began to feel a bit ominous, especially with Texas Pete's glare warming her back. She moved out of his view around the side of the house and into the back garden where more parts of a dismembered car lay abandoned, one of it's seats was propped against a wall holding a large dirtybrown dog. It blinked at her and snorted derisively as if to say 'I wouldn't bother love' before turning it's attention to its backside. The back door was open. She tapped and called 'hello' in a speculative spirit of enquiry. This action took her far enough over the step to witness a serving hatch burst open from the other side of the room to disclose a head and shoulders as if fired from a circus cannon. 'I'll need to adjust your plugs first.' Said the head, belonging to a young man in overalls wearing a well-oiled woollen hat. Before she could reply to this the head retracted as swiftly as it had appeared. Then a different voice, corncrake and querulous piped up from behind a door to her right. 'He's doing his best for you.' It said.

Cindy was badly rattled now and asked in a voice of frank alarm if there was anybody there. After a pause the second voice; female, elderly said. 'Come in duck.' Anxious that the serving hatch could burst open again she nipped across to the pantry door and pulled it open. Inside she found a small old lady sitting calmly on a wooden school chair. The rest of the space looked to be taken up by tins of dog food, empty bottles and piles of auto magazines, by the old lady's foot a picture of Jeremy Clarkson smiled up at her. 'Don't you worry about him, he's not as green as he's cabbage looking.' She said as she recrossed her legs.

.No.' Said Cindy. 'No, I'm sure he's not.'

She gave Cindy a look of Steptoesque scorn and sniffed. 'You're not here about the car then.'

'No.' Said Cindy again. 'No I haven't. My name's Cindy Watson, I'm a social worker from the Community Mental Health Team.' She reinforced this by flourishing her official ID card with mug shot and asked her if she was Mrs. Brestbohn. She didn't bother to inspect Cindy's' card but started to regard her with a baleful might-have-known look. Cindy wondered if she would pull the door shut and tell her to wait for the serving hatch to bang again.

Instead she said. 'Yes, of course you are. They said you'd be coming.'

'Yes, well, there did seem to be some concern about what might have been happening here last night.' Mrs. Brestbohn kept her counsel over this then there was an almighty thump that rattled the door followed by a muffled 'bollocks to it'.

'I think.' Ventured Cindy. 'That people were worried by the noise, that somebody might have been in danger.' Then a drilling sound started up and she thought it was about time the old girl explained.

She sniffed again, lit up a fag and said. 'Lot of fuss over nothing – the lad's only trying to make his way, nobody was hurt.' This was followed by a cry of pain and further

ASK ME NOW

'bollocks'.

'Well what's happening?' Asked Cindy, adding as an afterthought. 'And are you all right?'

'Oh, don't worry 'bout me – it's our Phillip. They'll call you from a pig to a dog if you don't work then come round mythering if you show a bit of gumption and try to make something of yourself.'

'Will you tell me what Phillip was doing?'

'See for yourself.' Said his Mother nodding towards the room beyond the serving hatch. Cindy went out into the kitchen and Mrs. Brestbohn pulled the door shut promptly behind her. Cindy knocked at the hatch. Almost simultaneously a door opened further down the hall and Phillip showed himself.

'I've a bit to do yet but you can come inside and have a look if you like.'

'I'm not here about … ' She said but the lad had disappeared so she wandered up the hall taking care with the oily cylinder head propped by the stairs, to enter a small garage where the living room should have been. The space was a largish undivided structure resembling Minty and Gary's workshop in 'Eastenders'. Apart from a beat up old Shakletons chair there was no furniture to speak of which at least clarified his Mothers flight to the pantry. What there was, which caused her to laugh out loud, was an old Austin Maestro taking up most of the space in the area by the serving hatch – she thought a donkey would have looked less unexpected. Phillip simply continued with his work under the bonnet while she admired the Aladdin's cave of tools, tyres and other such essentials of the mechanics trade, there was even a Linda Barker calendar where a clock would normally be. This month the gormless bint was draped across a cheesy leather sofa; 'get down on it' said the by-line. Get a life thought Cindy.

'Can you pass me that wrench love?' Asked Phillip. Cindy knew a thing or two about spanners and such like and passed him the correct implement.

'What needs doing on this one.' She asked.
'Ooh, what doesn't.' Replied the mechanic.

She was shocked when she looked upwards by an impromptu hoist rigged up somehow on the ceiling. Something boxy and electrical looking lay beneath the window. How on Earth had he managed to get the thing in? 'Were you working late on this last night?'

'Had to – said I'd have it finished by Christmas.'

'Whose car is it, Christmas is ages off – is your Mother comfortable in the pantry on her own?'

'It's a friend of hers. She was down the pub and our Mam tells her I'm set to become a mechanic so she says if he can put my car together by Christmas she'd put in a word with her brother who has a garage, a proper one on the industrial estate. Mam doesn't mind – she told me the family name depends on me, or something.'

'So the car was in bits?'

'Yeah.'

'But how will you get it out?'

'Don't need to. When it's done they can come round to see it, doesn't matter if it stops here does it?'

Cindy couldn't see how it did really. 'But the chap next door

ASK ME NOW

doesn't like you banging at night. That's why I've come round – nobody knew what was happening.'

'It's not me makin' all the noise, our Richard does grease while I'm working. Comes in from the pub with his mates, thinks it's a laugh.'

'What do they do with the grease?'

'Dance mostly – set of Herberts.'

'But that is dangerous, they could fall – not to mention the mess. It ruins your clothes.'

'Are you soft or what?' Asked Phillip. 'Grease – that film; one of them gets himself up as Olivia whats-her-face in a wig of our Mams and that's when I got mad and chucked a wheel at him. Richard pegged it back so we had a bit of a ruck – so what? Nobody got hurt, really. If you want I could tell you a tale of him next door, talks to the trees and goes to a cowboy club. It's not our Mam that's crackers it was just when they got a new gaffer in at The Man In The Moon that she got a bit doolally that time.'

Cindy felt she shouldn't pry and pursued a more pragmatic line, God only knew where they'd end up if she suggested an extended care assessment. 'Well it seems to me that if you don't want us knocking on your door you could let him have a bit more peace at night.'

'Easy for you to say, how would you frame this job?'

'I'll just have another word with your Mother before I go.'

When she returned to the kitchen the pantry was unoccupied, Cindy looked out into the back garden. She watched as Mrs. Brestbohn knelt beneath the back window to water a plant while through the window she could see Phillip donning a welding mask. She stood up carefully and smiled at her son who seemed to be grinning back from behind his iron mask. 'I'll see they keep the noise down Mrs.' She said as Cindy patted the dog on her way out.

'Well.' Said Claire Todgers. 'I suppose that so long as they pay the rent and shut up shop at normal hours no one needs to be bothered.'

'I'm amazed no one knows all ready. It's incredible what people get up to behind their front doors, if we're meant to be agents of social control this is something else we're falling short with. I basically just advised them to be a bit more careful.'

'What did you make of her?'

'Seemed right enough to me, hopefully we can leave well alone.'

Claire closed the office door and made herself comfortable on a beanbag. Cindy swivelled aimlessly for a bit on the big office chair and started fiddling with the ends of her hair. 'Well?' Asked Claire eventually. 'This isn't just your Mum is it.'

'It's Alan.'

'Right.'

'You know we've … well, you know.'
'Yes.'

'Well it's all getting a bit complex a bit quickly – I feel really mean saying this.'

'It's all right, you know it'll stay in here.'

ASK ME NOW

'Yeah I know. It's quiet in here today, is that self-harm bloke okay? I know how these things can affect the group.'

'He's fine but you're not, what's been happening?'

'Poor Alan, he's badly depressed. I don't know how long it's been coming on, probably he doesn't, but it really seems to be sweeping him off his feet and I can't help thinking it might be something to do with us getting together – it seems to have pulled him out of shape, knocked him off balance. I don't know – I don't know what to do.'

'What do you want to do?'

'He's off now, seeing his Doc. tonight. I think he'll have to go off sick for a while. I know it's not my responsibility but I want to help him get better, at least.'

'What do you mean by better?'

Cindy baulked at this. 'I could do without the Socratic dialogue Claire – I think we'd agree on what better means.'

'I don't want to tell you what to do.'
'You can if you like.'

'Well you've just said you don't know.'

'I know.'

'All right, how do you feel about Alan, what was it like when it all started to happen?'

'Pretty good. He makes me laugh, he's a bit odd but I don't mind that – I mean, why do you fancy somebody. We seem to be compatible in that area, which is nice after all that carry on with Steve. I suspect his melancholy side harbours a lot of good stuff. It hurts me to see him so scared.'

'That sounds worth hanging on to.'

'Yes, I mean we both know he'll get better but I doubt this is the first time it's happened to him. I feel I should be there but that's not the answer. I think he struggles with the responsibility bit, but he's not mine.

As Alan left the Rio Grande surgery lights were coming on below him along South Way, he watched them for a while and felt a momentary uplift. He could see the headlights of vehicles moving smoothly as if along setlines. Without the sounds of traffic the process looked ordered and peaceful; a benign rite calmly working itself out. He tried to stretch the moment, get his thoughts moving in harmony with the neutral bright shapes but it soon dispersed leaving him feeling empty and lost again, he didn't want to be on his own. Dr. Rose had spoiled him with a double appointment and another set for Friday. He'd wept when she'd done that and won five minutes injury time on the back of it – of all the related jobs in the world of welfare General Practitioners were the group he most admired. How did she do it? Stuck in her little office like that listening to the sad and the mad, the old and the cold and the Minister Of Health and expected to make them feel better. And a double dose of Dickie before day was done. Also, he wasn't one of those patients who saw the prescription pad as a signal to sod off and stop bothering me. What else could they do? Besides, Dr. Rose hadn't produced hers until the end of what had been a proper consultation, which had featured a close reading of his records. He'd been a bit damp eyed at this as they not only disclosed details of his previous bout of melancholia but happier associations like the inoculation before that fancy holiday or the day his mates had brought him along after an ill-advised post-lunch pollarding of somebody's wobbly lime tree. Then there was his Mum bringing him in for jabs and childhood illnesses. And now he

ASK ME NOW

was here on his own.

His Doctor had made sensible sober comments on not pondering too much on why, taking things step by step, gathering support and recognising that he was poorly, that it was treatable and would mend. He shouldn't be at work but they could make a decision about this on Friday. For him just the fact of her sitting there unfazed by his lachrymose presence, dispensing sturdy concern was enough and took him back to the wind swept moments of his withering Sunday with Cindy. If only a warm bubble could form around them and hold till he was better. Instead he was soon verifying his next appointment with the receptionist, as he shuffled out he noticed a tense looking woman waiting with a sick toddler and knew for certain he was a big girls blouse. As he got into his car he pondered on how Cindy saw all this – they hadn't even had their first Sainsburys squabble yet but they were at the tears before bedtime stage all ready, it was all moving too quickly. What time had she said to call? It was quarter past five, if he went through town at this time of day he wouldn't be there much before six, if he took the by-pass he could be too early. He sat for fifteen minutes trying to decide until a kid kicked a ball against the car and he took off through the town arriving at Cindy's forty minutes later. She welcomed him with a big hug and asked him how it had gone.

'The appointment? Fine, she's really nice you know – I was in for nearly twenty minutes.'

'Mmm.' Said Cindy. 'She's very interested in mental health, usually sends good referrals to the team. She didn't refer you did she?'

'No – eh?'

'Joke Alan.'

'Oh, very good. No she's put me on escitalopram.'

'Good, lets look it up, have you got them with you?'

'No, I'll take the prescription in tomorrow.'

'I'll get on the net after tea. What do you fancy?'

'Cindy?'
'What?'

'I'm scared, I don't know what's going to happen.'

'You're going to get better – you do know this don't you?'

'It's worse than an illness. If I had a bad attack of shingles or something at least I could live with it, you know.'

'Some people get shingles instead of depression – sardines again?'

'I dunno – yeah. I'm not very hungry actually.'

Cindy put their meal together and chatted about her day. Alan managed a solemn titter at Phillip Brestbohn and his neighbour from The High Chaparral but was very glad he hadn't had to pick it up. 'Are you sure they'll be okay?'

'I should think so. They've obviously lived like that for some time, here sit down while I dish up.' She said this in a mock wifey, slightly brittle tone. He decided she was just chivvying him along and meant no harm by it. The food tasted hostile and fatty but he managed to keep pace with her. This was definitely not normal for him so there was some grim reassurance that it wasn't all in his head. 'It's Monday isn't it. She said.

'Yeah, still.'

ASK ME NOW

'Right, so that's 'Eastenders' sandwiched by double 'Corrie.' What a lovely way to spend an evening.'

She's definitely taking the piss, he thought, but the days bulletins from Wetherfield and Walford unfolded nicely enough as he felt his happy hour come round; Minty's garage turned out to be haunted and Roy Cropper was off his food again. He tried not to dwell on this and by eight thirty was feeling slightly better. Cindy had rested her leg against his throughout and given him a playful dig when Deirdre had tried to seduce Ken with a Carpenters record ('I Wont Last A Day Without You'). Then there was an awkward interlude when 'Shed Swap' came on; neither of them was interested but they watched the first five minutes until she took his hand and said. 'Alan'. In a serious voice.

'Yes.' He managed as his stomach turned over.

'I don't think we ought to spend the night together but can I come over to yours with you for a while?'

'Yeah ... okay, but we'll have to travel in two cars though.'

'Yes, I know. Will that be a problem?'

'No, no of course not. Yes.'

'Right, is it all right to go now?' She asked with a kindly smile.

'Yes, fine.'

The return trip took much less time but his anxiety not to lose Cindy gave it a bit of an edge for Alan. There was never much trouble parking at this time and after she'd pulled in behind him Alan managed to time his exit from the car to coincide with hers and thus reduce the risks of kerbside indecision. They found themselves at the front door in unison and he opened it first go. 'You've got one of those time limited light switch things, on the left isn't it?' Said Cindy, who'd been round a couple of times but never to stay, all night anyway.

'Give it a good push – should give us three minutes climbing time.'

'Right, I'll push, you climb and lets hope for the best.'

He had them safely in his flat before the lights went out. 'Sit down, I'll put the kettle on, shall I?'

'If you want. I'd quite like a cup of tea.'

As he set to with the tea she had a look through Alan's enormous stack of CD's hoping to find one that wasn't on an obscure German label or bearing a title like 'New Music From Stoke-on-Trent : Vol. 2'. She flicked swiftly past 'The World Of Harry Partsch' to find an unexpected treasure; 'Hunky Dory' – Alan liked Bowie. 'Can I put some music on?' She called through to the kitchen.

An alarmed looking host appeared in the doorway to say 'yes' with two mugs of Indian Prince which he placed carefully on his prized Formica table. He stood and she came over to embrace him firmly throught most of 'Life On Mars'. 'Alan it's going to be all right – we'll get you through this.'

He started to breathe more deeply so they took their seats on his old two seater that was covered by a white throw. The place had a rather odd feel to it; thematically late 1950's with bakelite radio flying ducks and patterned rug, but put together by someone still living in the 1970's given the joss sticks bare floorboards and functional bookshelves. In it's way it said quite a bit about Alan and it suited the music, which always came over to her with a faint whiff of patchouli. It also made her feel they were both getting on a bit. 'You're a closet Bowie fan – an old girlfriends? Did you ever wear eye makeup?'

'Yeah.' He said and laughed without saying which.

He rested a hand on her leg as they sipped companionably along with the music. 'What's this one called?' She asked. 'I think I know this.'

He got up to fetch the case. 'Fill Your Heart'.

'I really like this one.' She said and began saying the words. 'Fear is in your head so just forget your head and you'll be free.'

'Nice idea.'

'It could be a cock-eyed CBT thing – you know, coming down out of your head.' She said.

'I think that's the worst of it.' He said. 'Stuck up with your thoughts all day, watching yourself like a hawk – I want to switch it all off.'

She didn't say anything and held his hand. They sat like that until the end of the record, then for a little while longer, eventually Alan said. 'It's nearly my bed time.'

'I can stay a bit longer if you want.'

'No it's all right, I'm starting to feel tired.'

'Okay. Can I come round tomorrow?'

'Of course, when?'

'Keep your mobile on and I'll phone you in the morning when I know what I'm doing.'

After her heartfelt farewell Cindy nipped off into the night and Alan went back in. He felt he might be able to read a bit before bed with Radio 4 on low; it was broadcasting a soothing late night sonata of thoughtful discussion, reasoned, well modulated and friendly. He poured a short glassful of cranberry juice to wash down his antidepressant and read through the side effects, which he knew about anyway. He snorted at the 'two to three weeks' before you could expect to feel a lift in your mood but what were the drug companies supposed to say? If you can bear another month of the collywobbles you might be in with a shout? No wonder half the prescriptions made out never saw the pharmacist. Another troubling thought wormed its way across his beleaguered brain – if they could give you a pill to make you better straightaway would he take it? He tried to stop this in its slimy track, what common sense he had told him it led down a dead end, a cognitive cul-de-sac. He needed a different kind of distraction. He fished out a book at random then put it straight back, it was 'The Quantity Theory Of Insanity', normally the kind of thing he was keen on but he knew the hook on this one and it perturbed him now. The proposition was that there was only a fixed amount of sanity in the world so when one person recovered another must become ill, and vice versa. The implication was that his ardent ministrations with Bill Clayton might not have been in his best interests because if Bill got better it increased his chances of falling off the edge. Was he jeopardising his sanity by doing the job he did? He didn't want to pursue that one now. Was it him and Cindy? She seemed so sane, and level headed, so content and capable, how did she manage? Did he want her here now, was he choosing to be depressed?

These and related reflections crowded his troubled mind. They were like his Mothers holiday snaps; he knew roughly what was coming but he'd have to sit through them just the

ASK ME NOW

same. With a bluffed up effort of faith he took his tablet, swallowed the juice and got ready for bed. He reckoned that if he could manage ten pages of a favourite book and left the radio on he'd get off. It was a toss up between Beryl Bainbridge and Dickens, Our Mutual Friend made the final cut and he was able to get something from it, only a sliver of what he wanted to feel but something. He tried not to crush the feeling by getting it to carry too much but he couldn't forget his head enough. He did his ten pages though and was interested enough to find out what happened next to read an extra two then curl into the bed.

Mike Pearson

MAKING PLANS FOR NIGEL

'Off it then?'

'Yes - maybe for a while.'

Graham didn't ask anything else. 'I'll just be with Val.' She said. 'If anybody wants me.'

'What about Alan? I mean if anybody wants him.' Graham asked reasonably enough. 'He must have some appointments and stuff.'

'Oh … come and find me.'

Cindy sat down in Val Meatings office and wept. Val waited then asked if it was Alan.

'Yes. He's really depressed – I'm sorry.'

'It's all right Cindy, it's not your fault.'

'I wouldn't be too sure about that.'

Val handed her a tissue, stroked her arm and waited for more. 'I did think there might be something happening.'

'We're consenting adults.'

'No, no something about Alan last week. He seemed in a right old tizz about that
carry on with daft Dave Bamber – think it's nice you and Alan have got together.
You're not responsible for his feelings though.'
'Oh I know but it really did seem to come out of the blue. He seemed all right – you know, just Alan.'

'Well that's just Alan isn't it – you never really know with

ASK ME NOW

him. Is he taking anything?'

'Yes he's been to his GP, I think she'll sign him off till the end of the week.'

Val made them tea and they sat for a while until Cindy asked her with a straight face if she should be at a meeting.

'They won't miss me this morning, it's only Department S and more capers with the computers, Tommy Pollard making it up as he goes along – come to think of it, we'd probably get better input that way.'

Cindy smiled at this. 'Yes, what was all that about with Dave Bamber. Did he really turn up for a placement meeting with no student?'

'Yes, there's a connection with the overall IT debacle. It seemed to reach crisis point last week when an especially aggressive virus called Vic was born out of the interbred affair between Health and ourselves. It's mischievous and quite resourceful and somehow lodged itself in the system at TAT. It ruffled Netty Kirton along the way but really bamboozled brother Bamber. He's come a cropper before – once let an entire placement go by before he realised he hadn't made himself known to the agency so he tends to err on the other side now. When Alan's feeling better you can amuse him with the tale. You know he'll get better don't you?'
'Yes – I don't know that he does though.'

'What have you got on this morning Cindy?'

'Not a lot. I ought to talk to Lyn about the Brestbohns and there's Alan's diary to sort out.'

'Well look, let's get together at lunchtime and get out of this place for an hour.'

'Yes all right, I'll just compose myself. I think I'll give him a ring as well.'

Val left her to finish her tea and went out to set Graham about his business. She'd taken lately to highlighting the job vacancies in Parks and Gardens and leaving them on his desk in a lightly joshing manner. It didn't do any good. Once the computer malarkey was bottomed he would hear more of this.

Cindy regarded Val's computer screen and wondered at the Faustian pact they'd all made with the powers that managed the information highway. She didn't understand a lot of it but used it all the time. What if they were simply biding their time? What if Vic was merely an outrider for a force that could only be guessed at? They were girding their gigabytes as she mused. All she could see in the screen was a muted fisheye reflection of some of the room. She had a memory of a bearded dog for some reason and decided it was time she did some work.

Back at her desk the phone soon buzzed. 'Oh Cindy, Nigel Culverhouse is here, can he have a word?' Asked Becky.

'Yes – I'll be out in a minute.'

Nigel was a sociable obsessive whom she'd been trying to offer some basic CBT to over a time limited period. He'd missed his last appointment and wasn't due another till next week. He rarely left his Fathers house in Milnrow. As far as the CBT went Cindy was pretty sure they'd made an ABC formulation between them so she had been intending to move onto the CSE ASAP. He could be said to be a man of fixed habits so an unformulated visit was big news.

He sat peaceably in reception and smiled when he saw her.

ASK ME NOW

Cindy felt more than usually sympathetic towards him and led him to a vacant interview room. 'I've bested those taps.' He said.

'Good.' She replied evenly and waited for more.

He smiled again. 'I managed to get out of the house without going back up. Straight through the kitchen and out into the street, I thought, if I don't come in to tell you, I'd go back to see them again. But I didn't.'

'That's good. You must be really pleased.'

'Yeah, well – will it last?'

'I don't know, but the point is you've made a change so you know it's possible. How do you feel now?'

'I'm not sure – bit anxious really.'

'Well that's normal.'

'Is it?'

'Yes, you've done something new and you're in uncharted waters.'

'Don't mention water.'

'Sorry Nigel. You asked if it'll last – that's where the worry comes in.'

'Is that to do with the ABC bit?'

'Yes, antecedent – belief – consequence but you've successfully challenged it because you've made a different consequence come out of the A bit, the bit that starts it off.'

'Right.' He said slowly. 'When you showed me the CBT stuff there was something about CSE – I won't have to sit an exam?'

'Coping Skills Enhancement.' She said in a now-we're-cooking manner.'

'Does that mean doing what I did this morning only more often?'

'Exactly.'

Nigel pondered. She could see him thinking 'is that it then'? 'What do you think made the difference this morning?' She asked.

'I don't really know. The old man had taken the dog out and I just thought I don't want to be in. I think I was a bit cross really – also, I remembered something you said.'

'What was that?'

'That it's all right to be angry, and I was, so I thought beggar the taps I'm off out, there's no-one to stop me. So I got the bus here – that went all right as well, apart from a bad moment with the automatic doors, but I've plans for them as well.'

'Cindy couldn't help but smile. 'I'm glad you came in.'

'Yes but I've got to go back now.'

'Not right now, not if you don't want to.'

''So how do I keep it up? Enhance the coping skills?'

'Doing it again and more often.'

ASK ME NOW

'Could this be the Steely Dan approach? You know 'Do It Again'.

This reminded her of Alan and she felt the fog gathering, this was no way to navigate those uncharted waters. 'Well, whatever we call it you've done it. I suppose the trick is to work out what made the difference and …'

'Do it again.'

'Yes.' But was it really this simple? Just level headed encouragement and grounded support, a bit of a challenge now and then? She knew though that if they left it at this he might forget about the taps but start fretting over the gas fire. 'But I think we should make some plans. I think we can build on what you did this morning so you can start tackling other things.'

'What other things?'

'You mentioned the doors on the bus.'

'Oh I've all ready formulated for them. I'll close my eyes till I hear them swish.'

'Right, well if that works stick with it.'

He thought for a while. 'I'm not convinced I locked that door you know.'

'Is the key in your pocket?'

He felt around in the numerous pockets of his cargo pants eventually fishing out a dull metal key. 'I probably have.'

'Almost certainly.'

'Only almost?'

'Do you think any of us can be certain of anything?'

'Well, a bit more certain than this.'

Cindy thought before countering this one, there were a few things she might say but she held her tongue. Nigel appeared to enjoy bearing coded witness to his inner world – the overall effect was a rumpled ruefulness where wit was a challenge to the presenting past. Definitely a coping strategy. 'If it were possible to be completely certain about something.' She began cautiously. 'It would remove all doubt, but wouldn't it take some of the fun out of things?'

'Fun?' He said.

'Yes, because it depends on not knowing – you might be surprised.'

'Unpleasantly.'

'Yes, that, but not always. Uncertainty lets you hope – you never know what's going to happen.'

'Yes, I know.' He said with a bit more emphasis. 'That's my problem. Isn't it?'

She thought again. 'What about this morning? You didn't know, when you got up, the way it was going to go. Not knowing helped you put one over on those taps.'

'They're waiting for me now. I'll be made to pay.'

'By who?'

'Those pissing taps.' He said with his bland smile.

ASK ME NOW

'But what if that doesn't happen?'

Nigel looked properly alarmed by this. 'Well, what happens then ... what if ...?'

Cindy cut in quickly. 'Lets examine the possibilities, how likely is it that ...?' Nigel's eyes had begun to glaze over. 'Are you all right?' She asked.

'Yeah. It's yeah it's okay – so what happens next?'

'Well I think it's great that you've come in this morning and it's certainly a breakthrough. I think we can be sure of that much.' She noticed the flicker of a smile. 'So I think we should build on it.'

'Do it again?'

'Yes, but make some plans, look at other things you could tackle, how you could do things differently to see what happens – over the next week say?'

He stayed put so Cindy spent the remaining twenty-five minutes of their time together identifying three areas to address with preferred strategies for challenging their concomitant heebie jeebies. She tried her hardest to avoid sounding too much like Mary Poppins directing a recalcitrant road sweeper and Nigel engaged as positively as he could. By the end of it all it had been agreed that he would continue his war on the taps, challenge his reactions to whatever arrangement his Dad left the breakfast pots in, and leave the front door mat to it's own devises.

'Right.' He said. 'I think I've got that. So, what happens next?'

'We get together here this time next week and see how it's

gone.' As she walked back with him through reception he asked if he could use the Gents. As he disappeared into the communal facilities behind reception she caught Becky's eye. 'Would you give me a ring if he's in there for more than five minutes?'

'Why, he's not going to …?'

'No, no. It's just – if he lingers it's a bad sign. I'll stay if you like.'

'No, it's all right. More than five minutes?'

'Yes. Thank you, I'll be at my desk.'

Not bad she thought as she sat back down at her desk. Which was about as good as it got, a feeling qualified with many a yes but and a side order of what ifs. She was aware of something else. She hadn't given Alan much thought despite spending the past hour with another storm tossed screwball. She pulled out her to-dos and put the kettle on, by the time her tea was cool enough to sip another ten minutes had passed and the only call she'd taken had been a message for Graham.

Alan had woken abruptly at ten past five and twitched till twenty past when he finally managed to turn over and switch on the radio. The cold plastic felt toxic but the effort required and the level burble of voices in the room kindled something like uplift in his mood. However, the closest he came to hope was the absence of angst. He couldn't be sure though, his thoughts were on a timetable set by the bad thing at the back of his head. And that was just biding its time. He thought about Larkin's last great poem; seeing something that was always there, light edging the curtains and decided the old git had got off lightly. Then he felt bad again. The poet had taken to half a bottle of sherry before breakfast at the end. If life was first boredom then fear was there something worse? He noticed how his lit-crit lamentations had distracted him;

ASK ME NOW

dredging up scraps of poetry did soothe him at tattered moments. The next thing he caught on to was 'to my own sad self let me be hereinafter kind, charitable/ not live this tormented mind, with this tormented mind tormenting yet'. Who'd written that? Rod McKuen, Hardy? At least he wasn't alone. He looked at his watch – five thirty-five. He knew he should get up but if he did what was he going to do then ?

This opened up a terrible two minutes. His stomach turned over like an old whale in some mud then he felt as bad as it was possible for him to feel; something awful that had been hanging around the room in grey kit form fell together and folded into him as he hunkered. He bunched into the quilt and wept till six, which felt slightly less bad than that moment which seemed to him afterwards to have been about as bad as it had ever got; something fixed but active, sticking him for ever in an accelerating point of pure horror – frozen but out of control. Something that was always there, an object casting long shadows with only one end.

When he finally got out of bed he felt drained, ashamed and, without consulting a mirror, knew his face to be fixed in a rictus of stupid found-out guilt. He should have got straight up and as soon as he spotted the Bowie CD he couldn't believe how he'd felt last night. He felt unable to see her again after this and tried to remember what they'd agreed.

Cindy made a few notes in the multi-disciplinary file then decided she'd better have a few words with Dr. Wallace about her visit to the Brestbohns. The consultant's door displayed the green 'vacant' slide but as this didn't always signify, as it should she checked with the medical secretaries first.

'Oh she's free right now, there was a cancellation in her clinic.' Said Ruby.

Her knock elicited a coughed 'come in'. 'Ah, Cindy, sit

down.' Said the Doctor as she shifted some files from the comfortable chair to the carpet. 'How are things?'

After a slight pause Cindy said. 'Fine thanks – you as busy as ever?'

'No as it happens, Mr. Gonnella my new patient cancelled so I've a double slot free. Who did you want to talk about?'

'Well, this Brestbohn business – you heard about my visit after the Police got involved?'

'Yes – an incident of some sort. It's been all quiet on that front for ages now, what did you make of it all?'
'Well it's hard to say really. I could see why the neighbours took umbrage but getting the Police and EDT out seemed a bit top heavy. I think they'll cop it though if the council finds out they're running a car repair business in their living room. From what I could see though that's normal for them so to be honest I didn't think we should be doing anything much. I just felt a bit alarmed coming away from it all.'

Dr. Wallace smiled to herself. 'What was the old girl like?'

'Well on first meeting she did seem a bit odd but then I came to see why she might take refuge in the kitchen cupboard. Would have been a bit daft not too, but I feel I must be a bit off message saying so after the three-ring circus I eventually caught sight of in the living room. I didn't get upstairs.'

'Mmm, I shouldn't worry Cindy – you did the right thing. Was there much in the cupboard with her?'

'Lots of dog food.'

'Good. She's getting out for her messages then.'

This seemed a bit cavalier to the social worker. 'Do you think

ASK ME NOW

she could benefit from some medication, will you be reviewing her in out-patients?'

'What for? There's nothing wrong with her that we can fix. I'll write to the GP – Dr. Wilson gets on with her as well as anyone. As for medication, it's best not to.'

'Has she had bad side effects?'

This drew another knowing smirk from Dr. Wallace. 'In a way. Last time I saw her I thought she might be a bit depressed so I put her on a low dose of Prozac. When she got home one of the lads – not the one you met, he's the responsible one – told her they were no good but if she swapped them for some stuff she had she'd be right in no time. God knows what he thought Prozac would do for him but the extra strong whiz he prescribed for his mother worked their magic pretty sharpish. I think she was speeding for three days before she crashed into the coalbunker. After that of course she was properly depressed.' This brought her to a pause for reflection. 'They're just an odd sort of family really. If they lived in Strathclyde no-one would notice.'

'Perhaps we could get them to do a housing swap.' Put in Cindy.

'Ah yes but we don't know what we'd be getting coming our way, better the dysfunctional you know eh?' She reached for her handbag and stood up. 'I could do with some fresh air – I will have a word with Dr. Wilson.'

Cindy made herself scarce while Dr. Wallace tottered at speed towards the rear entrance where fresh air met the smokers shed.

Val was back in her office with two capable looking men crouching by the computer talking between themselves with knowledge and authority. She heard her say. 'Well, I'll leave you my mobile number in case you need to get me. I've got an important meeting this afternoon but I'm disturb able.' Then she moved smoothly into the team room and suggested that she and Cindy take an early lunch.

Where shall we go?' Asked Cindy.

'I don't know, where do you fancy?'

'There's a new place Claire Todgers told me about. A craft Centre type thing with a café, fresh bread, homemade soup – you know the sort of thing. Not too disturb able.'

'Sounds good. Where is it?'

'Just outside town on the way to Oldham. It's a converted mill development; they're hoping to have makers renting spaces and eventually a gallery plus performance space. I know where it is.'

'I'll drive then.'

Val's car had just come back from the garage and seemed especially light and airy compared to her little Cinquento or Alan's mobile midden. She enjoyed the way being driven could make her feel looked after. 'Did it need much doing to it?'

'Clutch cable was too slack, some difficulty with the distribution – they did explain it all but it's gone.'

This made Cindy think of the responsible Brestbohn brother and how satisfying it might be to fix broken cars, or boot up a confused computer. Something achievable and useful, no need for ambiguity or faffing about. There were times when it seemed fair to pay social workers a pittance. 'Was it a big job?'

ASK ME NOW

'No, but you wouldn't know that from the bill.'

'What about the computers, presumably those men are setting them to rights.'

'Those men are Tommy Pollards crack team of I.T. troubleshooters. He tells me that Chubby Jackson, the smaller one, is the Red Adair of the information highway and as for his mate Pod, what he doesn't know about connections isn't worth storing in your trash bin. I'm therefore persuaded by Tommy with the laughing face that all will be well by tea time.' Cindy laughed herself and asked her how much faith she had in this.

'Oh I think it will be. I've heard that Tommy got a right seeing to over the whole caper – the word is that unless we're on line tomorrow his job will be.'

'Christ, they can really move in health when they want to. It's quite a culture difference isn't it.'

'Yes but as good social workers we embrace diversity and to be honest our lot could take some leaves out of their management book.'

'Do you really think so?'

'Oh yes, and it'll come with single line management. There'll be a few cherries needing a polish if they're to be picked when the day comes.'

Cindy felt the need to change course and diverted Val down another road. 'What's Tommy Pollard like? You seem to get on with him.'

'Tommy? You've never met him?'

'I've seen him now and again, Alan knows him a bit I think.'

'Basically I like Tommy a lot but I think he's a fish in the wrong pool. He was a charge nurse for years, and I should think a good one, he was always into computers too and moved across at the right time when it was all coming in. His career's taken off in a way it never would if he'd stayed on the wards but I wonder if he'd have been happier. Anyway, they've got five kids, two of them at Uni. So he's a bit stuck now and that's why I'm pretty sure our computers'll be back on by bedtime. You say Alan knows him.'

'Yes. They go to gigs sometimes.'

'I could see them getting on.' Said Val. 'About Ala …'

'Ah, now – turn off next left. Can you see the old chimney?'

'Oh, right. Come on mate – I think he needs his cable tightening, yes, take your time.' Val smiled winningly at the elderly motorist as he inched his enormous saloon out through the car parks only conduit. As he passed them he favoured the patient ladies with a lordly wave and vacant nod. The parking of the car and ordering of lunch left little time for conversation beyond the functional so it was only when they were seated by a sculptured pile of scrap machine parts with a view of the building site below that Val was able to raise Alan's name again. 'You're really worried about him aren't you.' She said.

'Yes, yes I am. It seems to have come on so quickly but thinking about it now he's one of those where you don't really know that much about what's going on. He may have been sliding into it for much longer.'

'Yes, I'd say you're right about that.' Said Val as she buttered a cheese scone and slapped on some coleslaw.

ASK ME NOW

Cindy stared at her bowl of carrot and coriander soup and said. 'When something goes wrong with someone you always look back.'

Val emptied her mouth. 'How do you mean?'

'I think now that there was something not normal for him, even by his standards, with some of the stuff he was coming out with. Just odd things, when we were together.'

Val gallantly set aside her scone. 'What kind of stuff?'

'Stuff about women on the telly and in films – actresses, really hostile things now I think about it. I mean its just stuff on the goggle box but Alan took it so personally – he went off on one about Julie Walters playing these warm hearted roles and what was she really like as if it mattered. Brenda Blethyn was another then there were the films – Billy Orton is it?'

'Eliot.' Said Val as she reached across to hold Cindy's hand.

'Eh, oh right. I realised I'd seen it but I didn't let on to him – he thinks it's bogus and cynical. I mean it's just a sodding film. Little Voice, that's another one, starring Jane Bollocks, he says.'

'Oh that is bad, but not in the way he seems to mean. What's your soup like?'

By this time it was cool enough to slurp and this enabled Val to dig in at her preferred rate. Cindy indicated that it wasn't bad but soon put her spoon down to look out of the window. She could see some substantial hills in the distance. 'There was something else. We went out for the day, afternoon really, up to the Moors. He got stuck on this theme about Myra Hyndley and the murdered children – we weren't far from Saddleworth. We all know about it but Alan really seemed disturbed and I got the uncomfortable feeling it was connected with sex in a dark damaging sort of way. Again putting himself into the picture in a totally inappropriate way. A bit grandiose. A bit mad really.'

'Is that what concerns you so much?'

'In a way yes. I mean I know he's depressed and that it passes with or without the medication. But you can go round the bend with it can't you. And it's just so awful for him; he looks so frightened all the time. I feel that I'm being so hard and withholding but I know I have to be. He's really going through it Val.'

'Well, he's taking his antidepressant – isn't he? – so he'll come through because he's properly depressed. It is very hard being close to it as you are, don't let your soup get cold.'

'Yes. I'm really fed up with him as well. Isn't that awful, we've only just begun.'

'The Carpenters.' Said Val, though she didn't mean to. 'You're not a fan are you?'

'I might be. I know it's normal, in theory, to get angry with them but I'm struggling in practice. Perhaps frustrated is a kinder word than angry.'

Val looked out over to the hills for a bit and Cindy picked up her spoon and watched as she sipped. She could see one or two black figures shrunken in the wet light, like flies on giant green scones. She tried to focus on them while Val looked over the ex-works figurine. As she was doing this she asked Cindy if she wanted some time off too.

'No, no. I don't think so; I'm better off at work. You don't think I should do you?'

ASK ME NOW

'No.' Answered Val firmly. 'I just wondered that's all.'

'I did consider taking some leave, you know, just till he's got through the worst but, like I was saying to you, I just feel it wouldn't be for the best. I can't nurse or social work him – mind you, if it comes to it …'

'Well.' Said Val. 'Let's open that fridge if we come to it.'

'His parents are both re-married across the Pennines somewhere and there's a brother in East Anglia – a teacher, also has something to do with an Art Centre like this I think. After all the business re wicked women I haven't asked about Mummy and he hasn't said. Directly I suppose.'

Val tore herself away from 'Oil: Oligarchy number 3' and mmmed empathically. 'I know what you mean about work when times are hard elsewhere, you can forget them and feel effective.'

'Exactly. I was able to do something with Nigel Culverhouse this morning, nothing too high falutin' but I'm sure it's helping him. And that's all right, it makes a small difference to him and if he keeps coming back for more it'll add up to something he might not have got otherwise – and that's not bad is it? It's about the best we can do but it's all right.'

'Yes. If it's not bad and it's all right you can be confident you won't go too far wrong. As Dave Bamber wouldn't say in a month of psychosocial Sundays.'

Cindy laughed at this. 'There must be some kind of relationship between the amount of bullshit that you speak and the lack of faith you feel in what you're trying to say. A symbiotic relationship I should say.'

Val smiled back at her. 'That's just what Bamber would say.

It's a bad road to go down and unfortunately the Health Service seem to be picking up some bad habits from us in this.'

'Oh, I bet I know what you're thinking of, that paper from POTI we got last week, a multi-disciplinary paradigm for inclusionistic practice. You couldn't make it up could you?'

'Somebody did.' Said Val as she cast a plaintive glance at her departing bun. The waitress returned swiftly for the rest of their pots in a way suggestive of early closure. 'Did you read it?'

'Did you?' Countered Cindy with slight alarm.

'Some of it – I decided it was more of same really; we can't afford Day Therapy services anymore so here's some evidence based practice to justify closing them while enabling service users to have what they're increasingly demanding. This, apparently, turns out to be unqualified volunteers who can be mentored towards responsive blah blah blah …'

'Do you think it'll come to anything?'

'Who knows.'

'What time is it? They seem to be closing and I should be getting back.'

'It's just after two, have you got much on this afternoon?'

'I don't think so – not much no.'

'Good. Well, if Tommy's troopers have got us on line you can show me round the system. It would be nice if we could access Dave Bambers interface.'

Alan's morning had been hanging in a limbo of just-for-now

ASK ME NOW

neutrality which frayed each time he decided he was feeling a bit better; 'want some more' it seemed to say if he mustered enough of what it took to think about it. That little man at the back of his head was just taking the piss, he'd be back with more.

He'd got through till about two by pouring over his books about depression. Much of it was familiar; grief without a pang, hidden in the bone and such like but it gleaned some slim pickings of cold comfort, especially Ursula Fanthorpe, a uni-polar poet who also went to bed with Andrew Marr when she was desperate. He recognised he refrain about the price you paid later for putting on a good show for someone. Elsewhere he was counselled to be not solitary or idle and to 'construct an image' for his angst. Alan had never been keen on the old black dog bit, being a dog devotee and seeing them as basically friendly, although he could see that if mans best friend ever turned on you then you really would be in trouble. He tried harder and envisaged a little man who lived in a house full of shit at the back of his head. He was in there now reading with gob-smacked disgust through a grey ledger of Alan's mad dirt. It was all there for those with the stomach for it; chapter and verse set forth in plain but stained prose. The room inside the house full of shit at the back of his head was dimly lit with a poky little table and chair and mucky looking sideboard just about visible in the background. There was no real colour, simply variegated shades of crappy brown. The sickly light oozed from somewhere over the table, then the little man was suddenly there, sat in the poxy little chair. Everything about him was stiff and static apart from his face, which, as he poured over a volume titled 'Alan's Greatest Shits', twitched and leered with something like lust. 'Aye.' He seemed to be saying. 'Much worse than we thought, there'll be a reckoning to come with this one.'

Alan wondered what the little man would be wearing then decided that was off the point. He now knew what he looked

Mike Pearson

like though – a kid he'd known at school, Nigel Harding. It was Nigel Harding hiding in his head and the important thing was to keep him out of harms way. He decided he ought to go out, head for Londis, then the canal path.

ASK ME NOW

HEAVEN KNOWS I'M MISERABLE NOW

Northfield Community Mental Health Team Wednesday 9.15am

'The thing about water is you can't impose a structure on it, it just leaks out – you have to be careful with it otherwise you're liable to get carried away, not waiving but … well, you know.'

'I wouldn't know.' Said Graham. 'Anyway sit down you look a bit rough, if you don't mind me saying so.'

'Don't mind if I do.' Said Alan and laughed at three times the volume he normally reached.

'I'll put the kettle on then.' Said Graham and gave Alan's arm a friendly pat on his way out.

He sat at Cindy's desk to watch Dr. Wallace sucking the life out of her last roll up before clinic. He became aware of someone entering the room behind him. 'You fuckin' arsehole – you twattin' shitbag shithead.' Shouted Cindy.

'Eh?'

'You.' She stood before him and let off a further broadside of lavatorial invective then hit him hard on the head with a large book; as she threw it onto the desk he noticed it was called 'Dealing With Difficult People'. He began to cry, Cindy sighed loudly and threw up her arms in a gesture of helpless fury. He said 'sorry' to her as she left the room and sat sniffing in a soft, slow motion spasm.

Graham stood in the doorframe. 'What do you want to do?' He asked.

'I don't know.'

'Only, you know … I need to get on.' He picked up his diary by way of emphasis but Alan took this as a signal for further rough stuff and cowered. There was an awkward pause then Graham said. 'You're not well are you mate? I'll give you a lift home eh?' Then Val Meatings door opened slightly before closing again as the figure on the other side changed their mind. There was enough time for him to hear Cindy say 'arsehole' with feeling. Alan hadn't a clue what to do, neither did Graham, he moved across to his own desk and felt pushed out; things weren't as they were. A random arrangement of coaster, computer hardware and paper clips returned a bemused thought-you'd-gone look. He knew they didn't mean it but it was all too late. He froze as his phone trilled, Graham picked it up. 'No, he's off today – not sure, I'll make sure he knows. Bye.'

'Who was that?' Asked Alan.

'Look.' Said Graham softly. 'It will get sorted – I'll just have a word with Ina then we can get off.' He left the room.

He didn't seem to be gone long before Cindy came back. 'You and I need to talk.'

'Right.'
'Not here, let's go and sit in my car.'

Dr. Wallace passed them on their way out and nodded absently, Becky was fully engaged with a querulous appointee who seemed to think she should know the bus timetable from off the top of her head. 'Reception gets all the hassle doesn't it?' He ventured. 'By the time they get to us they've usually blown themselves out.'

Cindy didn't respond in any way that he could see and by the time they reached her car he found that he was biting his

ASK ME NOW

bottom lip in sickly little-boy mode. She turned to him once the doors were closed on them. 'Have you any idea what you've put me through Alan?'

'Um, yes – I think so.'

She laughed in mock amusement at this and looked ahead through the windscreen. 'You haven't have you. Where have you been? You were supposed to phone me, yesterday, at six.'

'Right.' He said deadpan.

The controlled vexation gave way at this point to her earlier mode of unvarnished fury. 'Alan.' She bellowed. 'Where the fuck have you been? I came round, you weren't in, your phone was off – the bloke downstairs didn't know anything. I thought you'd done something even more stupid than you seem to have,'

'I'm sorry Cind. – I... don't know what's happening.'

'Where have you been Alan? You look terrible.' Then she burst into tears. 'I can't handle this – you need someone with you at the moment, and I don't care what you say, it's not going to be me.'

They sat silently for five minutes. Cindy's bollocking had cleared the air and as her breathing steadied and deepened he felt his own falling in line with hers. 'I went out for a walk.'

'What, all night?'

'Yes.'

'Well, where did you go?'

'I went down to the canal.'

'To the canal.' She said flatly and glanced at him.

'Along it actually.'

'You went along the canal all night?'

'Yes, I just went on walking – you can go for miles – and back. Then I thought I'd come in to tell Graham, he's interested in that sort of thing. If you get as far as …'

'Alan.' She cut in. 'If the fancy takes you for a lads club caper down the canal just remember to let someone know eh?' Stroppy cow he couldn't stop himself thinking but held his tongue for a further two minutes then asked her what she had on for the rest of the day. 'You.' She replied.
'What do you mean?'

'What I mean is that this can't go on; you need to be somewhere safe with someone you can trust and, because ... it has to be someone else. So, where to Alan?'

'I don't know … I mean …'

'Well it's either friends or family.'

He thought for a while. 'Well, family I suppose.'

'Right we're getting somewhere. Mum Dad or Brother?'

'Dad I suppose.'

'Okay, where does your Father live? It's over in Yorkshire somewhere isn't it?'

'Northallerton.'

'There's him and your step-mum isn't there?'

ASK ME NOW

'Yeah, Flora.'

'That's a nice name – Northallerton's near some nice countryside isn't it?'

'Yeah – they like it there.'

They sat on for another, less cross five minutes and eventually made contact for the first time since she'd clobbered him with that book as she reached across to hold his hand. 'You do understand why it can't be me don't you?'

'I think so, yeah.'

'Right, we'll stop off at yours to get some stuff then go straight across.'

'Are you going to drive me across now?'

'How else will you get there, the Liverpool to Leeds canal?'

'What about work?'

'I've talked to Val.'

She started the car and tuned into Start The Week where Melvyn Bragg was chairing a good-natured natter around the theme of Round Britain. Alan listened in vain for contributions from John Julius Norwich or Matt Lucas before a testy peroration by Polly Toynbee enlivened things. It was something to do with proximity and sharpening edges, as Hampsons Bikes hoved into view he asked Cindy what it all meant. 'It's very interesting actually, I was reading about this last week; apparently someone's written a book about boundaries being harmful because keeping us apart means that resources and individual capacities get diluted and undercut a natural desire to federate. It would therefore be better to see beyond surface details and embrace similarities, it's a more playful take on multi-culturalism – as Britain effectively gets smaller and denser it should get rounder and give us a more rounded version of what living here means. Of course it's stirred up a right old hoo-haa, Germane Greer's all ready been at it saying that obesity is the issue in Round Britain; men because they're greedy, women because they're hungry. I was hoping she'd be on this morning.'

'But she isn't even British.'

'See what I mean, she's very funny though.'

Alan wasn't sure that he did but he wanted to keep her from shouting at him again and prolong the happier path they seemed to have hit on. 'Wasn't there another hoo-haa she was involved with – she had a go at a fellow journo' – something to do with yucky sandals. Wasn't it Melanie Phillips?'

'It wasn't her it was that other one, and it was fuck me shoes. God if that's all people can remember about her they should try to get the story straight.'

Alan was interested now. 'What other one and how would you spot these shoes?'

'Oh I don't know. Maybe in a Rounder Britain these things wouldn't matter.'

Alan looked out over Gas Street and imagined a rounder Ridsdale as Melvyn made his even handed summing up, managing due deference to each participants position but spoiling it with some half hearted joshing about squaring circles. There was an audible groan from Polly then Cindy switched off. They reached the top of his street, Cindy said she'd wait in the car and he had another fit of the vapours. Up in his flat he felt a crueller version of the paper clips coldness.

ASK ME NOW

'You again' it seemed to be saying, who are you and what are you doing here? Didn't you know everyone's gone, it's too late? He threw clean stuff together and got out as quickly as he could. As he came down to the street he could see her through the car window pouring over a map. It reminded him of an earlier image of her watering a plant through her kitchen window but he felt much further away. If he knocked on the window would she see him? He got in beside her and planted his bag between his feet. 'Do you want to put that in the boot?' She asked without looking up from the map. He felt paralysed and realised that he hadn't phoned his Father to tell him he was coming.

'Can we stop on the way, I ought to let them know?'

'Phone him now. Here my mobiles charged.' She said handing it across.

He considered the neat little object and said. 'It's all right. Can we get going, I'm cold?'

Cindy was preoccupied with the route and hardly noticed. 'Okay, I've got it; M62 to Leeds then via York to the A19. Shall we stop off after Leeds?'

'Yes all right, after Leeds.'

By the time they were back on the by-pass Alan's mood had lifted enough for him to want them to just carry on moving like this for a long time, for long enough to make it all unhappen.

'Do you mind if I put the radio on again Cindy?'

'No sure, wouldn't you rather have some music on?'

'No – I can't listen to it at the moment.'

'It's what the text books call anhedonia Alan.'

'It's crap, Cindy.' He pushed on the car radio. Dr. Raj Persud was on evaluating the rising figures for diagnosed depression. Alan managed a snigger as Cindy moved to retune. 'It's all right, leave it on – he's got a soothing voice, reminds me of the only Spike Milligan joke I ever laughed at; a patient asks a doctor to say something soothing and the doctor says 'Largactol'.

'Well, soothing after a fashion in the short term.'

'What's wrong with short-term comfort? Why does everything have to take so long or be such a bloody performance – why can't I be in a nice white bed attended by respectful nurses as I pull through with aplomb? If I had something physical it would be like that.'

'You reckon?'

'Well, not exactly but mental illness is serious and it's there all the time. It's like trying to fix a car as it's running. I need a nice garage, one in someone's living room even.'

Cindy pointed out that they were heading for something similar as they beetled along the M60 and then asked him a question he found he'd all ready pondered, to no real effect. 'If they produced a white pill tomorrow that would take it all away – all the mad stuff and the biochemical kerfuffle – straightaway, how many of us would take it do you think?'

'What, how many of us were going through it at any given point?'

'Yes.'

'Well … everyone I would have thought.'

ASK ME NOW

'You would hope so, wouldn't you.'

'I don't know what you mean.'

Cindy paused just a little longer than would have been expected. 'Alan – you will won't you?'

'Yes, yes of course I will.' He said while reaching down discreetly to feel the outside of his jacket pocket. They were there although he couldn't remember putting them in. Then he became sure he hadn't taken them yet, something else to do after Leeds. He thought he might know what she was getting at though; a reluctance to take them could be about a terrible what if? What if they didn't work, what then? They represented the ultimate last resort because he couldn't for the life of him see anything else working. Or was it the madness telling him not to so it could win? Maybe when –if – they started working he'd feel differently, it was just that he couldn't remember feeling any other way. I t was like the paper clips at work or the smell of his kitchen; a him that must have been, things that were still there but lost, something bad in his head that represented the whole world. Could Tommy Smith tell him and if he could what happens then? Wasn't there some body in the bible that was lost and wherefore was he now or some such, hallucinations in the desert then ransomed, healed, restored, put on a waiting list. Jonah or Ezekiel – one of them anyway. He wanted to forget his head and be freeeeee or hear some words of wisdom and let it be. He looked out of his window; they were going up and over past Saddleworth Moor; suffer the little children he thought. Heaven knows I'm miserable now.

'What?' She asked quietly.

'I didn't say anything.'

'I thought you were about to.'

'No.'

He could see she was lovely but what did it all have to do with him? He couldn't believe they'd had sex, that they could again. Her hand reached down to change gear, he loved her hands – pornography got everything wrong – the most allusive part of a woman were her hands, leave the rest to your imagination. He felt pleased he'd thought that, nothing too bad on the old shit scale but now he'd gone and s(p)oiled himself, woken Nigel Harding up. Someone on the radio said 'Kittiwake' and before Nigel could do something obscene with it Alan asked Cindy what was on.

'It's one of those off the wall things with Bill Oddie – The Trail Of The Lonesome Pine Martin.'

'Ridsdale's own Bill Oddie – known in some parts of the town as Odd Billie.' She smiled at this even though it wasn't that funny, or even factual. 'We can't be that far from Leeds now.'

'No, fancy stopping soon?'

'Yes – tea, scone and citalopram.' She smiled again and stroked his knee. He noticed that whenever he spoke he felt slightly better and settled in his seat, Bill Oddie's voice wasn't really a soothing thing but he found himself unbending and at least thinking about not thinking. They couldn't be far from Elland Road – he remembered his Dad taking him there to see them play Manchester United. They'd all been on the pitch that day; both Charltons, Denis Law, Crerand, Billy Bremner – who'd been man of the match – Paul Madeley, of paint shop fame, and George Best. He could remember how Paul Reaney had followed him everywhere, kicking him blatantly, but Best had still scored both their goals in a drawn game, even the Leeds fans, some anyway, applauding him off.

ASK ME NOW

At least they'd be able to talk about football when he got there. Cindy hadn't shown the slightest interest despite her having someone in the family who'd played at one time - a cousin was it? Think about the seaside, the sea was soothing – maybe they could go to Scarborough. He came around with a start. 'Whe ... are, is this?

'Just coming up to Easingwold.'

'Easingwold – that's past York. We must be nearly there – I've been asleep.'

'For nearly an hour.'

'An hour?'

'You must be quite tired, you were up all night.'

'Eh? ... Oh yeah – shall we stop?'

'Yes, I need a pee and you should give your Dad a call.'

The main street became a long slope up through the village with a green, clustered shops, two pubs and The Copper Kettle Tea Rooms sandwiched by Sandra's Hairstyles and an electrical shop advertising 'Hi-Fi Equipment'. Alan's mood had slipped a fair bit since his nap and the whole place looked to him as if it was stuck in a Sunday afternoon of 1972. Cindy loved it. 'You're so lucky being able to come over this way, is Northallerton like this?'

'Just like this.' He replied. 'But they've a growing problem with the young people.'

'You what?'

'They knock on doors then run away – soon there'll be drive

by shootings on the High Street. It's time some social workers took them on holiday.'

'That's not your Dad is it?'

'No. It's just, you know this whole going home bit – it's all right really, Northallerton, bit like a boring version of Ambridge.'

Alan's wit earned him another laugh and she left him to phone his Father while she got their tea and scones. There was nobody in so he left a message saying he was coming to visit and would like to stay for a few days. Cindy returned with the refreshments. 'How is he?'

'Oh fine.'

'All right about you coming?'

'Yeah fine.'

'What time is he expecting us?'

'I said we'd be there by three.'

She seemed satisfied with this and advised him that the cheese scones were on their way. 'They're home made.'

'Aren't we all.'? He said in a tired voice.

She looked at him directly. 'You sound as if you want someone to blame – Larkin wasn't right about everything you know.'

'No – I guess tough love is what survives.'

'Oh for Christ's sake Alan.'

ASK ME NOW

'What?'

'I'm really not happy with the positions you keep trying to put me in … and all this heroic victim hood, it's … errrgh.'

He thought for a while before responding. 'Yeah … sorry.'

She nodded slightly without really giving much away and they got going with the home-made buns, Alan washing his down with some quite acceptable Darjeeling and remembering his little pill before draining the pot. The numbers of people he and the rest of them had had to persuade, debate with and cajole to keep taking the tablets and here he was fannying about. A familiar riff with ambivalent types was the one about how you wouldn't stop your insulin if you were diabetic or your whatever for your Addisons Disease. But depression wasn't diabetes or jungle fever, it was him and it was his, just like everybody else's was theirs. Or are we all less unique and 'special' as we'd like to believe and was his 'madness' his way of being special? Was this what she'd been getting at in the car? Cindy had been watching something through the café window. 'What time is it?' She asked. 'Should we be making a move?'

Christ, why does everything have to be a question?' He blurted, then felt terrible.

She waited untill he'd composed himself and said nothing.

'Ten past two – I suppose so. They've got plenty of room you know – I mean you could set off back tomorrow, if you want.' He said eventualy.
'I don't know, I've got a lot on tomorrow – I'll see.'

'You don't want to hang around here for a bit then – there might be a ducking or a wicker man. You never know.' He stood up as he was saying this making great play with his purse to signal his intent. She didn't react either way but he noticed her taking one of the local guides and places to stay booklets.She waited for him outside and gave him a neutral smile as they walked back to the car.

It was just past Thirsk before she said anything further so by the time she drew in some breath and sighed significantly Alan was experiencing a moderate to severe dose of the collywobbles. 'Alan.' She said. 'I feel that I want this thing we've started between us to go somewhere.'

'Our relationship?'

'Our relationship, but I think that for a while you really need to be somewhere you're around people – people who know you. I'm not pushing you away but I think it's best if its not me.'

'No, yes – I know what you're saying.'

'Good.'

'And thanks for all this. I must have been in a bit of a daze this morning.'

'It's all right Alan – you're not well, try to hang on to that. You deserve some care.'
They were passing through the last stretch of North Yorkshire as it prepares to meet Teeside and the places have French names like Thornton-le-Beans . Then Northallerton announced itself as faceless new bungalows gave way to older terraces. Alan pointed Cindy along a short by-pass via County Hall that took them to a newish estate at the northern end of the town. Alan's Father lived on a horseshoe called The Cuckoos, she stiffled a laugh given that she was bringing one home to roost, and who seemed unusually swift of movement, nipping out and up to the door before she could pull the handbrake fast.

ASK ME NOW

To Alan's great relief he could discern movement and muffled conversation as he pressed the doorbell, then a clearer 'that'll be him' as his Dad came up the hall. He glanced at his watch; it was twenty past three. Cindy was pulling his bag from the car. 'Now then.' Said his Father and clipped him lightly on the shoulder. Alan noticed his gaze settle on Cindy with the bag.

'Dad, this is Cindy, my friend. You've time for a cup of tea haven't you Cindy?'

'If that's okay.' She said and smiled at the older man.

'Of course it is – don't leave the lass there with your stuff.' Flora appeared and began to impose order on events. Alan moved back towards his friend who had set down his stuff just inside the gate and taken up a neutral looking position about a yard from it towards the house. To take the bag Alan stepped onto the grass and stepped in to a concealed pile of putty coloured cat shit. This put him in mind of the dog crap at Sweethaven and how he'd like to be there now – anonymous and looked after with nothing expected of him, anywhere really but here and now. For a long moment their placings had the feel of psco-drama or something from Scarborough; Alan Ayckborn directing the opening of a domestic four hander freighted with misunderstandings and darker currents. He dithered by the gate, Cindy looked back to him for guidance and his parents stood by an open door uncertain about which way it would go. He collected the bag, tapped Cindy on the elbow and moved towards the doorstep where his Father welcomed Cindy in and Alan removed his dirty shoe. 'I thought you'd cleared up the front.' Said his Stepmother.

'It's that tortoiseshell from over there – I've seen it, they never mucky their own.'

'It doesn't matter who, it'll need shifting Dave.'

'I'll see to it when I've done my shoes.' Put in Alan.

'Yes well.' Said Flora doubtfully.' What about a drink Sandra?'

'Cindy – can I have coffee please?'

'Of course. You two'll have tea I expect.' She left the three of them in the sitting room. Alan was intrigued by the new sofa and that it left room for his Dads old arm chair, an ever-present he could remember from childhood, there was still a polished over nick from his brothers home made Davy Crockett hatchet on one of the legs.

'Has Linda Barker been round then?' He asked.

'Eh?' Said his Dad. Alan nodded at the settee. 'Oh that was Floras idea, very smart isn't it? He thought for a moment. 'Whose Linda Barker?' Cindy smiled so his Dad asked her if she knew her.

'She's always on the tele.' Said Flora as she set down a plate of biscuits and smiled at Cindy.

'Eh … oh, I never bother.' Said his Dad mysteriously.

'Never bothers.' Said Flora with mock incredulity. 'Never misses 'Countdown' – and the rest.'

'Aye, now then, it'll be on soon.' He said with some feeling.

'They won't want to sit through that Dave.'

Alan said they wouldn't mind, adding that Richard Whitely could be amusing and had been a surprise hit at the Edinburgh

ASK ME NOW

Festival. 'Aye well, he'll not be doing that again.' Observed his Dad quietly.

'He died the other week.' Said Cindy. 'He wasn't very old was he?'

'No.' Said his Dad. 'Can't have been much over sixty when he rattled his clogs.'

Alan was greatly shocked by this revelation. 'So who is doing it now?'

'Nobody.' Answered his Dad in his World-gone-to-pot voice.

Beam me up thought Alan as his been-here-five-minutes-and-I-want-to die mood began to gather. 'Well why is it on now?'

'The Peoples Presenter – they're showing a months worth of classic shows as a tribute. They say Carol Vorderman can't watch them she's so overcome.'

Alan was unsure about being exposed to this degree of high expressed emotion, but on the other hand, what were they going to chat about over their refreshments. Also, it would open up a natural interlude for Cindy to have her coffee before setting back. 'Well, lets have a look then.' He said.

His Dad poked impotently at the remote control for a while then grasped that the set needed switching on first so he hauled himself from his chair, did the necessary then sat down to faff some more, to no great effect. Cindy caught Alan's eye and they shared a wry smile as Flora came in with the tea, nodded to Alan's Dad, who was becoming quite flustered, and said. 'Needs new batteries.' Certain they'd get the joke. She soon had the tele on and drinks dispensed then the ghost of Richard Whitely appeared and set the clock going for a classic. They soon became engaged by it all and began to chip in with their own answers – his Dad excelling himself. Alan decided charitably that the old man had forgotten it was a repeat. Flora opined that 'poor Richard' hadn't looked well when this one was filmed though it seemed to Alan that he was much the same, Carol though did look to him to be dangerously thin, perhaps pining in advance for her cheeky chappie of the blazers. God bless him anyway for being there in spirit.

Alan became aware, in the short time they'd all been together, how well Cindy was fitting in; a few questions to Flora about the garden and a winning way with his Fathers toy soldiers seemed to unbend them in ways he could never seem to manage. When the talk turned to the cutting of the grass at this time of year he began to see himself as the conversational equivalent of an old lawn mower; the kind you had to lavish time and attention on to get started then nurture while it spluttered into life for two minutes with a strange noise before making the best of as it kept conking out. But then, he thought, I am ill, then what time will Cindy go and what do I say to them? Countdown came to a close as the co-presenters wrapped it up with some cheesy banter which had the opposite effect of making them mourn, it didn't even seem much like immortality; you were here one minute shooting the breeze with some deferential punter too polite to tell you where to put your consonants, gone the next and who really cared. After one of the Bee Gees had snuffed it the 'Stayin' Alive' jokes were doing the rounds with indecent haste. It could be the kindest thing to be forgotten. Cindy drained her cup and stretched out. 'I really should make tracks.' She said.

'Oh, stay for some tea – eh Alan?' Said his Father.

'I'd like to but I need to get back to Ridsdale.'

'I'll pop out with you and make sure there's nothing left in the car.' Alan said and stood up.'
'Well, nice to meet you.' Called Flora as they headed back

ASK ME NOW

down the garden path to Cindy's car where Alan made great play with the careful searching of the back seat. As he straightened himself she simply hugged him and said to call her the next night, then she was off. He turned back in through the gate, his Father having come part way down the path to meet him.

'Long drive ahead of her eh?' He said.

'Yes.' Said Alan.

By the time Cindy was retracing her way past County Hall the remaining trio was seated in the sitting room. 'What a nice girl.' Said Flora. 'Have you known her long?'

'Yeah … we work together.' He was aware of his Father watching him.' We see quite a lot of each other really.'

His Dad didn't leave it too much longer. 'Well it's nice to see you any way. Would you like to stay for a bit?'

Alan felt himself filling up so he nodded and managed. 'I haven't been too well recently.'

'You look as if you've lost some weight.' Said Flora. 'What's been the matter?'

'I got this virus that wouldn't go away and it's left me completely worn out. I just feel pretty shattered.'

His Father perked up at this. 'Oh there are some terrible bugs doing the rounds. Mr. Shorter down the road caught a stinker – went to his chest, took him weeks to through it off. Is that where it got you then?'

'Not really … just all over.' Alan felt that Mr. Shorter was probably in his seventies and that he'd better begin sliding truthwards sooner rather than not. 'It's affected my mood as well – I've lost interest in everything. The Doc's signed me off.' That would do for now, and it was better out than in.

'Well.' Said his Dad. 'Your job must wear you down, listening to other folks troubles all day and it's not as if you got much appreciation for it either.'

Alan felt touched again by this and took refuge in the downstairs loo where he sat and wept as silently as he could for fully five minutes before flushing and washing his face. Would Cindy be at York yet he wondered?

'Are you all right in there?' Called his Father.

'Yeah.' He called. 'Just waiting for another consonant.'

His Father laughed at this and Alan heard him say 'he's okay' to Flora who sounded as if she was still on the settee. He gave it another minute then rejoined them, making passing reference to lingering viral difficulties, leaving the rest to their imaginations. 'What do you fancy for tea? I could make something light.' She asked.

This caused him to see the things he'd not considered. Naturally they would feed and water him, and he would get them a nice present, but what if they'd planned to go away? They might be expecting other visitors, how would he get back to Lancashire, when the time came? Then there was Flora. He'd come to assume that she liked him but what if she didn't? The home would be mostly shaped to her tastes, knowing his Father the old settee would have been there still – he felt horribly aware of the ambiguous nature of his intrusion. Then there was his old man; was Alan exploiting some sense of obligation – knowing he couldn't be turned away because his Father had been at fault, an adulterer, despite the generally held belief that few 'would have blamed him' and that his behaviour had been 'out of character'.

ASK ME NOW

Tellingly no one, as far as he knew, had critised Flora apart from his Mother.

He wondered what Flora thought he thought, perhaps she saw this as her punishment. He was felt to take after his Mother in some ways – there was a strain of melancholia on the Poskett side, old Nanny Pos would take to her bed for the week of a new moon and it was known that she could levitate kitchen tables at will. She had been a truly terrifying figure causing Alan and his brother many an anxious afternoon, as likely to put them in the back yard because she 'could tell what you're thinking' as she was to dandle them fondly in turn on her sparrow shank knees and run her fingers through their hair opining that there was more in there than lice. Either way, the pair of them would kick up the most heartfelt fuss whenever a visit to Newton Aycliffe was mooted where she and Granda lived out their days in an old coal board house. He had succumbed to emphysema, and possibly a flying table, when the lads had been toddlers and had formulated the most arcane coping strategies, which enabled him to be out of the house most of the time. He was thus a potent absent presence and the subject of Family myth, though Alan was blowed if he could remember much of it now. The only image he could recall was a photograph taken at the colliery of him singing to one of the canaries, the photographer had contrived to make it look as if the bird was inclining its head in Granda's direction, in the background several unfocussed figures could be made out puffing on cigarettes and smiling – he didn't fancy the canaries chances but it did imply an off the wall gaiety he liked to think had been bequeathed and he regretted not knowing him better. Had some of this found its way into the mix of his own temperament and did it grow from the same root as the jitters? One way or another you could always blame your family. As far as he knew, which might not be very far admittedly, his brother Peter seemed all right; wife of eight years standing and new baby wreathed in smiles last time he'd seen him – hard working deputy at a high performing secondary school in Norwich. He was a good bloke and Alan had been thinking that he'd like to show Cindy off to Pete and Phoebe. Moreover, if they knew what was happening they'd be concerned, accepting, keen to help. When Cindy had asked him about boltholes he'd very nearly nominated them but the new baby and the distance had made him choose here.

'What?' Asked his Dad.

'Eh?'

'I thought you said something.'

'I was probably thinking aloud.'

'About what you want for tea?'
'Oh, umm – what are you having?'

'Quiche and salad.'

'Oh that's fine, I'm not that hungry really.'

His Dad popped through to the kitchen and Alan found himself thinking about Bill and Betty Clayton. The lines of communication were subtler here, les angst ridden but the principle was the same – what someone in a another place had dubbed 'The Ballad Of Sexual Dependency' Was this what his brother and partner had, where he and Cindy might go? His Father must have been so fed up. It was true that unhappy families were more interesting – but he knew where this particular soliloquy was heading; they may not mean to but they do te tum te tum te tum. It was all very seductive but he wasn't interested. As far as he was concerned if they didn't mean to then that lets them off the blame, and that meant that you could forgive them. And if you can forgive them you might forgive yourself.

ASK ME NOW

He didn't like being on his own, even for two minutes and was glad when his Dad poked his head through. 'Ready round six.' He said.

'Good.' Said Alan.

'Home And Away' had come on and his Dad switched it off. ' Right load of old rubbish that is.'

'You don't watch it then?'

'Nah, 'Coronation Street's on later though.'
'Good.' Alan found himself looking at a photograph placed on top of the television, a group of six in foreign looking parts. His Father and Flora were present in the picture and when he asked Alan learned that the other four had made up the party when they visited Rome in September. His Father explained that they were all laughing because the passing Jap tourist they'd roped in to take the shot hadn't been able to work his Dads ancient SLR camera, it being too simple. His Dad had called out instructions and in the end it had made a great picture. 'You should get a digital Dad.'

'Pfwaah – you must be joking.'

'Talking of photographs, do you remember that one of Granda Posket?'

'Good heavens, what made you think of him?'

'I dunno – he was a miner wasn't he?'

Mr. Duright smiled wryly at this. 'He was a few things in his time, basically anything that kept him out of the way by the time I met him. You haven't got a picture of him have you?'

'No but I've remembered one from when we were kids for

some reason. I suppose because it was so odd – he was covered in coal dust singing to a canary, the bird was either stuffed or stunned. I suppose its an image of iconic proportions in its way.' His Dad just sniffed and Alan remembered that he didn't read The Guardian, more to the point he might find the Posket family archives an unwelcome topic. 'I suppose I remember it because it was so funny.'

'Oh he was that all right – they all were , known as characters, a bit potty really.' His Dad laughed more openly at this and continued. 'I actually knew of him before I met your Mother – he used to be a general dogs body at Feethams, sold the programmes, kept the fans off the pitch – that was a cushy job. O f course he puffed it all up later on; drinks with the players, tales from the dressing rooms, the inside line on the great creosote scandal of '51.'

'The what?'

'It was a big story in it's day. It was never properly understood how a vast amount of the stuff that was destined for Catterick Camp disappeared from sidings at Shildon and reappeared on Darlington's main stand for the start of the next season. The club claimed ignorance, which everybody believed of course, but what was harder to fathom was why half the players developed breathing problems that summer and had to be hospitalised – Army strength creosote is powerful stuff, you need masks and stuff if you're going to be slapping it about in warm weather. The official line about the breathless sportsmen was a mystery bug that had incubated at the cricket club where they trained and that two of the new signings were also prone to asthma. I mean, whoever heard of asthmatic footballers – even at Darlington?'

'And nobody got done for it?'

'No. The creosote dried, the trail went cold and somebody at Shildon depot got the push but the really interesting thing is

ASK ME NOW

that season the club finished third in the league and knocked West Brom. out of the cup. Remarkable, especially for a team with an asthmatic midfield and strikers in poor health.'

'So they were as good at knocking off creosote as knocking out the big boys that season?'

'Well this is where old Geordie Posket comes in.'

Alan was intrigued by now, the prospect of a lineage to the lighter side of North Eastern criminality appealed to him. 'So he was in on it then – I suppose he'd have been useful with details of shunting time-tables, security and such like.'

His Dad snorted at this. 'Perff his tallest tale was about the players sudden transformation into decent footballers – they beat one team 8-0, he swore that they were made to sniff a diluted mixture of what was left of the hot creosote before the games and at half-time. He claimed it made them fizz like rockets and shoot like canons, reckoned they'd have won the league if the stuff hadn't run out by March.'

'What happened the next season?'

'I don't know. There ought to have been some sort of investigation by rights, if only on the grounds of our lot finishing third, but football was different then.'

Everything was, thought Alan. Then he thought about how much he'd enjoyed his Dads little story but here he was watching himself again – all what ifs? And please nots. He wanted some more of the creosote. 'I hope you don't mind me talking about all that, you know – Mums family, and all that.'

'No, it's alright.'

Berk, thought Alan, forget you're a social wanker for five

minutes. Remember who you're talking to.

His Dad got up. 'I'll just see how Flora's doing with the tea.'

Idiot, arsehole, how very like our own dear Alan. Back to the shithouse with you where you can sniff your own farts with Nigel Harding. You're going to shit yourself at table; Flora all flustered saying it doesn't matter, Father looking out of the window with a sneer of familiar disgust. Shite on the carpet, Dirty Alan in the room – just can't help yourself can you? … he thought it would never stop, and even if it did the damage was done. How could he go on with stuff like that in his head – unforgettable, that's what you are, you're going mad tra la la. And there was always more to come oh yes. He didn't want to be here, he wanted certainty, safety. He held his breath and tried to stop thinking but it went on … creosote looks like you know what, footballers in the bath. Then he felt cold and still and stuck on a point of cold imploding chaos, it took his breath away. He went to sit in the downstairs loo again and heard his Father call 'ready in five minutes'. Then it started to happen, it seemed nearly funny really – he could actually see the funny side for a bit; the accelerating release of madness in his head while somewhere in there a quiet, appalled voice was saying 'no, no'. He was going to scream then he moved his hand onto his knee and it all rolled through and out of him.

'Alan are you alright?' Asked his Father.

'Yeah … I don't know.'

Are you not well?'

'I don't know.' The exchange had diverted him and it was beginning to fade, he knew enough to make some kind of movement, go through the motions, appear. 'I won't be a minute Dad.' Then there was another split second of cartoon terror; diahoreah seeping out through his pores like creosote

ASK ME NOW

as they ate. Dirty boy, knew you were full of shit. He told himself that they were just thoughts, that he had a choice and opened the door, flushing the chain just in case. He made it across the hall and into the back room where the table was carefully laid out for three with baby tomatoes in bowls, potatoes in mayonnaise, celery but no dog muck on sticks or cold piss in a jug. Just non-alcoholic fruit wine and a smiling Flora urging him to dig in, making sure the men had enough. They set to in silence. This seemed to be how they did it but Alan soon felt tension gathering and ventured an observation about how Cindy would be home by now but you could never be sure with all the road works on the motorways at the moment. He was rewarded with a knowing grunt from the old man and Flora asked him if the quiche was all right. He realised that he hadn't eaten anything and that he was crying. 'It's okay.' He muttered. It's not the quiche.' They looked so concerned, maybe a bit embarrassed but clearly sad for him. The last thing he wanted was to hurt them.

'It's alright son.' Said his Dad. 'Doesn't matter, it can't be that bad.'

This didn't really help Alan. 'I'm sorry.' He said. 'Really sorry.' He noticed how still he was feeling, how it was tears that were seeping through and at that moment nothing seemed to matter too much. All that mad business in the toilet couldn't hurt anyone but him, couldn't happen outside his own head. He had no genuine interest in asking how often Flora had sex or if she was to dish up her special cold sick pie for afters. He remembered David Bowie and another song he'd heard somewhere; sometimes my mind plays tricks on me / sometimes I give myself the creeps. Who sang that? The Carpenters? Robbie Williams? Andy Williams? Val Doon … anyway they'd been through it too, and that helped. He noticed that they were waiting for him to say something. 'I'm sorry, my mind's not right.' (who'd said that?)

'Eh?' Said his Dad. 'You'd like some ... there's beer in if you … '

'Can I go and sit through there again?'

'Of course.' Said his Dad, as Flora watched him. 'I'll come through with you.'

Alan sat down first on the settee then his Dad joined him and rested a hand on his son's knee. 'You can stay here, we'll get you through this.'
And that did it properly, he wept like a water pump for twenty minutes while his Father sat with him and when it was all over he fell back completely washed out, and more peaceful than he could remember feeling in months. He wondered too if Linda Barker might be brighter than she seemed and that her soft furnishings held deeper designs for living conferring real therapeutic affect. You wouldn't need social workers with psychosocial sofas. The next time anything bad came along he'd block it out with this moment. His Dad asked him if he wanted anything to eat and Alan nodded. It hadn't occurred to him that he might be hungry as well, had any of them eaten anything yet? He came back in with two platefuls and settled himself in his chair, after a little while he switched on 'Emmerdale Farm' and they munched away contentedly. By the time 'Coro.' Came round Father and Son were pulling on cans of Co-op light ale then Flora joined them bringing tumblers with her. Roy Cropper had become bed bound and Hayley felt he might be depressed. Alan laughed dryly and made a poor joke about buying himself a Littlewoods cardie from the town tomorrow.

'Are you depressed too then?' Asked Flora quietly.

'Yes … yes, I think I am.' He answered.

'We thought you might be.' She said.

ASK ME NOW

It came to him then that he was liable to underestimate people; they usually knew more than he thought. Usually the women, the watchers who held their tongues, waiting for the right moment. He wondered if he had what seemed to be seen as a feminine side and looked across at his Father tussling with the crossword – three parts done he noticed – half an eye on the tele the rest on higher things. The same he thought, just the same. 'This ones giving me trouble.' He said.

Flora turned away from the screen. 'Read it out.'

'Patio extended in wartime, we hear. Four words; three, three, four and five.'

'Any letters?' Asked Flora.

'I've got some but it's stumping me – first word must be pat or pit, then off maybe? I dunno.'

Alan piped up. 'Put off something.'

Flora laughed and said. 'Put out more flags.'

'Eh?'

'It's war Dad – Evelyn, we hear.' Quiet amusement for three. The curtains were still open and outside Alan could see distant warmth from other windows. I want some of this he thought and tried to remember when he said he'd phone Cindy again. His Dad finished the crossword then folded it over to the sport section for Alan. 'Guess what?' He said.

'What?'

'Darlo. Are at home tomorrow night – re-arranged game. That's almost a local derby.'

Flora looked at Alan. 'Why don't you both go?'

Tomorrow night. That's when he said he'd phone her, he could do both, multi-task.. 'Do you fancy it Dad?'

'Why not.'

'How're they doing?'

'Better than Ridsdale.'

Tomorrow eh? He'd managed to keep the mad stuff at bay for nearly twenty minutes now – but you couldn't be too careful, he was bound to pay for all this pleasant banter. What times fuck off? 'What times kick off?'

'Quarter to eight, could have tea out.'

'Yeah yeah, I'd like that.' He hoped. So, here for another two days at least. Then what? Cindy had asked him to imagine what he would say to someone else in his position and this had shocked him because he couldn't not see how much kinder or accepting he'd be to anyone else but himself. He would tell them that none of it mattered, the only person they were hurting was themselves, that they were poorly – it happened to lots of people and you got better. Or, if they preferred, normalise their experience, reinforce their coping strategies to work with them collaboratively from a recovery perspective. Or maybe not. Either way he'd certainly advise them to persevere with their pills, which reminded him. He'd noted his gippy tummy as a side effect so, only another three weeks to go before they'd 'kick in properly' as Dr. Rose had put it. He knew that coping strategies tended to boil down to the kind of common sense folk wisdom, which was the flip side of singing to canaries. To taking things one day at a time (sweet Jesus), diverting yourself with people you liked, eating properly and getting out into the light.

ASK ME NOW

'We've put you in the back bedroom.' Said Flora as the weatherman wrapped up his forecast – uncertain with some bright intervals.

'Thank you.' He took his cue and went up first. After getting the hang of another unfamiliar bathroom he soon found himself settling to the sounds of a home arranging itself for slumber; muffled voices becoming clearer through a suddenly swished door, water falling through to it's lowest level. He stretched and felt his breathing deepen, outside in the garden a cat shat by the red-hot pokers.

Mike Pearson

FOOTBALL AT FEETHAMS
(BIG NIGHT OUT)

Alan sat on the bottom stair watching the light play against a patch porridgey anaglipta and persuaded himself he'd just dialled a wrong number. A cold voice had taken forever to tell him that Cindy wasn't in/had dumped him/was in bed with Nav but could do with a good laugh – so could he leave a message. This threw him badly; if it was a wrong number he could hardly leave a message, but what if it wasn't and he didn't? The connection finished so he replaced the thing on its daft little plinth and sloped off up stairs to flop down in the back bedroom. The phone went. 'It's for you Alan.' Called Flora. 'Shall I bring it up?'

'Yes … no, I'm coming.' He retrieved the phone and took it back upstairs, waiting till he reached the top before saying 'hello'.

'Oh hi, it's me – did you just call?' Said Cindy.

'Yeah – I thought you were out, or something.'

'I was in the bath so I rang call back. I thought it might be you.'

He pictured that bathroom; spare and functional but full of her if you knew where to look. 'They've got one of these cordless phones here, I'm lying down now. Flora told me it took my Dad ages to get used to it – he used to raise his voice if he got too far from the daft little stand it lives on.'

'You sound a bit brighter, did you do much today?'

He decided to gloss over the first couple of hours when he'd lain in a blue funk but putting on a middling show of a nice lie in. She waited for more. 'We all went to a garden centre this afternoon and I'm off with my Dad to see a footer match

ASK ME NOW

tonight – Darlington versus Bury so I may feel divided loyalties.'

'Bury are the Shakers aren't they?'

'That's right and Darlo. are the Quakers – the local press generally rise to the occasion next day. Have you been busy?'

'Yes and no, one of those days where you're rushing around to no great effect. I spent all morning trying to get a warrant to enter and search an old blokes house because someone had heard him shouting 'unhand me sir' and 'quit the room else I shall trample you to atoms' then heard no more or seen him for several days. I eventually got there with a very nice Policeman in tow to be met by the neighbour waiving a postcard from Porthmadoc. He was on a tour of Wales with a local theatre group and it seems that they sometimes use his home for rehearsals – they're doing some restoration whodunit.'

'Was this chap – the actor – known to services at all?'

'No but once we couldn't find him registered with a local GP we started to wonder and then, you know how these things snowball, well, you can't just leave it can you. I don't think we'll have to record it or anything do you?'

'Probably not, probably best not what with the computer situation. How is everyone, Nav okay?'

'I haven't seen him, everyone I have seen sends their love – our little secret being common knowledge now, which I prefer to be honest.'

'Yes, yes ... so do I. I was thinking about Nav because the weatherman on local TV here is a lookalikey.'

Mike Pearson

'Oh, right.'

'Are you doing anything interesting tonight?'

'I'm going out with Val – off to see a play.'

'Val Meating, what play?'

'Yes, that Val, you know what a culture vulture she is on the quiet. It's by one of those grumpy old git types – I think he did one of those 'has the modern world gone mad' books, The Smirking Diaries or something. Val's a big fan and the play is reckoned to be one of his best, she told me that the original production had Alec Guinness in drag and plenty of incorrect material so she's keen to see how the Preston Players handle it.'

Alan had been interested in much of this but then found himself wondering if he'd ever be able to enjoy anything like it again. 'Sounds really good, tell Val I hope she's got the computer crisis under control.'

'Hmmm that could take some time, anyway, you take care and phone me tomorrow. Enjoy the Bakers.'

'It's Quakers – or Shakers – bye Cindy.' He went downstairs to put the phone back. His Dad was busying himself in the kitchen and Flora was in the garden noting what was coming through. He asked his Dad if they should be setting off but was assured that there was plenty of time. His earliest experience of proper football had been the traditional Saturday afternoon games but the ones he'd really liked, once he was old enough, were the evening kick offs in Spring when more people went and the floodlights came on before sunset. Also, the ground seemed to be full of blokes with pipes and he'd been surprised by the number of older looking women who went along to shout out loud and how cross they seemed to get with the referee. The men simply wished their team to

ASK ME NOW

win but for the women perceived injustice was worse than a game lost, they tended to single out one or two players, usually the smaller nippier ones, to favour and defend whenever they were dealt roughly with by the opposition. As far as he knew Flora had never shown an interest but he could imagine her there; she would know all the players names, express views on their temperaments and want them to do themselves justice, get involved at a level the blokes, including her husband, would think odd. Then he remembered that that was just how he'd been as a boy; wanting to know if the manager gave the players a lift home, who was the centre forwards best friend among the players, why the man behind them had sicked up his tea.

Alan's childhood had been right enough. It all got a bit bumpy when his Dad and Flora became a known phenomenon but he and Pete couldn't really claim victim hood on the back of it. Not really, he knew well enough how kids, boys especially, just turned aside from it all and absorbed themselves in other things; school, mates, the football team then girls, work and you were out of it. His career choice had been, at the time, a case of sounds like an interesting job and a slight feeling that trying to do well in the world was his tiny contribution to making it a better place. But you didn't need to be a social worker to do that, and was that really what they did anyway? He thought about that boy, the 'taking it too seriously' that tended to get him teased. He felt like shouting out loud that there was nothing the matter with him.

'Eh?' Said his Father.

'Oh, I was thinking it's different from Saturday … going to an evening match.'

'Aye well we'd best look sharp, I didn't realise what the time was. I don't think we've time for tea, Flora says she'll put something up for us when we get back.'

Alan had noticed the new car, a discreetly flash saloon type model in cold grey steel. Had they made it to the comfort zone? God knew they deserved some peace in old age but he couldn't stop himself thinking they'd got jam on it too. They must have spent around £80 at Greenacres Garden world and the mortgage finished years ago. He resolved to pay them both in when they got there as he buckled his belt and stretched out beside his Father. By the time they'd reached the A19 some non-committal chat about the new estate at the end of town being below the flood plane and Phoebes Father's driving ban ('in his cups again') had petered out so Alan put in a sterling fifteen or so minutes with an embellished account of Cindy's morning. He fleshed it out with a thoughtful review of the pros and cons of assertive interventions in the lives of others, taking care to edit out Cindy's reflections on 'the fucking magistrate' which brought about a dodgy moment, but, no nothing came. Anyway he carried on with more in the vein of it shouldn't happen to a social worker. All told, he thought it wasn't bad going given the circumstances. His companion gave it due consideration before musing aloud that. 'Well there's one thing, you're lot will never be short of work.'

And that's it is it, he thought. Well I've done my bit, lets see what you can come up with, I'm sure Shula Hebdons lardie cakes are drooping again. His Dad offered him a polo and pointed out the late daffodils, by the time they'd passed through Croft to reach the outskirts of Darlington there was a settled feeling of something like ease between them and Alan looked outside. It was a beautiful evening; the sun had nipped out beneath the cloud line to throw down the kind of light he liked. Hedges and lumps of farming ephemera picked it up, one or two early lambs shivered next to their Mothers, not ready to separate. He noticed the ruthless violent lunge one of them made to be fed, how it fastened on and sucked for life. His Father surprised him. 'That one'll be a survivor.'

ASK ME NOW

He tried to carry on enjoying the view, thinking that not everything had to mean something. They were in the outer environs of the town; lovely looking semis then three storey late-Victorian terraces. It was true that much of the place appeared more characteristic of the region generally, i.e. dog rough, but the place was only just in the North-East and really had more in common with the farming towns of Teesdale than the craggier districts of Cleveland.

'Not much left to play for at this stage of the season.' Observed his Father.

'Weren't they doing quite well at one point?'

'They've fallen away since Christmas, the usual story; couple of injuries, players up in court for fighting in the town. The tale I've heard is that they want the manager out but they can't afford to pay him off – and they wonder why the players won't try for him.'

The delinquent ghost of Granda Posket laughed on the back seat as they parked up by the cricket pitch. After a kindly jostle over the buying of the tickets, won by Alan, they joined the straggle of penitents drifting stone-faced towards the grandstand. When they took their seats the floodlights came on as the players took the field to Rick Astley belting out 'Never Gonna Give You Up'.

'Do you believe in Ghosts?' Val asked Cindy.

She bought some time by sipping thoughtfully from her half of Fosters. 'Not literally, not in the sense of phantoms, spectres – all that palaver, why?'

'Well it's partly to do with this play, how we're haunted by experience and loss and sometimes by not knowing where we're coming from, or even when we know – or we think we know, never being sure. That hidden crack of doubt suddenly expanding as we fall down it.'

It was at times like this that Cindy drew from a deep well of affection for her friend and knew that as long as there were women in the world like Val she'd be all right. It didn't matter that she hadn't a clue what she was getting at. 'How does that translate into what people generally mean by ghosts, you know – vaporous visitations from the other side?'

'I'd say it's about the wish for guidance and the fear of having got something wrong.'

Cindy thought for a while. 'Do you think there'll be many there tonight – playgoers I mean?'

'Oh I should think so, they're building quite an audience base in the region. The Guardian reviewer was came up last month.'

Big deal thought Cindy ungraciously and wondered if they had time for another drink, Val was driving and there had been a hint that she could stay over. Maybe in the interval. 'Did that chap you called Cal after do plays?'

'No, only poems though there is a connection – the chap who wrote his biography was a big mate of the playwright and I think there is also some vague northern connection. The biographer went to school in Darlington, or somewhere.'

Cindy felt her mood sinking and thought that for a small town it had spread it's spores far and wide, like dry rot. 'Alan's there tonight with his Father, for a football match.'

'Oh well, let's hope they win, come on we'll have another one after if you want.'

ASK ME NOW

Val was the best kind of companion for the theatre; sat quietly, no surplus prattle and so obviously focussed on the stage that Cindy couldn't help but be drawn into the spectacle despite an earlier wish for a nice nap instead. The first half, which covered two acts, amused and alarmed her by turn and when the curtains came down she was full of questions. Val sat for a minute then patted her knees and said 'brilliant'. Cindy wondered if she could follow with anything which wouldn't seem trite or off putting, Val was probably one of those people who enjoy coming along to these things by themselves. Her own interest in the theatre didn't really extend beyond the tele., she could see that Shakespeare was good but sometimes wondered about the rest of it. She could never really get past the theatricality of it all. This reminded her of one of Alan's funny stories; a German dramatist was keen that his audiences should never forget that they were before a stage and had directed a number of diversions to remind them. During a play windows could be opened onto a busy street outside and the actors could be observed making up for the next scene at another part of the auditorium. All most folk needed to know where they were was to walk through the cloakroom and buy their ticket. Val wasn't like that of course and offered some helpful comments that made some difference to Cindy's grasp of the thing and enjoy the second half even more. Apparently at the time when the piece had been written in the late 1960's there had been a bit of a debate because the BBC wouldn't do it, perhaps because part of the story featured a young black girl being rebuked and called 'nigger'. This would have caused more tugging of chins today and the Preston Players got round it by replacing her with a homeless person called 'sniffer'. In the pub afterwards they found themselves in accord about this. 'Well I thought it was bad Val. Presumably the writer gave permission.'

'It seems he takes a world weary well-this-is-the-way-we-live-now view. I would bet he's privately pretty fed up.'

'Do you think a black person knowing this would be cross? I think I would.'

'Why?'

'Because it shows another kind of racism – the black girl has to be made invisible or else people will become uncomfortable with the issues. Which was probably what the writer wanted them to be. Also people were more apt to say that then, what is it we're concealing?'

'But even if you got the point would you still accept 'nigger' on the stage?'

'I'm not sure but they could have said something else – cow or black cow.'

'Wouldn't that be as bad as cutting her out altogether?'

'Mmmm maybe dressing things up differently lets us off the hook. I know the arguments against PC go on at the most abysmal level. You know – haven't you heard they've banned 'Ba Ba Blacksheep'. I mean that story's never been true but people want it to be. But PC is cobblers isn't it, just eases bad consciences.'

'Well it gets people going. I fancy another tonic, can I get you another – you might as well stop over tonight?'

'Yes that would be good.'

As Val got them in Cindy looked about the pub. There were a few black faces and it was possible that some might have been in the theatre, they looked happy enough and the scene was definitely something you wouldn't have found in a Preston pub forty years ago. It wasn't just race, there was an

ASK ME NOW

openly gay couple at the next table and the beer was drinkable. Perhaps things just evolved if you gave them time and tried to do the right thing, nobody liked being told what to do.

When Val put down their drinks she said. 'At least they took care with the period details.'

'Yes.' Laughed Cindy. 'You don't see many bedspreads like that now.'

'Bye, look at that little black lad – he goes like stink, they're full back doesn't know what to do with him.'

Alan had totted up the number of athletic black frames, out of the twenty-two on view nearly a third were Afro-Caribbean or African. Darlington also had a Dutchman called Kaak in attack. He'd already missed two sitters and the prat in the hat behind them had bellowed 'you're a pile of shite Kaak'. Alan was certain the player would have heard.

'You still get the usual clowns down here.' Said his Dad. Then Bury scored.

'Fookin' 'ell Darlo. are you crap or what?' Queried the cap, who turned out to be seventy something when Alan sneaked a look.

'Good question.' Said his Dad.

Alan registered a rising level of anxiety but this was surely normal given that he was amongst a baying pack of senile delinquents watching a football match. Would his Father lose his restraint and start a fight? As it was he was watching carefully some funny business unfolding near the far corner flag. It seemed that one of the Bury players had become embroiled in a gentleman's disagreement with one of the fans in the sparsely populated paddock. It was now becoming more heated as several of the fans friends took up the cudgels and only the waist high barrier stood between them. The referee's assistant had come bravely between them but the Bury player – Blair he'd learned later – had become very upset, pointing to his head. The other players, friend and foe alike, stood around chatting with hands on hips and little apparent interest until the ref. intervened to lead the player away amid scornful rebukes from the fans. Alan noted that none of them seemed young and that a number were women in headscarves. His Dad nudged him gently and said. 'Hey now just watch this.' The ref. listened tolerantly to the Bury man's heart-felt account then produced a red card. An enormous cheer went up then Jimmy Noone, the 'colourful', i.e. bonkers, Bury manager entered the fray and the fun really started. It was at least five minutes before order could be restored and five policemen escorted Blair, who seemed to be holding something carefully in his hand, and his manager beneath the stand. Just before they passed out of view it could be seen that Blair spoke to a policewoman, opened his hand and passed her the bottom half of a set of dentures. Alan also saw that one of her colleagues was leaning against the barrier chatting quite amicably to an old man with a headscarf wrapped around his lower face.

'Has he just …?'

'Yes, I saw the whole thing. Granda Posket couldn't have made it up.'

The pantomime had taken up around seven minutes and Darlo. equalised in time added on to the first half. A shot going wide struck Kaak on his hip and went in to predictable tributes to the man behind them. Alan offered to get the teas and joined a queue of chattering supporters. He began to chatter within but he felt this might be his own chance of an injury time equaliser; he had a good feeling about those teas. This was empowerment, this was coping, this was …

ASK ME NOW

'That was some let off eh?' Proffered a deep voice behind him.
I'm not going to let off thought Alan but said. 'You mean the old fella?'

'Aye, 'im an all, no I meant our lot. What a bloody shambles, Kaak's a looky booger – sticks his fat arse out and in it goes.'

Alan was very keen not to let this one develop. 'That wingers having a good game.'

'Who?'

'That smallish player on the left.'

'Oh the little black lad – yeah, got him on loan from 'Boro, too good for us. Junior Blenkinsop.'

'Eh?'

'The winger, right mouthful isn't it. The lads all call him Wilf - player like that's wasted down here, who's he got to pass to? Kaak? You know what the lads'll call Kaak if he doesn't smarten his ideas up …'

Fortunately Alan had come to the front of the queue by this time and walked back to his seat like Hercules after a particularly trying labour, feeling all the better for it. His watch told him it was ten to nine and it seemed that his happy hour and a half had gone into extra time.

'Would you believe it eh?' Said his Father as they sipped reflectively while scanning the corner of controversy. 'Someone was telling me while you were away – apparently it all started when the ball went out of play and the Bury lad asked for it back. The old chap bent to pick it up and stumbled so their lad said something to the effect that he'd fit into our back line and why didn't he take his teeth out and get stripped off, you know him being so nimble. Well after they'd called him a cheeky beggar, or words to that effect, he complained to the linesman and it got serious, then the dentures started to fly.'

'And then he called the ref a daft beggar?'

'Aye, like as not – mind you he is. Kaak was yards off-side when our goal went in, you could hardly say he was interfering with play, it was the only time he got his backside into gear all game.'

'Still.' Mused Alan. 'I feel Darlo. merited an equaliser. They came back strongly and that winger had their back line in all sorts of trouble.'

'Maybes.' Sniffed his Dad in a seasoned footy fans don't-get-too-excited way. Alan could tell he was enjoying himself though, as were the rest of them – you knew how much it meant to the blokes by how much they pretended it didn't. As he'd anticipated there were a number of women around them who were not fettered by such bluff insouciance, chatting openly about how smart the little black lad looked in his white kit, how the Bury supporters – a straggled group of thirty with a paddock to themselves – had got behind their heroes even when they'd let one in. They also felt that people were being hard on Kaak and should give him some encouragement to 'lift the lad'. Alan and his Dad shared a smile at this.

'I'm enjoying this – it's good of you to let me come home for a bit.'

His Dad touched his elbow. 'Here they come, just keep the ball out of that corner.'

Cindy heard the bell ring out in the crush bar as people came

ASK ME NOW

back through in twos and threes. She and Val stood to let their fellow play-goers along the aisle – one man stood on her foot then another pushed his bottom in her ribs making her think of Alan at his football match. All the women skipped past with practiced poise. 'Did you see that great ape stick his arse in my face?'

'No.' Said Val. 'Perhaps it's an invitation to make yourself known to him.'

'Well he can practice a more roundabout route if he wants to mark his card. I honestly think that as far as the arguments for being female go one of the best is the quantity theory. I mean, with men there's just so much of them; feet like boats, great long shanks and once they start filling out. Alan takes a size ten shoe, when he parks them next to mine I feel like Esmerelda.' Val laughed at this but bringing Alan into their playful nattering made Cindy a bit sad. His big hands could be gentle as well, they'd warmed her on the draughty moor and, when she wanted them to, they would fit wonderfully round a buttock each, and, when she didn't, he generally got the message. She wondered what he'd make of this play.

'He's a hopeless hunchback though.' Said Val knowingly, then the curtain swished up again.
The rest of the drama developed skilfully the themes hinted at earlier and passed into the audience's imaginations during the break. It came as no surprise to Cindy that co-dependence, hate and abandonment crept out of the shadows as the story darkened and amusing quirks curdled to booze raddled terror then murder. She sensed the mental health connection too but it was so much subtler than any 'academic' article could be. People really did drive each other round the bend with their clinging and closeness, like bindweed it might seem attractive but if you looked harder it could stifle – and kill.

'When was the last time they went up?' He asked his Dad.

Mike Pearson

'They year they landed on the Moon.'

'1969.'

'Correct. They came back down in 1972, the year the last man left the moon – Christ, he's put it in.' Darlos. Own dark star had curled in a beauty and seemed to be leading off a minimalist Moon walk of his own in celebration; holding his left leg up in slow motion as several of his fellows knelt in genuflection to kiss the golden boot. The ref – 'fussy beggar'- was having none of it and pulled out his yellow card in an absurdly theatrical flourish for overly jubilant goings-on in a Northern sports arena. Alan decided he hadn't really heard his Father shout 'miserable get' and asked him if he'd kept his telescope.

'Somewhere about I should think. Have I to fish it out?'

'If you wouldn't mind – fuck … he's going to put another one in.' His Fathers reaction to this was drowned out as all hell broke lose and old men jumped for joy. 'Straight from the kick off, did you see him? Took it off their number fives toes.'

There really was no holding young Blenkinsop now. He lay down in Bury's goal area with all fours in the air twisting in pleasure from the neck down in perfect simulation of a dog on a carpet. His teammates seemed uncertain how best to participate; should they clap their knees or venture a friendly sniff? The matter was settled when the affronted number five kicked him quite hard. The lads then found themselves on surer ground and pitched in with gusto for a two-minute brawl. When it was all over the two main protagonists could be seen chatting casually by the corner flag and the ref. -'seen sense at last' – was content to restart the game without further ado. Alan found the last half-hour fascinating. The football was okay – Darlington managing a fourth goal at the end

ASK ME NOW

when the ball hit Kaaks head as he slipped to much general jollity – even Bury's keeper managing a smile and walking off with him at the end on friendly terms – but it was the theatre of it all, the atmosphere which seemed so remarkable to him. Something between a crowd of warty yokels in the year of the plague and the audience at the first night of a Stravinsky ballet, except that this lot were really enjoying themselves. His Father, flushed and stirred, was heard to say 'eh what a performance' as they all stood to clap them off at the end. As far as Alan could see Nijinsky himself could have got his game for Darlo. on this showing.

From the car as they drove out of town Alan could see lads and Dads walking home together and he looked forward to the next days Northern Echo. He tried not to think about how he might be feeling when it plopped on the mat in the hall. He thought about Cindy instead, how he might polish up the whole thing to make her laugh.

In another car in another part of the north she was watching a different kind of play going on between a man and a woman, both youngish and dressed for a picnic in the rain. At first sight it appeared that he might be waiving his arms about to keep warm then she could see that he was shouting something too. It conveyed the impression of thwarted entreaty to the woman who stood regarding him with fed up disdain before casually clocked him one. Cindy gasped when she hit him again and her T-shirt rode up to reveal an elaborate tattoo covering the small of her back. Her bloke fell back as another couple paused briefly on their way past. When she looked again the girl had gone. Cindy felt shaken by this, she hated violence, especially her own. The worst part of yesterday had been when she'd set about him with that book, how right then she'd hated him and getting him weighed off to his parents had seemed the best way to not wring his stupid neck. It was their own fault, they always asked for it.

Mike Pearson

'Something happening out there?' Asked Val.

'Just a bit of a ruck across the road.'

'Funny place Preston.' Said Val.

'How do you mean?'

'Well it's got one of the best provincial theatres after Newcastle-Under-Lyme and it's not what you'd call rough, but I'd feel safer on the streets of Oldham after the pubs shut.'

'Do you think an interest in the theatre should rule out blood in the street?'

'God no, think about ancient Rome, not to mention North Staffordshire– worse than Ridsdale I shouldn't wonder – it's just that Preston looks such a nice place and … well nicer places should make nicer people.'

Cindy was tired and wondered why on Earth Val didn't know better by now, she could also see another spot of bother taking shape right in front of them – one lad was on his knees while two others danced around him shouting 'carrots' then he was extravagantly sick all over the pavement. Val seemed to be blithely unaware of it all and continued wittering on about the social and the inner landscape. Cindy would usually be happy enough to listen and respond but just then she wanted her to shut up and let her have a nap. After some more discursive mulling from the drivers seat about fences, neighbours and some other barmy American poet they reached open country and Cindy composed herself in an attitude of repose. Val took the hint but Cindy was too tense and uncomfortable to go off, she also felt rotten; Val was only trying to help. She sat up and asked if they could have the radio on. Val nodded keenly and twiddled into Late Junction where Hortense Poshvoice was introducing a live set from Klangfarbun; before the music could start Hortense explained that this would be an

ASK ME NOW

exceptional performance featuring elements of music concrete, Latin rhythms and popular British dance music of the 1930's – 'a sort of fabulous musical concatenation where Stockhausen meets Jack Hylton in a Cuban tea-shop.' I bet I know who'd enjoy this thought Cindy, although Val surprised her by pouring scorn on 'the cobblers some people spout' which made Cindy smile to herself. The music sounded pleasant though, interesting but not that original. Like much of the 'new' music she'd heard via Alan it sounded unique but very similar to other stuff. She made this point to Val who reverted to form. 'Ah.' She said. 'You've been reading Eliot.'

This decided Cindy to say nothing more till they got home and to turn up the volume. Klangwhatsit gave way to another track from the Rotherhithe Rappers new cd – 'Do Agnes Of Bingen'. This took her back to the discussion with Alan and Melvyn Bragg in the car, if the world was getting smaller would it also get dafter? The round lights of Ridsdale eventually signalled home and Cindy asked if it was still all right for her to stay. 'Of course it is, Cal might keep you company.'

Yes, of course, Cal – Vals great mutt, famous for lifting his leg against the reception desk. In the event he approached her with care to give a few cursory sniffs before prancing around Val with his tail ablur. 'I'll not be long.' She said as she slipped on his lead. 'Make yourself at home.' She hesitated over filling the kettle and considered the best way to secure an offer of something stronger. She went through to the sitting room and settled herself in a comfortable corner of Vals settee (pre Linda Barker but post Jack Hylton). She sat for a while but being in Vals house alone wasn't helping and a big dog like Cal might need a big walk. She tried some square breathing and thought about the play, remembering a lot more than she'd thought. By the time Val ambled back in she'd come up with a number of things to talk about but when Val asked her if she was warm enough Cindy burst into tears. Val locked up, dimmed the lights and came over to her. Cindy fell into her ample frame and sobbed for five minutes before she worked out that the warmth gathering around her bottom and thigh was being given by Cal who'd curled himself perfectly into the sofas last third. She propped herself to get a better look and he sighed with the shifting arrangement of his pack. He was a good looker and his thick tan gave off a nice whiff of damp dog. She'd have liked the position to continue but could sense her friends posture giving her some difficulties. 'Here, I'd better get up.' She said.

Val perched herself on the arm of the couch while Cal stretched. 'Shall we have a drink Cindy? A drink drink?'

'Yes I think so – just the one though.'

Two glasses of malt whisky later and without referring to him by name they'd shared their views on co-dependency, depression as passive aggression and the victim as persecutor and how charity shop shirts should never be sold to anyone over 35. 'It must be love then.' Said Val.

Cindy smiled ruefully and pushed her fingers deeply into Cals coat. 'He's like a bear, do you have to get him clipped often?' 'I let him grow it through the winter – he's about due for a spring clean.'

'Where does he sleep?'

'With me usually. Why don't you join us tonight – there's plenty of room.'

Cindy felt glad that this had come about. She knew what was meant and what wasn't and when Val sent her up first she felt quite safe. The actuality, of course, turned out differently; she'd had too much to drink and couldn't get off, Val was a terrible fidget and Cal wheezed and spluttered like a soggy football. In the end she got up for a pee and found the spare

ASK ME NOW

bed where she dosed off eventually wondering how much an Airedale would cost to keep.

Mike Pearson

LEAN ON ME

'Well, you're looking better.'

'I don't look any different ... do I.'?

'Christ, you were yellow that day I dropped you off at your Fathers.'

'Yellow.'?

'Yeah, dead peaky – your Dad remarked on it.'

'Oh well, I don't remember too much about that. They're talking about coming over soon, did I tell you? They're keen to see you again.'

Cindy nodded then pursed her lips tightly. 'Then it's back to work next week I think I can say you've been missed.'

Alan expelled a quick puff of air from his nose. 'I'm actually seeing Graham tonight for a drink. I can catch up a bit then.'

'Oh, right. Where you off to.'?

'Up the Cocky Sailor.'

'Where'? She asked in a mildly horrified way.

'We're meeting at the Trafalgar. It's known as such to men about the town there being a slight incline at that point on the High Street.'
'How charming – don't forget your compass. I'll see you as soon as I know a bit more about what's happening at home.'
They had a nice hug and playful peck on the cheek in the style of a long married couple then Alan waived her off from his doorstep.

ASK ME NOW

Back up in the flat he fell into his resurrection shuffle via the breakfast pots, some light tidying and putting straight, all the while setting out in his mind his stall for the day ahead. As it was a Monday and the weather was bright he decided on a power walk to and round the park, back for a shower then lunch at Green Judgements before a gentle stroll up to town to read the papers in the Central Library. He could get the bus back home and talk to Steve for a while. He was crying more now but it was all right and hadn't someone pointed out that tears wash the eyes? Yes, he thought, but how am I doing?

He clicked off Sonny Rollins in mid-squawk and hit the street striding. By the time he chugged paunchily through the brown gates of Jubilee Park he was wheezing nicely with a fine sweat on. He stopped to enjoy the scene; there was blossom everywhere, the conker trees swayed gracefully, heavy with candles, a little dog scampered for a ball. Once round the block he thought, then a nice sit down before another go. He wanted to be happy, happier than he was but the best he was getting was less bad than he had been. He wanted to be free of himself, wanted not to be bothered but thought he must be getting better, or maybe he was levelling out of free-fall. He was watching himself so much that he didn't notice that the little dog had fallen in behind him, it's stout little body borne along by busy legs. It broke into a canter and managed to edge ahead to drop a dirty grey tennis ball on the path. It was an odd terrier type production with flappy ears and a stumpy tail atwitch with anticipation. It looked at the ball then at its new friend. Alan bent to ruffle behind those out size ears but the little dog pulled back then pounced at the ball yapping. Alan shaped up to kick the ball one way and as the dog haired off in the direction he'd signalled, he turned neatly and wellied it the opposite way. The dog heard the aqueous contact of Matalan trainer with small ball and slowed in a wide circle to pick up speed and sprint after it with its ears catching the wind like Piglets. Alan smiled and walked on, and where was he? What happened to your thoughts once you took your eye off them? 'Shut the fuck up' he said to himself. Trust to the ice and it might hold you. An old lady with a poodle watched him stride past and pulled her dog off in another direction.

He picked up enough speed so that by the time he passed the bandstand he was breathing deeply. He wondered if there were any evening concerts planned for the summer, it might be nice to come down with Cindy and Steve with his new girlfriend. A nice idea, on he went – over the bridge of sighs, through the arboretum then the home stretch all the way to the bench of rumination, which he was pleased to find unoccupied. He flopped down to meditate with the conker trees while his breathing steadied. After a while he noticed that he wasn't quite alone; several scruffy pigeons were pecking at stuff on the path, one of them had other ideas and began to push out his belly and sweep the path with his tail feathers. This seemed to annoy the others, possibly as his prancing about had scattered the crumbs or whatever. Alan noted that he had a bad limp as well, which must undercut a pigeons chances in the leg over stakes. Nobody seemed much bothered either way so he gave it up as a bad job to join in with the rest, then they all peeled off suddenly towards the bandstand. The next thing he was aware of was the sounds of a damp plop by his foot and eager panting. He looked to see the dog he'd met earlier grinning back at him, it moved closer and this time permitted Alan to fondle it's ears as it sat against his foot. As they got to know each other better he felt a collar and worked it round to find a silver name disc; 'Beeswing' from 25, Gas Street. There was a phone number too but he didn't have his mobile to hand. When the dog got up for a stretch and waggle Alan saw that Beeswing was a bloke. 'Good lad.' He murmured fondly and stroked him under the chin.

They sat for a while but the only other people to pass by were a couple of youths talking intensely about a car, and a smart looking woman with a Weimarnier on a lead. Beeswing bared

ASK ME NOW

his teeth and growled at the large grey dog so Alan was forced to feign ownership and hold him steady. This set him thinking about dogs, hadn't there been another one, something to do with Mr. Clayton? Probably another tireless tickle addict with sawn off trotters. Then there was that great daft lump Val Meating kept. A dog would make the best of any situation it found itself in, find itself a new companion, or sleep alone in a shed. Drink dirty water from a hollow log – they were just so determined, optimistic ... dogged. Beeswing looked up at him with his big tongue lolling and Alan sensed that the dog was anxious. He didn't know for sure where Gas Street was but he had an idea it might be nearby. The dog had now parked the edge of his backside against Alan's foot and was still panting. He remembered a short course the Health Trust had paid for him to go on concerning psychosocial interventions, one of the main topics had been the moving of people 'from dependent to independent relationships'. A dog would see through all that pretty quickly. He moved his foot then put it back as the warmth began to fade – Beeswing wasn't bothered; a therapeutic alliance was in the making. Alan decided to get him to walk in the first instance, they could review things at the park gates. Alan stood and stretched. 'Right mate, someone must be missing you.' He took a short walk then looked back. Beeswing had stayed put and was licking a front paw, for comfort or had he stood in something nice wondered Alan? A feral looking Chihuahua toddled into view and he sensed trouble brewing as his pal clapped eyes on it – he managed to scoop him up as the runty miniature made its move. There had been no doubt in his mind who would have come off best and was relieved when the smaller dog took no further interest after a dismissive sniff of his ankles and took itself off. Where was its owner? He didn't want to be lumbered with the pair of them and why was he bothered in the first place? He should table this in supervision. The canine Billy Mitchell reappeared to leave a stringy coil by the bushes and busy itself with a discarded burger box, then to his relief a teenage girl appeared with a plastic bag to spirit 'Samson' and his gift over to the red bin by the bogs. Alan waited a while then followed.

The lad at the garage across the main road confirmed that Gas Street wasn't far and gave directions taking them down past the canal and over some old industrial ground to a little community of terraces. It turned out to be a cul-de-sac opening onto the waste area. He could see how a dog could break free from here but he'd been lucky with the main road. Beeswing seemed quite content in Alan's arms, which were aching a bit. He liked the warmth though from his firm little frame and stroked his sides with his thumbs. It was the first time he had felt anything like this since the last time he and Cindy … he felt himself twitch against his boxers. This was good stuff and it was only just coming up to lunchtime. There was nobody about in the street and one or two of the houses looked abandoned, he felt his mood dipping. It all looked a bit sad – a documentary photographer of the 1930's would have found women scrubbing steps, white shirts billowing on lines, kids hoolahooping in the back alleyway. Now it was in its end state, full of things in their farewell – ancient brick and glass that had seen too much. It hadn't been built to come to this.

Number 25 was about halfway down one side and appeared to be mid-way along a continuum of decline; the paint wasn't peeling but it had been a long time since anyone had knelt to whiten the doorstep. He put the dog down and it scampered down the passage forming a bridge with next door. Alan wondered whether to knock, the back gate looked shut and Beeswing was snorting into the space beneath it. He went down to join him and called 'hello' over the top as the dog gave up a few half-hearted yelps. He got a restricted view of the back room, it looked lived in but there was no-one about as far as he could see. He could hardly lob Beeswing over the gate and was just about to try his luck at 27 when a figure appeared from the street to ask 'can I help you'? He moved towards the light and saw that the voice belonged to an old lady. 'Oh, I found this dog across at the park so I thought I'd

ASK ME NOW

better… you know. He didn't seem to be with anyone, and it's a busy road.'

'Eh'? She said, then. 'Oh, have you been off on your travels again'? The dog had joined her and was stretching up against her pale blue housecoat.

'Has he taken off before'? He asked as the dog hopped across the doorstep and into the house.

'Twice this week. I think there must be a bitch on heat somewhere – I didn't even miss him this time. If he sees daylight through that door he's off, the lass from the social must have left it open. I thought he was in the back.'

Oh dear, thought Alan; lass from the social, rickety recall span – lives alone. 'Wont you come in'? She said. Beeswing reappeared bearing an enormous and much-masticated chewing thing which he managed to waive at Alan, this decided it. He was shown into the front room. 'You go out on your own as well then'? She asked.

'Yes – day off.' This opened the conversation up along predictable lines. When she asked him he took a deep breath and said. 'I'm a social worker, over at Northfield.'

'Oh, I see.' She said. 'Well I'm glad you brought Twinkletoes back anyway.'

He decided to be bold. 'Was your visitor able to help you with anything'?
It turned out that the lass had been an Occupational Therapist sent by Mrs. Thorpe's GP to assess her capacity to undertake activities of daily living, or as the assessee had put it 'manage in me own 'ome'. He reflected in passing that some sort of multi-disciplinary identity must have been forming if all the occupational groups arrived on your doorstep from 'the

social'. She got him to call her Nina and let on that she'd not long been in The General to have her knee done and wondered why she'd need help if they'd fixed it like they said, she'd waited long enough as it was. It went on like this for a while as she chuntered on in a tone of plaintive belligerence he'd come to know via contact with folk from her generation. The landscape on their journey was beginning to look different to what they'd been led to expect, what was it coming to? Perhaps where you were going seemed unfamiliar once you neared the end of the line. He scanned the settee for fallen cream crackers and wondered what he thought he was doing there. 'Is your knee any better then'?

'We're getting there.' She said casting a baleful look at the dog. He'd crashed out beneath the bay window, his little paws tapping through dreams of his trip to the park. Alan wondered if he'd saved a life and how many good deeds there were to redemption?

'He's a bit nippy then'?

'Oh yes, likes his turn out. He got spoiled when I was in – went to my friends – took him out three times a day then fed him from her plate.' Beeswing stretched and sighed. 'She'll come down most nights to take him and the little girl next door likes to walk him round the block but he played her up last time – reckoned to run for his ball but wouldn't come back.'

Alan was pretty sure by now that Nina lived alone. He'd already spotted a small framed photograph on top of the tele – it displayed a sternly smiling man in a cardigan who would be the significant other. He looked to be a classic Jack Russell owner, bluff and beery, fond of his garden, soft with his dog. Beeswing might be her last link to him; did his twinkle toes know what powerful stuff they were messing with? 'Is he good company then'?

ASK ME NOW

'Never says a dickey bird.' He realised he'd been looking at the photograph as he spoke. 'Not that he came out with that much when he was here.' This was said without rancour and made him think about other moments like this he'd shared with older people. How 'in my day' glanced back to a different world they felt cut off from. This woman had come to a place where it was good to talk (as long as you were careful not to say the wrong thing) where things that had happened without much thought now had titles and people paid to do them. A time now when someone who'd chosen you and put you first, a man who had been just the job could be seen as 'uncommunicative' and of his day, as if you could be anything else. And this, he was coming to see, was his generations great illusion, that you could somehow fast forward the world to a better place you had in your head, that you could bypass evolution. It was like taking drugs, taking a trip from one state to another without having to do anything tricky or time consuming in between. Until it all wore off and you had to see it wasn't real. It was like cosmetic surgery or men who wore wigs, you always knew, no amount of wishful thinking could make it otherwise. Things would take their own time. Wigs set him thinking, he'd noticed that it seemed to be fashionable to be bald – young men with beautiful thick locks would now have it all shaved off, and what did it all mean? Were they rehearsing a better life in age? Would theirs be the generation to get it right, to gather in the sun boiled sitting rooms of Sweethaven like wise Greeks who would refine their wisdom for the respectful young.

'He's made you think.'

'Eh.'

'Twinkletoes, you were miles away. It's always a mystery what goes on in their little heads – if only they could talk eh'?

'Well, they certainly seem to get the best from whatever spot they're in.'

'Cottoned on to you quick enough – must have known you were from the social.'

Must have known I was soft in the head, thought Alan. Why can't I be the Sam Spade of social work? A knowing hipster from the mean streets of North Lancs. Cognisant of tough love and durable advice, a mercurial mix of Humphrey Bogart and R. H. Tawney – 'see ya around kiddo and remember to apply that recovery paradigm'. But such things could not be wished into being; he was what he was and even a foot loose Jack Russell had his number. 'Maybe he sensed I liked dogs.'
'Well, it comes to the same thing.' She replied a bit enigmatically.

He was enjoying his Blue Ribband and decided to pursue this. 'Do you think my job makes it more likely that I'll pick up stray dogs in the park?'

'Oh I should have thought so, trying to be helpful.'

'How did you get on with your visitor, was she helpful?'

Nina sniffed. 'Fair enough – she was right, I'll need something to help me in and out of the bath and one of those mobile telephones would be a good idea, just in case, but, well …' Alan nodded and she thought for a while. 'We had a visitor from Northfield once, one of your lot I should think, came out to see Eric not long before he died. He was all right; nice chap but there wasn't much he could do. We all agreed it was natural for someone with cancer to feel depressed – there'd be something wrong if they weren't. As I remember Eric took to him so he did well there, invited him back a second time to show him his rabbits. He certainly got him started, but he still died.' She looked directly at him then but there was nothing to say.

ASK ME NOW

This had taken him out of the tenuous loop of his big-boy-now coping strategy and he was pretty sure she'd had enough of him. Why was he prone to underestimating other people? Was it a sour tendril of his weedy self-image? He knew outsiders weren't bound to get on and this woman seemed to dislike self-pity as much as he did. Something was hovering between them, somewhere near the back door step, which threatened to open up more than either really wanted. The dog decided it again; one minute he was dead to the world, the next half way up the passage before Nina could execute an uncertain swivel to cry 'little beggar'. Alan managed to head him off at the top of the street where two lads were tinkering with a car. Beeswing had taken against them and was barking furiously – one of the lads had a wrench in his hand and didn't look to be a dog lover. Alan apologised as he scooped up the dog, the young man simply looked at him and gobbed extravagantly on the pavement before turning to his mate who said 'fuck to it'. Thug thought Alan, cock o t'school at St. Retards and look at him now. Which, as it was safe to, he did, the boy was leaning into the engine and Alan could see that he had a blue tattoo on the back of his shaven head. It was an elaborate composition in dotted lines, perhaps it instructed the curious where to insert a thumb to lift a flap. He scolded himself for this unkind thought, he could recognise a useful skill when he saw one – for all he knew they might be fixing his grannies car.

When he'd returned the dog for the second time he lingered by the back door and made free with sage advice about a catch for the gate, going so far as to offer his services. Nina thanked him but was sure she'd manage. He was reminded of a similar exchange on Cindy's back door step; it wasn't that he'd outstayed his welcome but it was clearly time he was off.

On his way back across the waste ground he tried to overlook the stink and splatter of detritus; dog shit gone furry under glass, paint stiffened weeds and fly tipped pornography, to pin down another line the morning's capers had stirred up.

Something about if you must do good to another, do it in minute particulars. It sounded odd but reachable so must be Blake, which made him think about the young boy beneath the bonnet and his snooty attitude to him. For all Alan knew he might have a couplet from Swinburne inked somewhere about his person. Stop it he thought, stop it now you overeducated smirker much more of this and you'll be heading for trouble. He kicked an old wooden chair, shouted 'fuck to it' and ran all the way home, jogging on the spot like a twit till it was safe to cross the main road.

Safely home he collapsed into his old wing chair and focussing on his breathing till it began to steady, concentrated on his framed photograph of Lester Young laughing at something Count Basie was telling him. 'So' he thought 'how'm I doin.' Well, not so bad considering – made most of this mornings deadlines, he was all ready starting to feel pleasantly tired, no more news from Nigel, and what about all that business with Beeswing? He decided to have some Lester, in Alan's considered view the greatest jazz musician who ever lived, and an occasional visitor to the dark side himself. Basically he knew he was on the mend, knew 'objectively' that things were tons better than they had been eight weeks ago when Cindy had driven him across the Pennines for his tea time of torment. He reckoned to have hit bottom at some point during that afternoon. And it wasn't coming back; he couldn't care less if he'd have to take tablets for the rest of his life, not now they were working. You wouldn't tell a diabetic not … lets have some Lester.

His CD player had been getting more use recently and there was a scattering of jewel cases on the floor – mostly chamber music or minimalist piano stuff but he wanted jazz today and soon found what he was looking for, Lester's 'Chronological Classics' volume 1. He dropped it in and sat back waiting for the little steel box to give off its watery fizz then track one flashed up and Count Basies allusive tinklings ushered in Lester's solo on 'Lady Be Good'. Everything about the record

ASK ME NOW

seemed spot on, even 'Tatti' Smiths cackling trumpet part, it was pure chance the record got made at all – they must have been playing like that all the time then, in 1936, in Chicago when they made what could have been the first modern jazz record. Alan thought it might still be the best with every subsequent effort falling a little way short of the same sense of discovery they'd found that day. Lester's solo was a simple thing – 'just notes' as Ronnie Scott had said, wonderingly – but it was blown with such joy and certainty and spring that it made you smile inwardly. By the time 'Taxi War Dance' came on Alan's feet were tapping. Yes, there was no doubt he was getting better ... but; would it last, what if he lost it, did he really want to get better at all (depression being a great get out)? He wasn't without common sense but, as Frank Sinatra had pointed out to him only the other day 'what good does common sense for it do'? Ol' Blue Eyes had been singing about the vagaries of the human heart of course and it was here that Alan felt most in need of wise counsel. She'd been fantastic throughout, right from that heartfelt bollocking at work to last night's tendresse over the phone. There'd been trips out during the day, a couple of films and plenty of talk, even an afternoon in each others arms listening to Richard Burton in an old recording of 'Under Milkwood'. Generally speaking a level of companionability and communication the stuff on which proper relationships were made, but what did it all mean - did it amount to anymore than a hill of beans in a crazy world?

He was sure they knew it was one day as it goes and all – but he couldn't help remembering Betty Clayton and playing some of his own anxieties onto her pursed and long-suffering image. How cross she'd looked from behind as she'd paused in a doorway that day, the tired acceptance that looked close to 'who cares'. Bill had been wary of her and that level of dependency was generally bad news for a troubled twosome. Was she there because she couldn't go? Was this what did Bill's head in? Cindy seemed to be the last person to be up for that kind of thing – so would she bin him as soon as she decently could? He knew enough not to ask and it was tacitly understood that while love was a many splendoured thing, it often showed itself in forms of restraint, deferred gratification and airbrushed gestures of respect to build the backbone of astringent romance, which was might be lot more fun than it sounded. He also missed the sex. He took this to be good as it signified renewal but bad because he'd forgotten how to do it, and he could hardly ask her.

Lester was honking his way through 'Upright Organ Blues', part of a lesser-known recording session with an awful organist who thought he could squeeze out the right stuff on an old fairground calliope. The saxophone made it listenable but jazz was littered with strange meetings in obscure recording studios; 'Rubberlegs' Williams warbling the blues with Charlie Parker, Sonny Rollins plus bagpipes, Tiny Grimes and his Rockin' Highlanders. Reflections of 'Rubberlegs' – so named because Parker had become fed up with him and spiked his coffee – put him in the mood for something by the master so he pulled out his favourite, a live date with his friend 'Fats' Navarro and 'Bud' Powell at the piano. An ill-starred triumvirate who always managed to serve up some of the most wonderful music he'd ever heard. He settled back and as 'Cool Blues' unwound he felt a pleasant stiffness in his legs and eased himself into a more comfortable position in the chair, his breathing deepened as the music took on a friendly intensity. Nothing mattered but the moment.

Alan fell awake abruptly to a diminishing trace of doors slamming and trumpets blarting but Bird and Fats had blown their last some time ago. As his five second stay of grace fell away he saw that it was seven o' clock and realised he'd arranged to see Graham at seven thirty, whatever the dress code would be running gear wasn't required. Shat, showered and shod in smart casuals he hit the street at seven twenty and made for the bright lights. The Trafalgar was a standard repro. job in the towns developing 'café society' sector – there was

ASK ME NOW

still open invitation fighting at the week end but the Police got there earlier now that the trades council was promoting responsible drinking. And who better to fly the flag for this than two social workers out for a pint and a good natter? He'd been lucky with his bus and was only ten minutes late, Graham was sitting by the inglenook toying with the Mail crossword while Santana seeped out from somewhere above him. He was about two thirds of the way through his pint so Alan did the decent thing though Graham limited himself to a half of the guest ale – 'Cutpurse' which they were asked to believe had been brewed in Abingdon since the days of busty wenches in three cornered hats perched astride snorting stallions.

'Probably concocted by a drug company.' Said Graham when Alan expressed his doubts. 'Not a bad drop though.' He allowed after drinking his fill with the air of one who knew a thing or two about such matters. Alan sipped more carefully, it wasn't quite the first strong drink to pass his lips since he'd become ill, he had a trial run the previous night with a bottle of 'Auld Neds' and it had slipped down easily enough. He therefore took a more confident draught then paused, as with the opening moves of a chess game or military campaign, what happened next would shape the rest of the evening. 'So.' Said Graham. 'What's it like round the bend'?

He knew what his old friend was up to and appreciated it. He was setting him at his ease, clearing the decks and dispelling anxiety. Graham at his most incorrigible, drawing from the days of old school social work before PC had furred up people's thoughts and glued their tongues. He noted that he'd not got very far with the crossword and helpfully filled in one of the trickier ones for him. 'Not addled your brains then.' Said Graham having been helpfully put in his place.

'No, but we'd better stay off the darts tonight.'

Graham smiled then opened up a new front. 'Had the most awful assessment today, one of those where they phone you at the eleventh hour to say 'there's a section needs doing' and you say 'you mean an assessment' and they go 'well … yes.'

'Who was it – who phoned you I mean'?

'Cath Furnace from Motherhood and Baby, in a right tizz.'
'She's usually alright isn't she'?

'Yes well, they've a new manager now with a new risk assessment policy so their boundaries are suddenly much tighter. First we'd heard of it, Dr. Wallace went doolally over the phone to them apparently.'

'They can't just do that can they. It's like UDI'?

'Well they have and if Sector Management don't do something that's it. You know how it works; the longer it goes on the firmer it is understood to be part of the 'official' procedure. Then when you question it people go thick on you, can't remember how it started but tell you they've been told M&B don't carry any level three risk stuff anymore. Though they will make themselves available for support and advice to those taking it on. Been missing work then Dicky'?

He laughed softly through his nose. 'I think I must be.' Then gave Graham a condensed version of his morning, taking care to frame his contact with Nina in suitably kitchen sink terms. It turned out that her late husbands man from the social hadn't been Graham. He seemed intrigued anyway and observed that it was probably time he was back at work, where at least he'd get paid for it.

'But I am getting paid, for being not there.'

'Well that's fair enough being as how it was work that did for … sent you off in the first place.'

ASK ME NOW

'Was it'?

'Wasn't it'?

'Oh, I don't know. I don't believe it's that straightforward – the main thing is I'm feeling better. I try not to look too far in any direction but, you know – one day at a time.'

'Sweet Jesus.'

'Don't take the pee Graham.'

'No, no I'm not.' Said Graham quietly into his friend's ear. 'I've just clocked who's walked in with his new doxy – look, over there in the lounge. No, up there at the bar getting them in.'

He thought Grahams conspiratorial approach absurd – he'd actually put up furtive hand to hide his lips as his urgent whisperings were communicated three inches across to Alan's ear – so he got up to visit the toilets. On his way back he managed to notice, quite naturally, Nav carrying a pint of lager and a snowball over to his companion in the corner. She caused him to stop in his tracks and gawp like a booby. Nobody but Graham saw this, though he did laugh out loud. He sat back down. 'Christ you know who he's with don't you'?

'No, I didn't get a proper look.'

'It's only Briony Prince – Mr. Prince's daughter.'

'Well', I suppose she would be unless Nav does the decent thing and she becomes Briony Bhattacharya – has a nice ring to it actually. You know her then.' Graham asked with mild interest.

'Yes, yes I do know her – she's practically a service user, sees what's her name, Nav's colleague. It was a right to-do with her old Dad – he's the jazz fancier I got into Sweethaven. Do you remember me telling you about it, had this great pile of CD's at home, in fact there was also a copy of that incredibly rare vinyl issue of Hans Donkers last session from Denmark, original pressing I think …'

'Yeah right man, all very interesting, I can see now that you're getting back to your old self so get them in eh'?

'I can't go up there, what if she spots me'?

'Well, what if she does, you can ask after her old Dad.'

'Look you go then we'll head off somewhere else.' Alan said this with mighty conviction as he slapped down a fiver, which swung the argument his way. Graham seemed to be a while ordering and it seemed as if he was talking to someone out of view who was not the gormless youth in charge of their requirements, then the penny dropped as Graham nodded in Alan's general direction. He was inviting them through. He came back over with his bland smile and two more pints of Cutpurse. 'Thought it might be interesting did you'?

'Something like that, we could talk about jazz.'

'You are taking the piss now. I don't want anything to do with this, you don't know what you're messing with. Nav could get struck off – anything might happen, what if …'?

Before he could puff up any more wind in the way of righteous affront the door between lounge and bar swung open and in walked Nav, alone. Alan's relief dispersed when he learned that 'she' was in the ladies and would be joining them shortly. Graham asked Nav where he'd met his friend.

ASK ME NOW

'At work actually.' He said as Alan took a prolonged slurp of Cutpurse. Nav turned to him. 'Nice to see you mate.' And rested a friendly hand on his shoulder. 'If you're back on it you must be on the mend. 'The cheek of him thought Alan, the sheer brass faced effrontery, sitting there like a grinning monkey – no not a monkey – sitting there like a posturing peocock after a big strut. No, that wasn't right either and he had been touched by Nav's open friendliness. Where was the harm in it eh? He felt the wind leave his sails, how ridiculous was he? Spluttering inwardly like Lord Queensbury facing dear Oscar. What the devil did he think he would do? Thrash Nav, denounce him as a seducer of vulnerable women, a bad hat? Besides didn't the fair Briony deserve some light in her troubled life? Still, it was all a bit much.

Graham got out his wooden spoon. 'Is she a new worker, student on placement'?

'No, she came in to see Estelle but she was tied up and we got talking.'

Alan could contain himself no longer. 'So you just asked her out, like that?'

'Yeah, it is the usual procedure. She could have said no.'

'And does Estelle know?'

'Shouldn't think so.'

'Anyway.' Put in Graham. 'She's coming over so all pals together eh'?

Alan felt silly blustering like Captain Mainwearing while Graham played the liberal, Nav sitting there like bloody Imran Khan. And Briony drifting across like Isadora Duncan just off the last bus from Woodstock trilling. 'Hello Alan, how are you'?

'An oh fine thanks, better in fact … how's your Father'?

Graham coughed into his drink and Nav looked puzzled but she said. 'I can't believe how well he's taken to it at Sweethaven – he's made a friend who'll listen to Evan Parker with him and copped off in the first week.'

'Life in the old lad yet then.' Said a red-eyed Graham.

Alan wondered if the internal world of dementia was much like an Evan Parker record then decided to play along with the bizarre four-part improvisation unfolding around him. 'Off somewhere nice then'? He asked.

'Yeah, at least I hope so.' Said Nav. 'There's something doing at The Arts Centre – we'd best drink up actually.' Briony knocked back her Snowball while he took off the rest of his Khakenleider smoothly. As they were preparing to go Alan asked what they were off to see. 'A feminised version of 'Oh Calcutta', should be good.' And then they were off.

Graham waited till he was sure they'd gone then laughed out loud. 'You're priceless you are – how's your Father.'

'Well what could I say. It didn't seem to bother her'?

'I shouldn't think much bothers that lass. I only hope she gets her moneys worth.'

'It's refreshing to hear you taking a reconstructed line on that.'

'Oh lighten up mate. It's not so different from your mission of mercy this morning, you and him are both chipping in your two pence to the sum of human happiness – in an ideal world and all that.'

ASK ME NOW

Disgusted of Darlington was forced to concede the moral high ground on this point. 'Yes well, put like that … what do you think of this beer anyway'?

'Had better, fancy moving on to The Blacksmiths'?

'Good idea, should be quiet in there.'

Graham looked at him and shook his head slightly. Apart from the visit from Briony and Nav and an outrageously underage couple in the corner, they'd been the places only customers. The Blacksmiths Arms was parked on one corner of the Market Square and dated from days of yore thus lending an ideal watering hole to the local branch of CAMRA. It was also therefore the pub of choice for social workers, teachers and the like but the beer was reliable and Dave behind the bar had elastic opening hours. There were occasional 'incidents' when middle aged men in corduroys would set about one another in the back room while oath edged debate spilled onto the square. There had been a memorable one over a UNISON initiative concerning the pea harvest in Paraguay. The whole thing had been hushed up and it had been agreed that fraternal gestures to the oppressed of Central America were best left to the National Executive. Alan and Graham often went half-hoping for more of this but tonight the usual crowd were in; solemn looking forty something's smoking roll ups and playing dominoes, the women sitting separately in a group laughing over a bottle of white. At the bar the resident character was going on about Tony Blair to anyone daft enough to hover within two yards of him. Surveying the scene Alan's spirits rose, he felt at home. He sauntered up to the bar and ordered two pints of Sloans 'Lineament'.

'It was my round you know.' Said Graham as they stood near the dartboard.

'Oh it's alright, you get the next ones.'

'Are you sure? That'll be at least five pints before we're square.'

''Yeah I think so.' Said Alan, taking a full mouthful to show he meant business. The character – Freddie Hubbard from Housing – downed his own pint at this point and declared that he was 'going looking for Prescott'. Dave behind the bar gave him a wan smile as he swept out into the night.

'I'm glad he's gone.' Said one of the women.

'Tosser.' Said another.

'Probably his wife.' Mused Graham as they moved to the seats which brother Hubbard had rendered off limits by standing near them. 'No, what I meant was are you okay to drink so much Alan'?

'Probably not but I'm not bothered.'

'Right.' Said his friend. 'But if it's your first proper session for a while … well, I suppose we should get some chips on the way home.'

'Yeah, try that new Chinky down Stubbs Road.'

'Keep your voice down mate – don't want to be blackballed from our favourite club.' One of the dominoes players glanced across to them so Graham suggested they move across to the snug, which had become empty for now. He told Alan how glad he was to see him looking so much better.

Alan sat thoughtfully and gave a rueful sniff. 'It's been a bit of a rough ride.'

ASK ME NOW

'It usually is.' Said Graham. 'I mean, it seems to be a pretty clear illness process but different for everyone. If you see what I mean.' Alcohol had an ironic effect on Graham making him nicer, more thoughtful, less ornery, he dropped his mask of gone cold bitterness and seemed to forget himself. Probably it's depressive properties thought Alan.

'Yeah, I think so.' Said Alan. 'I got most of the DSM stuff but then some extra, just for me.'

After a pause Graham said. 'How do you mean'?

'Well, I think you do go, or I went, a bit bonkers. You know, what Beth Wallace calls treading the borders of psychosis. Things in your thoughts you know aren't real but which bother you anyway and are real in a way if they're in your head, in a way – you know, if you can think them. It's the shit pit at the back of your head, you can see why drilling a hole seems like a good idea only I think they ought to do it at the back bit. I think the difficulty is that I can see it all as a symptom of an illness but it's also a symptom of me. So, if it is an illness then it's not like any other.'

'But it is if it's treatable – and it is isn't it'? Parried Graham.

'Oh sure and I know I'm on my way back to being my normal self, but what if it's part of my normal self to be depressed'?

'To fall ill – which is normal. But it's not normal to accept staying ill, isn't that depression talking, isn't that more than a bit bonkers'?

'Well, whatever.'

'No Alan, I think this is important. Do you remember us talking to Tommy Smith about this once – Tommy called it depressions double whammy. He's no big fan of psychopharmacology.'

'Not since they kicked Liverpool out of the Champions League.'

'No.' Laughed Graham. 'But Tommy knows his stuff and he was on about how hopeless it is trying to do any sort of therapy with someone who is depressed until you could sit on their symptoms chemically. You need to work against the illness in two ways because it works against the person that way – on two related fronts.'

Although beer appeared to make his mate more sensible, Alan was struggling to think straight in any related way. 'How do you mean'? He asked.

Graham warmed to his theme. 'Well one slides into a mood disorder by degrees, some days you don't really notice it happening and when you do it's soaked in a bit deeper. At that point the illness has robbed you of the capacity to think your way out of it or see what's been happening … then the guilt bites, it's all your fault and you don't deserve to be any other way. That really is mad.'

Alan was impressed and touched by this but his attention had been taken by a woman he could see through the door. She had her hair cut and coloured like Cindy but she was facing away from him. Her companion slid a hand into the rear pocket of some green jeans stretched tightly across her bottom and left it there. When she turned to kiss him lightly he could see it wasn't her. 'Yes.' He said. 'Double trouble.'

'Anyway, all I'm saying is, you've been very poorly but you're getting better and it's more complex than chicken pox.'

Alan considered this. 'Maybe if you got spots with it the world, and you, could see it come and go.'

ASK ME NOW

'You're talking about acceptance aren't you. What would you sat to me if our positions were the other way round'?

'Eh'?

'Listen, stop watching that pair in the bar, depression is ubiquitous, part of being human yeah? So it could easily be me sitting where you are and struggling with something similar – you're not you you're me, what would you say to you'?

'Have you been at the RD Laing again'?

'Come on Dickie, do the right thing.'

Alan sat up straight and concentrated. 'Right, okay. It's horrible, it happens, it's not your fault, and it gets better. Try not to worry about why, be with other people you trust, try not to turn inwards. Most of all, remember you're poorly so keep taking the tablets, they'll work. Also, when you're lying awake with the jitters at ten past five you are not alone – all around the world there are millions of you doing the same so imagine joining hands to contact the living, as Ronnie Scott said. And he would know, God bless him.' Alan raised his glass out of respect and saw it was empty.

'Well.' Said Graham. 'A bit bracing but I wouldn't fault you on any of it. So, if you can prop me up can you help you'?

'I don't know – it's the old problem isn't it, it's so much easier dishing out advice to other people. With me it's all the familiar what ifs; what if it gets worse, happens again, can't stand up without a tablet. What if I wear out my welcome'?

'Alan we can't live without what if's – a world without uncertainty is a world without hope.'

'I was reading this book where they said that one reason some people get depressed is to deal with uncertainty, more uncertainty than they think they can cope with. The depressions bad but the not knowing is worse – at least in depression nothing changes. Sounds properly bonkers doesn't it.'

Graham drank enough to catch up then patted his jacket pocket. 'All right, you're keen on theories – why did you get depressed when you did? Think about that while I get them in.'

This was something he'd managed not to ponder despite the unmapped trips down the highways and byways of his recent affective state. As he watched his friend beckon confidently in the barman's direction some traces made themselves known on his neural pathways in amongst the cobwebs and gathering serotonin. He liked to remember a comic strip he'd enjoyed as a boy which he would try to imagine himself a part of. It was called 'Georges Germs' and most of the action happened at various sites inside the body of George Jaundice; fabulously imagined microbes in battledress and boxing gloves would do battle with his long suffering immune system. Fiendish viruses would plot in secret then launch campaigns of attrition at both ends of his body. The drawings would draw on a rough understanding of native history; sometimes the invading hoards of a miscellaneous fever would land as Vikings and do battle mightily with anti-bodies clad in 'Dads Army' ARP uniform. Another week a troubling headache would be depicted in terms of Scotch mist blown about George's brain by Robert the Bruce. He could picture his own brain in a similar vein. A place of much conflict and strange incident where little men whizzed about making mischief before being caught and dealt with by plucky piles of reserved hormones who'd been massing discreetly like a loyalist resistance force. He had come to think of the footie match with his Father as the first significant victory for the home

ASK ME NOW

guard, sure there'd been some reverses since but he had to admit he'd been giving as good as he'd been getting. But who started it all though?

Graham had been nattering with Dave behind the bar, sharing a joke at something, and came back over chuckling. 'What'? Asked Alan.

'That woman who called Hubbard a tosser is his wife. Apparently they have an agreement that if she's out with her mates he either stays at home or visits his cronies in Warrington, which is her preferred option as it involves an over night stay for him.'

'He'll be getting his chips tonight then – typical local counsellor.' Snorted Alan to no obvious purpose. Graham sat down and waited, he hadn't forgotten the little test he'd set his friend. Alan dully piped up. 'I think I first noticed something wasn't right one Sunday when Cindy and I were out walking on the hills.' He hesitated and looked confidingly at Graham.' You know Cindy and I have been seeing a lot of each other'?

'Yes Alan, I think it's generally known.'

'Is it? Oh well, anyway, we were up there and I got a whiff of an odd awful feeling – the only way I can describe it is as an apprehension of something rotten and shameful breaking through inside me. Too late to do anything about but that I'd have to pay for, it would come back – I could depend on it. You know when a cat toys with its prey it has a really cruel way of letting on that it's lost interest and the worst has past, well the mouse or bird knows the awful truth, it goes into this sick swoon. There's really nothing more certain that Sylvester will do for Tweety Pie. It's almost a relief when he does. I knew then I was done for.'

Graham thought about this.' Certainty, something you could

depend on … Sylvester never does get Tweety Pie though does he'?

'Yes, well, you get the general idea.' He slurped his real ale and realised he was three parts pissed already, any more and he'd be well and truly, on that he could depend. 'But I really love Cindy.' He cried up suddenly.
Graham patted Alans elbow as Dave poked his head through the serving hatch. 'Yes, I think the general idea as explained is that this odd kind of feeling, this harbinger of melancholia, brought you some certainty at a time when you felt the winds of change were a gathering.' He was the worse for it too but Alan knew he meant well. They seemed to reach an understanding at this point that the time for serious talk had passed and found themselves focussing fitfully on a large poster nearby showing details of some forthcoming union business. Two black nurses grinned back at them stoically as if to say 'some folk don't know the half of it', behind them a tatty looking oldster gave the thumbs up from his reform threatened wheelchair. 'Do you know that song by Jack Bruce Alan, 'A Letter Of Thanks'? Pete Brown wrote the song – it's on Harmony Row.

'No, is it about Harbingers'?

'Sort of. There's a line 'love gives me indigestion/when they bring up the question/I walk into a solid brick wall'. Then there's Joy Division – it tore him apart alright.'

'Not the happiest of links Graham.'

'No but you know what I mean.'

Alan didn't really, what did Graham know about love anyway? They talked about football for a bit then he became aware that Nav was with them and seemed to have been there for some time, without a companion. It was also late because he'd referred to coming 'for t'last one'. Graham was by now

ASK ME NOW

in more familiar blokey mode. 'Hey mate have you heard there'll be a shortage of electricity in the premiership next season'?

'Oh yeah'? Said Nav

'No Leeds.'

'Clever twat, they're not down yet.'

Graham leaned into Alan amid the shared titterings. 'What else isn't down yet eh'?

Alan smiled without having much idea why and suggested a 'last one' to Graham reasoning that it wasn't going to make much difference now. He usually enjoyed hearing of Nav's capers and wished to know more of Briony. It turned out to be his round so as he passed Nav on his way back from the bar he asked if he'd enjoyed the show.

'Weren't my idea of a night out – tell you all about it when you get back.'

Alan waited his turn behind Barry Bishop, the elected member for Cindy's ward and one who knew a thing or two about dog muck. He'd paid for his pint and peanuts but was keen for Dave to understand that people couldn't just take their air guns to the offending dogs. Why didn't they 'take out' the owners instead? Committee was standing firm on the muck bins – no more were in the pipe line, there was nothing more he could do, what Tony Blair needed to see was …'What'll it be Alan'? Asked Dave with an unusual degree of warmth. He ordered but sensed a resentful Bishop skulking just behind, Cindy had told him an amusing story about the prospective counsellor being harder to shift off her back door step than some of the stuff he campaigned on. As Alan moved off Bishop returned to the bar to chunter on from where he'd left off but Dave was not behind the bar anymore and everyone else within earshot was spoken for.

'What a set of wazzocks.' Said Alan as he sat down. 'I don't know how Dave stands it every night; Bishop Bullshit on dog dirt, Freddie Hubbard on life in the local government fast lane.'

'Aye.' Agreed Nav. 'Neither of them'd give Hazlitt a run for his money.'

Graham laughed at this and Alan tried to stifle a resentment of Navs presence. 'Did he play for Leeds'? He asked then wished he hadn't. 'What was 'Oh Calcutta' like then'?

Nav savoured his bottle of Rott then said. 'Well I reckon if Ken Tynan were still here he'd have been outraged, which would take some doing.'

'Go on.' Urged Graham

'Well he was a man not easily outraged.' Said Nav blandly. 'I think what you want to know is am I shagging a service user'?

'Yes.' Said Alan.

'Right,' Said Nav.

'Eh'? Said Graham.

'Don't you start coming over all coy – it's quite straightforward … '

Nav was unable to offer further intellegence because a distraught Freddie Hubbard blew back into the bar and stood with beery belligerence looking about the room with an air of unfocussed menace. For some reason he fixed his troubled gaze on Alan's party. He then appeared to fasten onto an

ASK ME NOW

understanding, something that had to do with Nav. He bent forward and steadied himself on a table. 'So it's you then.' He bellowed.

Nav looked astonished. 'I'm sorry, do I know you'?

'You will be sunshine.' He stood to address the room. 'So here he is then, your fast bowler from the sub-continent.'

'Better than no-balls from the incontinent.' Answered a familiar voice from the room to scornful female laughter.

'If you're talking to me pal I was born in Leeds.' Said Nav quietly.

'Same difference.' Replied his challenger dismissively.

Alan felt Nav stiffen beside him so he stood up to say. 'I think we're at cross-purposes here, can I help you'?

Graham had moved off to say something to Dave who was back behind the bar and Sue Hubbard moved across to the space he'd left. 'Come on Rocky, let's get you home.' She accompanied this with a wifely but firm hold of Freddie's arm. 'Sorry about all this – bit of a misunderstanding.' This was directed at Nav and Alan with a long-suffering look, which seemed to be winning some time for calm reflection. But fiery Fred was having none of it. 'Leave me alone you ridiculous woman, there's a gentleman here thinks he might be able to help. Why don't we take him up on it? I'm sure he could help clear up the matter – let's have some audience participation while we're about it, this mutley crew of public service layabouts could shed light on our little difficulties. Might even tell me who you've been concertinaing with you old slipper.' He tossed a defiant head into the main body of the room to deliver this and was rewarded with a degree of laughter he seemed to find puzzling. Dave had disappeared again and it seemed to Alan that chaos was round the corner. Nav was very angry. He was quite still and breathing deeply – bad signs in Alan's experience, he felt he should act.

'It's alright Mr. Hubbard, I was just trying to … '

'Just trying to put your oar in.' Sneered Fred. 'Well it's not wanted thank you very much – you'd do better to mind your own if you don't mind me saying so.'

'Come on dear, this is becoming embarrassing.'

'Take your hands off me you absurd person.' Fred then amplified his thoughts for the audience. 'She won't touch me without her gardening gloves on at home.. Can't get enough of me now, I can't think why. Where does Dave think he's taken himself off to – I want a drink.'
'It's too late, for Gods sake Fred lets go home.' Then the tired and emotional husband pulled away from the frayed wife and lost his balance to tumble in a crumpled pirouette towards Alan who offered himself to cushion the larger mans fall. Tousled and beery, the emotional counsellor was too much for the recovering melancholic who lost his own balance and hit a window ledge with the back of his head as he took a blow from Hubbard's forehead near his right eye.

'Ooh, pull the stupid fucker off me.' He wailed, he also felt compelled to thump him as hard as he could. This was difficult as his assailant had softened his bulk against him and seemed content to stay put.

'Who're you calling bad names'? He murmured into Alan's shoulder then reached up to stroke his hair.

Alan was appalled. 'You, you bibulous cuckold, and get off me.'

'You've got a silver tongue you have, weren't you going to

ASK ME NOW

help me'?

'Yes but not here, not like this.'

'Where then? – I like you.'

Nav and Sue helped them to part and Alan was able to see Graham smirking with the ladies. Then another man helped Nav to settle Fred down on a two seater by the door. Sue Hubbard rested a warm hand on his shoulder throughout so Alan took a bit more interest in her. Fred's wife was a well preserved fifty something and he realised that more than anything, he wanted to sink into a bosomy clinch with her – a sort of antidote to the one he'd just had with the husband. Then Dave reappeared as someone else said 'taxi for Hubbard 'Come on then Hubbie.' She called fondly to her partner. He had lapsed into a light stupor but was easily roused and led happily in to the taxi where he sat smiling regally through the window while Sue nipped back in for a word with Dave behind the bar. Alan was by now very much the worse for his evenings experience and a bit concussed but the intimate quality of Dave and Sues tête-à-tête still registered with him. He heard Dave say quite clearly that Sue should give him a bell later if she needed to. She gave him a tight little smile then their taxi bore her and her 'Hubbie' off into the night.

The stragglers sloped off too and Dave offered Alan and Nav a scotch to steady their nerves, Graham loitered hopefully, but neither of them was that bothered so after some desultory small talk about nothing in particular the three amigos bade their farewell and hit the road where subdued streetlamps picked out puddles of black water. Alan tried to get a Charlie Parker soundtrack going in his head to stop thinking about how he might feel tomorrow, or how to get to Cindy's house from here. The best he could do was to rekindle the flickering embers of Lena Martell. It was like psychic hiccups and put him in a bad mood. The whole evening had been a bad idea;

how often did anybody really, truly enjoy a piss up? The tripe that got talked, the anxiety of it all, the faux-naïf blokiness – you leave my bubble alone and I won't prick yours. Nothing truly takes the piss like alcohol or cannabis – who said that?

'Who said what mate'?

'Eh? Oh nothing Nav, my voices are coming back.'

'What's he on about now'? Asked Graham.

'Oh found your tongue again have you, now the furs stopped flying.' Barked Alan indignantly. 'Leaving us with that twat – fat bastard's a racist too, did you hear what he said to Nav'?

'Yes well, what else can you expect from an old social democrat. He took to you though didn't he? If you take my advice you'll leave well alone though, someone's giving Sue a seeing-to but it's not Nav.' Said Graham in the manner of a-man-in-the-know.

'Thanks for that.' Said Nav. 'And you're right Alan, he is an ignoramus – so who is shagging Sue Hubbard'?

Alan was staring blankly at the cars on the by-pass. 'Dave behind the bar.' He said to no one in particular.

'They must be getting careless if you've noticed.' Said Graham.

'Dave.' Said Nav. 'Behind the bar'?

'Dave who is normally to be found behind the bar.' Answered Graham. 'I imagine they reserve their tender moments for somewhere else.'

'The sleazy beggar.' Said Alan with feeling. 'He's told you all about it hasn't he? The smirker, the smooth talker, the

ASK ME NOW

loathsome lothario – he wants a slap.'

'Or a slip, as fearless Fred would say.' Said Graham to Navs amusement.

Alan was still peering out towards the traffic but had become very upset by all this. 'It's all so sordid, no good ever comes of it and what's it all for? We're not just monkeys in a pond, frogs up a tree.'

Nav shared a knowing look with Graham who put an arm round Alan and held him close. 'Come on champ, you've had a heavy bout tonight – I think Sue appreciated your shining armour though .. you never know, maybe …'

'Stop it Gray.' Said Alan as Nav chuckled.

'Listen chums it's been a night to remember, see you soon mate.' Said Nav to Alan as he separated from them and disappeared down Cherry Street.

Graham kept his arm round his mate and steered them off towards his house, though Alan didn't get this until they'd ambled companionably for ten minutes then they disengaged and Graham said thoughtfully that Fred Hubbard had always been a berk.

'Do you know him then'? Asked Alan.

'Used to, he was a charge nurse at St. Cuthberts for years then when they closed it he opened his own care home. It was a bit like Sweethaven without the sweetness – Tommy Pollard knows him from then, even Tommy considers him a tosspot. Talking of Tommy …'

'I'm sure he was trying to feel me up after he'd nutted me – he isn't running a care home now is he'?

'No, sold it years ago – now he can concentrate his talents on the council. He was on the Social Services committee for ages, I think that all ended in a great falling out, but now he's the chair for equal opportunities.'

'Sounds about right.'

'You've not heard the best yet.'

'What, is he punching his weight there too'?

'No, not about him, the latest stop on the redeployment roundabout …'

'Did you see that bloke over there – I'm sure he was laughing at me.'

'Yeah well, you have been up the town fighting.'

'But I wasn't fighting, I was only trying to help. I didn't notice you trying to do anything constructive.'

'You wouldn't. I was sitting on the sidelines having a good laugh – some of his wife's mates wanted you to offer him outside. I'd have come between you if it had gone that far.'

'You're a good mate.' Alan said with a straight face. 'But why are we off to your house, its miles out of my way'?

'You can stay over if you want – I'll make you a cup of tea.'

'Cheese on toast'?

'Yes.'

'You're on.' Alan then began to feel a bit queasy after saying this. He was also fed up with the street lamps dancing about

ASK ME NOW

but they soon reached a spot with less light and some gently rustling trees. He also noted an open gate and derelict shed beside a nice old green bench and a large white board setting out the municipal allotment regulations in Proustean detail. 'Can we have a bit sit Graham'?

'What is it with you and park benches? You don't have to sit on them just because they're there, they wear out you know.'

Alan thought this was very funny and sat down on green slats beneath a frame on which someone had carved 'Never Cut A Friend'. Graham joined him and they began to enjoy the sight of shifting seeding grass, an owl hooted then Alan leaned forward carefully to vomit at speed over a pile of manure. 'I'll scratch the cheese on toast then.' Said Graham. Alan stayed in position for a while then straightened himself with a sigh, wiped his eyes and walked over to the gate where he stood to be sick some more. Graham had taken a tactful interest in the shed. 'I think this ones open, come here.'
'Fuck off.' Said a third party from inside the shed. So they did.

'The good old days eh.' Said Graham when they were back on the public highway. 'A skin full, a barney and a chuck up on the way home.'

'Yes.' Said Alan. 'Why don't we do this more often'? He wanted to sit down in the warm and felt pleased to recognise the bail hostel at the top of Grahams street. He also realised that he didn't have his anti-depressants with him. 'Have you got any nice strong painkillers Graham? I'll have them with my tea if you don't mind.'

'I'll see what I've got.'

Once across the doorstep of his friend's semi Alan started to pick up and sank gratefully into one of Grahams nice armchairs. The place looked neat enough but a few stray details gave the game away; it had been cleaned recently but in that kind of rough and irregular way that Alan could see signified a special event. And there was the pile of newspapers set aside on the just-in-case principle that told the tale of a man living alone. It hadn't always been so at Grahams house but this was never talked about. He came in bearing steaming mugs in each hand and a box of Sainsburys Nurofen beneath his chin. At least I can run to a tray thought Alan. Graham got the gas fire going then they sat in mullish repose with the light off till Alan remembered something 'What were you telling me about Tommy Pollard on the way home? Something to do with someone else … somewhere …'

'Eh? Oh yes, Tommy's got a new job.'

'Why, where'?

'Have a guess.'

'Well after the debacle over the new computers I'd expect him to be counting the paper clips for Doris Bonkers over at Rookery Nook.'

'You're not far off actually. Doris got the bullet because of the overspend – which wasn't helped by Tommy's lash up with the computers – and he's got her old job.'

'You're kidding – Tommy's the new El Supremo'?

'Beat off some strong challengers according to my man on the inside.'

'You're what'? Scoffed Alan. 'Oh, don't tell me – Nav.'

'That's right. One of Mr. Pollards first tasks was to address the issues raised by Nav's new relationship – Nav had done right by her and gone to Tommy at an early stage – he was

ASK ME NOW

advised to use his common sense.'

They laughed long and loud at this then Alan took his tablet and opined that Tommy would go far in higher management. It was all very convivial and soon the play of the gas jets began to emphasize the warmth of the armchair, the affable bulk of his mate in the other one and the blessed absence of any of the cartoon horrors of his borderline bonkers potherings. He held a cushion tightly and thought of Cindy in her nightie.

The next thing he knew was a terrible stiffness in his neck and the shocking presence of a steel football where his bladder used to be. He had the room to himself and Graham had left the fire on, thin light limning the curtains told him it was morning so he pulled them and went for a piss. Grahams toilet was upstairs so he went thoughtfully into the garden where he made free use of some scrubby looking bushes by the back door. Back inside most of the ingredients for a hangover began to announce themselves as he put together a tea tray in the kitchen; grimy water tank head with internal drip, dirty cracked cup in his throat and a little man with a hammer running between these two sites scattering shards of shame and piss coloured porcelain. As yet though no Nigel or early morning jitters, they would no doubt call at their leisure.

He didn't feel too bad though considering and took a gentle rummage through Grahams shelves as he let the tea mash. He found an old Classics edition of Martin Chuzzlewit and flipped through to a bit he could remember; Nadgetts unbelievable denunciation of Jonas concerning his father and the pennorth of poison. He picked out an earlier passage at random – young Martin in America where he shows himself to be a bit of a drip and struggles on a road less travelled. Are people much different now he wondered? For all the gothic jiggery pokery the book told a familiar story; daft lad falls for fair maid who shows herself wise and tolerant of his whimsical ways, fate separates the lovers and many trials and teases must be borne before two hearts beat as one. He wondered how Cindy might look in a bonnet. This was good stuff though, it had been a while since he'd been able to sit and speculate early doors, he thought he might be able to see his way ahead. All that kerfuffle last night with Freddie Hubbard would soon settle into a fixed part of their blokey folklore to be brought out and puffed up over further pints. Just like that night Sean Pluck from the vulnerable adults team had borrowed a powered wheelchair for the night. The plan was to disclose the depths of discrimination in Ridsdale pubs against the disabled but Pluck had ended the evening in A&E after he'd lost control of the thing. The Police had been involved but he'd been let off with a bollocking once they got the story straight. Alan was sure his black eye would be seen in a similar light by Cindy, all very amusing and he was only trying to prop up old Fred.

He felt another pee coming on, and a poem too. It was ten to seven, as far as he knew Graham was due in at work so he went upstairs this time and flushed. Back by the fire he thought about his poem – something suggested by Freddie Hubbard that had returned him to a strange goings on in Corro. There had been a mass murderer on the street but nobody had noticed till he bumped off gormless Maxine, Ashley's partner, in Aunty Emily's parlour. He called his poem 'The Ballad Of Ashley Peacock' and the first lines came to him quickly; 'Uncle Fred Maxine's dead/ someone's hit her on the 'ead' but dried at this point. Was Wetherfield to him as daffodils were to Wordsworth? He noted that his headache felt much worse then the flush went again. Give me half a chance he thought, and all the old crap comes out again, Martin Chuzzlewit – Dickens would have got Dickies number all right. He'd been all ready to show Graham his poem, after he'd watered his hedge. Which was the greater insult?

He busied himself in the kitchen putting together some breakfast in a just-got-up sort of way, washed the pots afterwards then it was time for the off. Graham slipped him

ASK ME NOW

home on his way in and while they shared a chuckle or two en route, Alan knew he was on borrowed time and could feel his mood sinking. It was an effort to get out of the car when they got to his place. 'See you soon then champ.' Said Graham.

'I think I'll be retiring after that one mate.'

And then he was gone and Alan was alone again, outside his house at eight thirty in the morning. He closed the front door behind him and stood in the hall, outside the sealed off sounds of traffic seemed part of a space he'd lost his place in. Inside was a dead place, the hall was like every other hall in a divided house – something everyone used but which belonged to no one, quarry tiled and unclaimed. He picked through some letters left on a table beside Steve's door and found a boring brown envelope with his name on. He stuffed it in his jacket pocket and stayed put. It was possible that there was nobody else in the house. He sat on the bottom stair to listen, light flumed across from the dusty fan light over the lintel, a car door clapped outside. He started to weep. All that stuff last night, he thought, he hadn't felt right, not really, he was just playing along hoping it would come out in tune. He felt cold blank and scared, even Nigel Harding had abandoned him, for now. He looked at his watch; it told him it was eight thirty six. He hadn't felt this bad for weeks, what had happened to this mornings vagabond aesthete? Yesterday's salesman for the happier life? Everything inside him inside the empty house was on the edge of an awful shape that would turn to him soon. The big bad thing knew where he was, knew he was going nowhere, Alan would get seen to, he could depend on it. He forced himself to stand and climbed to his flat where he stood inside the doorway and tried to distract himself by thinking about a weird film he'd seen set in a boarding house of horrors where a baby explodes slowly in a corner and large maggots fall out of the ceiling. Then he couldn't keep it back any more, great caulking gobfuls of rage and despair came up and out of him. He managed to arrange himself on his couch with a cushion on his lap then bent himself forward to bawl into it. At one point he screamed with such force and depth that his shirt button popped like the Incredible Hulk. Better hulk than sulk he thought and sat back holding the cushion as the storm passed through him and his breathing steadied. His head throbbed but, for now, he felt freer and safer. He pulled the cushion closer and felt himself letting go in another way.

He came round again very slowly, managing to put himself back under again for a while along the way. He wasn't going to make it work a second time though and stood up straight. It was eleven forty so he went directly out of the room and down into the entrance hall where he patted his pockets, left the house and made for Londis where he bought a scotch egg and the Independent. Then he went to the park to spend an ordinary lunch hour in proximity to the other normal people who would be there doing the same thing. They amazed him sometimes; how they did it, kept their ends up, bought new clothes and drove their cars – walked down the street, went away on holiday. Graham had gone to work that morning and would do so again tomorrow after he'd been back home again. Cindy couldn't possibly like him anymore. He knew he used to do all that out there business but he didn't really believe it, it had all been an elaborate extended cover up for what was really happening. 'Shut the fuck up.' He said to nobody in particular and headed to a vacant bench by the duck pond where he opened out his paper with the air of a man as comfortable booking a holiday as he was mowing the lawn and tried to choose between a feature on Fathers and Sons by one bloke and why Lambeth's libraries were totemic of municipal blight by another. He looked in the obituaries (never heard of 'em) and settled on the sports pages where there was a feature by yet another bloke on the England managers' wife. The piece pontificated about how contemporary coverage trivialised a once wonderful game. The article was illustrated by a large snap of her looking glam in a nightclub. Set of berkes thought Alan, you'd get more

ASK ME NOW

sense from Dud Fivers on Neasden FC. He'd often fancied himself as a journalist so was all this easy cynicism envy dressed up as contempt? He ploughed through the Dominick Lawson column and decided it wasn't.

His head still hurt and the morning's horrors had shaken him badly but he had enough sense to see that last nights indulgences had played their part in that. It was stupid to drink so much but it shouldn't rub out the ground he'd made – just a few steps too far, that was all. He needed to be as right as he could be for Cindy when she got back from seeing her Mother at the weekend, she wouldn't be wanting tears before bedtime here too. He decided to phone her about six when her brother was likely to be out of the house. He knew that in families the eldest girl generally copped for it and it was so with Cindy's lot. He'd gained an impression of Adrian the brother over time; a drug damaged charmer with a girlfriend who housed him and worked full-time while he taught Tai Chi and wrote poems. Sounded like a right waister but where did they find these women to look after them? She and Cindy got on apparently. He unwrapped his lunch and felt the inside flopping about against his thumb and forefinger. Scotch eggs, especially big ones, often generated an erotic charge for him – tactile, pap like – but nothing was doing today. Sex could trouble him at the best of times, hinting at chaos and anger. He really liked going to bed with Cindy but he'd rather be undepressed, was there a connection? He thought he was thinking too much and bit into the thing, the first mouthful was mostly meat casing so he got that down and extracted the rest of the cold egg. It was slimy to touch and when he reached the yoke the contrast and the coldness put him off going any further so he swallowed what he could, stuffed the rest of the meat into his mouth and chucked the remaining bits for the birds.

It did take his mind off sex with Cindy, as he had to focus hard on how to swallow his mouthful without choking. He felt like Dizzy Gillespie after an intake of breath and hoped no one could see him. He gradually emptied his mouth in the normal way and found his attention settling on the whole half egg that had come to rest near one of the chestnut trees. The birds weren't bothered but someone else was, an ancient boxer with a brindled coat and semi-prolapsed backside had lumbered onto the scene. He was sniffing with an almost carnal engagement at the base of the tree, and then paused to gaze absently into the distance with the obvious intention of peeing against the trunk. The best he could manage though was to hoist one rear leg about six inches to rest against a knobbly growth and aim absently in the general direction intended. It was an extended performance as the dog caught site of the egg and took up a rough yoga pose, unable to move until he'd finished but unable to take his eye off the egg. Once he was all done he ambled stiffly across to sniff at his prize. Alan noticed that a plucky sparrow had signalled an interest but hopped to a respectful distance as the dog snorted, snuffled and rolled the egg with his flat nose. Then a man wearing a trilby appeared and asked 'Pugwash' what he'd found. The dog gave him a wonderful wall eyed look, which said in more than mere words 'a cold boiled egg you daft sod'. Then they were off. Alan moved off too in the general direction of Gas Street.

Now that he knew where he was going the journey didn't seem long at all and he soon found himself threading a path across the waste ground beyond the main road. He wasn't ready to get there yet and lingered awhile to take in the flora and fauna growing around the concrete and fly tippings. Weeds could be plants in the wrong place but this lot seemed suited to their setting; small ratty growths with dirty leaves like lettuce on a budget, tall toxic looking pampas grass swaying with intent. Even the grass was feral and unruly, the sort of stuff to clog a lawnmower and snag its axle. Alan liked this, the notion that streets and houses were kidding themselves if they thought they'd got topside of such unfenced anarchy. If you left your own back garden for long

ASK ME NOW

enough it would soon go native. He came across a smart new notice climbing clear of some bloated bin bags, it informed him that an exciting development of affordable town houses would soon be going up here. A straggling clump of seeded rose bay willow brushed his knee as if to say 'we'll see'. He left the spot to wander down the opposite side of the street to number twenty-five. After he'd been up then down, then up again he knew he would either turn into the passage or carry on back to his own side of the tracks. He turned into the passage then dithered by the back gate. He could see over the top; the kitchen light was on and Matt Monroe was singing 'let's get the party started here and now' He took heart from this and let himself into the yard and knocked at the back door. He heard sudden accelerating scampers and ardent panting from under the door, then it opened and Alan said. 'Oh, hello, er, I was in the park again and I thought I saw your dog. I was a bit worried in case he'd got out again.' She looked down at the dog then they both looked up at him. 'Yes, well obviously not ...' From behind the door Matt was giving a mercy killing to 'Blue Velvet' and Alan was feeling a proper Nellie then Beeswing planted his front legs up against Alan's cords and stretched against them.

'You'd better come in.' She said. 'He's inviting you.' She looked at him as they stood in the kitchen. 'You've been in the wars.'

'Yes, I had a slight accident.'

She looked at him again as if to say 'yes, you're just the type'. 'Well, as you can see his lordship hasn't been out on his rounds today. In fact since you brought him back I've minded that back gate. He knows as well, little beggar.' Beeswing looked at his visitor again and twitched his tail hopefully. He knows he thought, he remembered me. Then he remembered he'd smeared eggy fingers on his trousers in the park – his friend was only out for what he could get. His headache was on its way back and he was thirsty from the dehydration and damp meat, it had been a long morning. A second after the silence had become uncomfortable she moved across to fill a kettle and nodded towards the front room as she replaced it on its base and clicked the control down.

He moved through and sat down on a rocking chair, he was feeling anxious and a bit foolish. What on Earth was he doing here, what did he want from this woman? If this had been an official encounter they would both have known – generally speaking – what the form was, even returning the dog had given them enough of a frame for some kind of contact. Which had as he remembered it opened out into quite a bit of personal revalation from her. He really should have left it at that though, now that he'd come back for more where would it lead? He knew from long experience that a freshly poured cup of tea took about fifteen minutes before you could decently get it down then make your excuses. With fellow chaps you could always talk about their record collection. He spotted some vinyl in the corner resting against an ancient hi-fi and reached to flick through; apart from the oily songbird he'd heard on his way in there were some brass band compilations, The World Of Val Doonican (naturally) 'Bless This House' with Harry Secombe and Deep Purple 'In Concert'. Further flipping was curtailed as he heard her coming, the dog followed, as there were biscuits on the tray and jumped directly onto his lap from a standing start. He rubbed his chin near his nametag. 'It's a good name, you must have known he'd be a fast mover.'

'He's really Beeswing the second, the original was a racing greyhound – you wouldn't have caught him. What was your accident then'?

Alan had all ready decided that this woman had a fully functioning bullshit detector and that people like him caused her to put fresh batteries in. He played a straight bat. 'Someone bumped into me. I cracked the back of my head as

ASK ME NOW

well, it still hurts.'

'It didn't happen in the streets then'?

'No, not in the street. It was all a bit daft really, I shouldn't have got involved and left well alone.'

She poured their tea and considered this. 'Well maybe we should get a bit more involved sometimes. You're forever hearing folk say somebody should have done something whenever a funny do goes off.'

'Hmm, this was between man and wife though and he was pi .. the worse for drink.'

'Was he lifting a hand to her though'?

'I think he may have been about to – it was all a bit complicated really.'

'A man like that should be ashamed. Just big babies really, they generally turn the water works on when it's all over.'

Alan recalled Hubbard's demeanour in the taxi and his wife's well-practiced air of clearing up after him – more like mum and boy. No wonder she took her adult needs to Dave behind the bar. He wondered about Nina's late husband; he'd decided without any real thought on a quiet man, not given to much in the way of expressed emotion – taciturn but decent. A good provider. This seemed to him a clichéd impression based on nothing more than a muddled view that this was how that generation were, reinforced by a few crappy radio plays he'd caught recently. People of a certain age living quite respectable lives – stoical, unfussy, shaped by unbudgeable values formed in the days before 'the social'. So where did that Deep Purple album fit in? He knew he had a lot invested in the mythology – the Thora Hird history of England –

because it offered a grim certainty. If we were all struggling through the aftermath of some slowly unfurling fall from grace then all we had to do was try hard enough for as long as it took to be good enough, then we might get back, healed, restored and forgiven. His favourite poem, by Douglas Dunn seemed to be on about this. It was called 'The Worst Of All Loves' and was full of hallucinatory stuff about missed ways and separation ... 'what great thing have I lost ... ' He knew as well that his own small torment was to do with loss, the personal meaning he'd put on it. It might be hard to spot as it happened but you always fell for a reason

She'd been watching him. 'How does your head feel now'?

'Eh. Oh, it aches, my cheek aches as well – this bloke fell against me. He was a great lump.'

'Caught you off balance'?

'Yes.'

The warmth of the dog across his groin and the sunshine through the sash window made him want to sit there indefinitely as she pottered about the house. For as long as it took to be better – he wouldn't be any trouble. 'Are you not at work today'? She asked.

'No. I'm off at the moment – off sick.'

'Your accident'?

'No. Stress.'

'Ahh, lot of that about.'

'Yes. I've been pretty run down with it, a bit depressed actually.'

ASK ME NOW

'Lady up the street's bad with that. An Indian chap comes to see her, nice mind.'

He rubbed the dog softly behind an ear, Beeswing snorted softly and stretched. Alan had begun to feel like stretching himself so when she left the room he put the dog down. He simply stretched again and padded through to the kitchen where the nametag chinked against his water bowl. Alan's own drink was about ready for knocking back in one go but he felt like leaving it just for now. He could hear the stairs leading up from the kitchen creaking, being a salaried nosey parker suited his temperament and he speculated about what was happening or about to in a detached manner he was familiar with. She came down with a shoe box put it on the floor between his rocker and her Shackletons prop-me-up, took out an old print and placed carefully on the mantelpiece against her carriage clock. 'Morecambe 1955.' She said and sat to see it better. The picture showed a holiday couple on the promenade – the standardised composition and formal smiles told the viewer that it had been caught by the kind of seaside photographer who plied his trade then. Couples were happy to buy them and they were often the only other record apart from the wedding album of partners together. What struck Alan as well was that such pictures were unusual in that the subjects were snapped being themselves outside their normal circle. Nobody else knew they were there, they could be anyone. This particular image showed a handsome pair in their twenties; he was carrying a canvas beach bag, she had an arm through his and there was plenty of life just going on in the background – an old man was pushing a cart across the road a bus leaned into the kerb, further back out of focus faces crowded like frogspawn.

'We'd just had a big row then flash bang wallop comes along – you wouldn't know from looking would you'?

Alan had to smile. 'No, did you row again after'?

'No but I remember that when the thing came in the post it reminded him and we had another set to. I can't remember for the life of me what it was all about though. Anyhow, that's him in his prime God bless him, he could be a moody beggar though.'

Alan didn't have a clue where this was going or what to say so he looked carefully at the picture. He was struck by how smart they looked, the man was wearing a white cotton shirt of the type Alan liked to buy from Oxfam, except this one would have been carefully saved up for not dressed down to. He was beginning to see the picture as an iconic image; two people walking into the unknown before the photographer, looking ahead. 'You both look really smart.'

'It was our first time away together.'

'Was it – would that have been your honeymoon'?

She shook her head slightly. 'No, we didn't get married till the following year.'

Right, so, thought Alan. So much for reveries of ration book restraint, this might be more information than he could accommodate, it jarred with what he thought he knew or what she could tell him.

'You're shocked. We weren't so different then – we knew we'd marry so what did it matter? People had done all kinds of things during the war round here.' She took down the print and picked about in the box for another. He wondered what was coming next, the Salford Swingers of 1961? He was relieved to see a dog eared snap of a lean looking greyhound wearing a ribbon surrounded by grinning blokes in caps. He recognised the man from the earlier picture, he was grinning again but this time with more conviction.

ASK ME NOW

'He looks as if he's enjoying himself there.'

'Who'? She said. 'The dog'? No, he was happy enough that day.'

Alan decided to push his luck. 'You said he was moody sometimes.'

'They both were but at least the dog couldn't speak .. anyway the dog track's been built over and …'

'I'm sorry, I didn't mean to …'

'No, it's all right, he generally pulled round – he was fine then. We found out later on that his Father had taken ill a time or two when Bob was little. He couldn't remember much about his Dad and he fell under a bus when Bob was quite young. Their Mother told me that he'd been in St. Cuthbert's when Bob was a baby. It was a shame for him never having much of his Dad. Loved his own kids mind, dead soft with our Phillip. Funny thing was – he seemed to go in on himself when Phillip was a baby, I found him crying one time up the yard – he got better though.'

Christ, thought Alan, he'd have had to. 'I'm just coming through a difficult time myself – I've been badly depressed really.'

'I thought you might be.'

The rest of his afternoon on Gas Street drifted along in a tea rinsed reverie. She mashed another pot, told him about the Deep Purple album ('our Phil's, used to drive his Dad mad') and even put it on for him leaving him with the dog to listen to it while she 'did' upstairs. Early seventies pomp rock wasn't really his cup of tea but the day had taken such a left turn that it all seemed to fit. He'd taken his leave around four thirty; Beeswing had watched him through the front window. On his way across the wildness he felt torn by what he'd done. Had the afternoon been a slice of the better life where people took a proper interest in each other, where we all moved together through the same air? Or had he sponged his way into her front room, leaving her feeling pissed off? She hadn't seemed that way, a bit bemused maybe but it had been all right he reckoned. He should have offered to walk the dog though. The tall grass whispered in his wake not to tell the trees about it.

By the time he was back in his hallway he was remembering a joke Nav had told him last night. It would do for Cindy when he phoned her. He braved the stairs and addressed his door with a brazen air slotting in the key first time then plumping up his cushions. The fridge buzzed on, someone else in the building made the water move in the antique plumbing with a soothing woosh then he got the fire on and made himself comfortable with his mobile. As the crow flew there wasn't too much distance involved but Alan had felt pretty edgy whenever he'd talked to Cindy on the phone recently, as he tapped in her Mothers number he told himself this was to be expected. Almost immediately a reedy female voice said 'yes'. 'Oh hallo, it's Alan Duright here. Is it possible to have a word with Cindy'?

Reception grew muffled but he heard a less forthright version of the same voice calling for 'Cynthia'. He smiled at this then picked up some miscellaneous shufflings and an intake of breath.

'Hi.' She said brightly. 'How are you'?

'Not bad really, an interesting couple of days one way and another. How about you'?

He heard her laugh softly. 'I suppose I could say the same really, anyway, I think I'll be able to get back before the week

ASK ME NOW

end.'

'Good, good.' He said. 'Is your Mum picking up then'?

'Not exactly but I finally managed to get someone out from the adult care management team yesterday so it looks like things should be clicking into gear soon.'

'How did she take it'?

'Oh all right. She wore her woollen hat throughout, smiled at the social worker no matter what he said and the place stank of burned chicken. I think he went away with the right idea.'

'Burnt chicken'?

'Yes, last nights tea. I was bored stiff so I went for a walk, you can get down to the river from here but I got lost so I was very late getting back. Mum was supposed to be doing the tea but I could smell it from the bottom of the street. God knows why she hadn't smelled it, perhaps she had. I didn't feel like chicken that night.'

'That reminds me of something Nav said – how do you turn a duck into a soul singer'?

'What'?

'Stick it in the oven till its bill withers.'

'When did you see Nav'? She asked neutrally.

'Last night. Graham and I went for a pint and bumped into him.'

'Oh right, yes I think you'd told me you were going. Anything interesting.'?

'Nah, not really. Oh I heard about Tommy Pollard – bit of a turn up there'?

'Do you think so? Anyway, good luck to him.' She didn't sound much bothered. 'Yes I won't be a minute. Sorry Alan, I might have to cut this short.' He could hear Mrs. Watson wittering in the background about something not working right. 'I'll have to go – I'm looking forward to seeing you soon, I'll give you a call when I get back.'

'Yeah, me too.'

Before the line went dead he caught some more of her old Mums importunings and wondered what on earth they expected Cindy to do, the whole lot of them seemed to want her to prop them up. He watched the fire for a bit then put the tele on. The next thing he knew was that Steve McDonald was a lying bastard but before he could understand why two women in blue candlewick dressing gowns began brawling in the street. He'd slept all through 'Emmerdale' and missed most of 'Corro.'
DON'T LET ME BE MISUNDERSTOOD

'Right, best foot forward, one day at a time. I'll be in about eleven but I can't remember if I signed out on Friday so could you check the board for me.'?

'Yeah of course – see you in a bit then.'

Cindy softened the mood of brittle gaiety with a heartfelt hug by the dustbin and told Alan how nice he looked in the brand new corduroy jacket she'd helped him buy on Saturday (soft brown shortie with split rear). 'I love you Cynthia.' He said. She gave him another hug then he toddled off to his car feeling like young Master Davey, off to see the world.

Her house was nearer to Northfield than his flat but the

ASK ME NOW

journey in took longer due to a combination of road works, clogged by-pass and his unfamiliarity with the route. He soon found himself stuck at the top of a street of scruffy Edwardian villas behind some grumbling vehicles. He put on his chosen tape of the week; Duke Ellington's early forties recordings – every one a winner with just the right cocktail of poignancy and punch to sustain the comeback kid. As the band sashayed through 'Jack The Bear' he caught sight of movement in a window of the house over to his left. A tiny hand was struggling to pull open a closed curtain; it waived briefly then disappeared allowing the curtain to fall across then a young woman with a buggy backed out of the front door and looked over again at the window laughing. She stood briefly with the buggy on the street then called something into the house through the open door and stood watching the window. After a while she closed the door and went up the street, looking back once. As soon as she'd passed out of site the hand reappeared and waived again. Then the traffic began to shift and he remembered Cindy's hug and how much he meant what he'd said. He started to fill up but it was all right, she'd cried a lot recently, mostly about her old mum but she'd told him some other things too. One of her uncles had played as a semi-professional for Bury and probably had depression; she'd seen him jump off the roof once when she was small. He'd told her it was part of their special training but even as a child she could tell he was facing the wrong way.

By now the Ellington band was stomping out 'Cottontail' and the wonderful world of Northfield CMHT could be seen on the horizon. He switched off the music as the gaudy swoon of 'All Too Soon' announced itself. The traffic began to build up as soon as he entered the hospital complex and unofficial overspills slowed up his route to the car park proper. He drove through slowly stopping twice for puzzled old folks still vague from surgery, brandishing dull grey walking aids as they rattled around the place. He couldn't help wondering if someone was looking after them. He carried on past the mortuary and dog crap corner then in through the barrier. Someone was leaving a space on the way out so he slid straight in, unclipped, got out and took one small step then stopped to look at the building. The first thing he spotted was Nav's face in profile at a window talking to someone behind him. Nav turned to face whoever it was, even from behind Alan could tell he was chuckling. He made for the entrance where he met Beth Wallace on her way out. She stopped and had a friendly chat as she rolled up a cigarette. 'What have they got you on.'? She asked and when he told her said. 'Excellent, that's what I would have prescribed – you'll do all right on that. Come for a chat later if you like.' Then she disappeared round the back of the car park.

He needed things to be as they were and in a world of many changes Dr. Wallace stood for certainty and settled ways, there was even something comforting about her cigarettes, he hoped she'd never give up. Becky on reception was in the middle of a phone call but nodded to him as he passed a couple of glum looking out patients. Once he was through to the office area he felt his stomach turn over so he went directly to the toilet and sat for five minutes. At one point two voices he couldn't place came in and talked about waiting lists as they peed. Then someone else clacked the door shut on the adjacent cubicle and undid their trousers, the clasp on the belt hit the floor and Alan held his hands to his head in a partial attempt to block it all out. His mystery guest eventually went and Alan was cross enough to act. He washed his hands and strode off to his office. He encountered Val Meating on the way. 'Ah Alan, there you are. Becky said you were in.'

'Yes.' He said.

'Well, look, if I give you some time to catch up with your e-mails and generally get your feet back under we can get together about eleven okay? Come straight across I should be free by then.'

ASK ME NOW

'Yes, fine – see you in a bit.'

A new coat was hanging up on Grahams peg, a stylish blouson type so was it Grahams? His colleague's desk looked as if it had been used that morning but there was no sign of him. He went across to his own which was pretty much as he remembered it from the day Cindy had set about him with the hard backed book. His guts trembled again so he made himself boot up his computer and do something. There was a lot of stuff to be getting on with in his tray involving diary work and thinking ahead, by the time Graham appeared he was surprised by how quickly he'd fallen back into role; hard-pressed social worker setting about his papers before the days main business could begin.

'Ah, they've let you out then – the police I mean, last I heard Fred Hubbard was arguing for an ASBO.'

'Eh.? Oh I'm surprised you can remember much of all that. Have you been back recently.'?

'No, it's not the same when you're not there.'

'Yes, well, is there much I need to know, I'm seeing Ina later on this morning.'?

'She'll fill you in. I can't think there's that much.'

'You've got a new jacket.'

'There is that ... also, you might need to know about the Stanley Clarke situation.'

'The what.'?

'You remember, about four years ago it must have been.

Mike Pearson

Caused no end of trouble at the time but it was all thought to have been put to bed, a bit like old Stan. Now the family are kicking up again and there's a feeling the local press might take an interest so Ina's in a right tizz about it. Anyway, I'm off see you later champ.'

And he was off, in his Ken Barlow look-a-likee smart-cas. zip up with a spring in his step. Alan wondered if this was new too and why? Now that he came to think about it the Stanley Clarke thing did ring a distant bell, a harsh sound heralding a roll call of shame glossed over. Something that definitely didn't ring right, to do with the mental health act and idiosyncratic practice from an esteemed colleague who'd been placed with them for 'approved social worker' training having practiced for several years without his full ticket and who had a fund of colourful stories. Larry was it? He'd ask Val later. He returned to his e-mails with a will, reading each one carefully even though most were the kind of irrelevant internal broadcasts public services sustained themselves with; he'd been invited three weeks ago to an area wide social care forum to ruminate upon how to 'preserve the social work ethos'. He typed in formaldehyde on the return but didn't send it. County Supplies had a new telephone number and Terry Towlyn would be on leave for most of June. Then an easily overlooked item caught his attention; a brief note from Sweethaven asking him to contact them about Bob Prince. It was from last month so he thought that what ever it was must have been seen to by now. He jotted down another thing to be checked with his line manager and continued with his work, adding to the list as he progressed. By ten twenty he felt he'd earned himself a coffee and looked for his Count Basie mug but the Count had stepped out and he had to make do with a drab looking vessel from Wilkos' in pea green with the price (59p.) still stuck underneath. Trinny and Susannah smiled mockingly from the coffee jar; there was no milk either.

On his way to the kitchen he bumped into Angie Boona from workforce development. 'Alan, I've been trying to get hold of you for ages – I think it would be a good idea to start a psycho-social interest group and you were one of my first choices. Would you be interested.'?

He thought about this, it could be called PSSIT. 'Yeah, sounds good, anyone else interested.'?

'Smashing, I'll e-mail you when I know more and yes, Nav. Have you seen him, he's another one I keep missing.'?

'I spotted him at a window when I came in.'

'Probably watching out for me.'

'Well if I see him I'll tell him you're after him.'

She smiled blandly at him and made for one of the offices where Nav could usually be found. Perhaps she wanted to tap his knowledge of links with carers, get him to form a support scheme. There seemed to be so much going on around him and everybody else looked to be so much a part of it all, how did they do it? He felt panicky again then Mr. Wilson from Estates came out of the kitchen and sited a stern metal-framed sign by the door. 'Can I just pop in for some milk.'? He asked.

'I don't rightly know.' Answered Mr. Wilson. 'Might have to decommission this part of the building.'

'What do you mean, what's happened.'?

'Been a nasty spillage, we need to seal off the danger zone for the rest of the morning and do a full risk assessment before I can tell you any more, could be a long job. I'm down on numbers you know.'

How many people does it take to …thought Alan, couldn't

someone just dab it up? 'Oh I see, couldn't somebody just pass me a carton.'?

Mr. Wilson, a fifty something pedant in a brown overall and trouble shooter for hospital hazards, poked his head back into the danger zone to ask 'Junior' if he could get the gentleman some milk. Alan reflected that it must be a mighty spillage if two men were stretched like this then a black hand appeared in the no-mans land between door frame and Mr. Wilson holding a fresh carton of milk. Mr. Wilson looked with due gravity at the milk then Alan and indicated that he was authorised to reach across and take it. Which he did then took his prize back to his billet where he decided to stay for as long as he could. He could make a couple of phone calls before dinner time, maybe get out to Sweethaven for a while, he generally found it restful over there. He switched on the kettle by the computer. 'Good, lets have a drink first.' Said Val from across the corridor.

'Do you remember that old mental welfare guy we had here about five years ago, had to come and get his hand in before re-training. Larry somebody wasn't it.'?
'Barry Weatherall.' She said sharply. 'Why what's he done now.'?

'I don't know – nothing I should think, it was just something Graham said.' Alan put down their drinks and seated himself by the new computer.

'His name's come up again because of a trail of havoc the gormless Herbert left in his wake back then. He took early retirement of course and works in the private sector now on behalf of poor souls who've been handled roughly by the system and need a voice.' This was expressed in a tone of sardonic nay-saying he'd never heard from her. 'Honestly.' She continued. 'I could wring his stupid neck.'

'Barry Weatheralls.'?

ASK ME NOW

'Yes. I'm going to have to see him you know, now this bloody Stanley business has come back to life.'

Yes, he thought, I knew there was something, something to not talk about. 'Cindy said she'd be in later on. What is this carry on in the kitchen.'?

'I don't know aren't Estates sorting it out? Stanley Clarke was minding his own business one fine Wednesday morning in Dr. Laubrocks waiting room in 1999 or thereabouts.' Alan decided to let it come and pick the bones out once she'd finished.'He'd only gone along to have his holiday jabs or something; by mid-afternoon he'd been detained at St. Cuthberts under the mental health act by brother Weatherall who told him his section would run without limit. Then it all started to unravel once he saw fit to contact the nearest relative ... who turned out to be?'

'Who.'?

'Colin Clarke, the son. Colin Clarke the investigative reporter, the self appointed hammer of incompetence in the social services.'

The penny dropped. 'Oh him. Didn't he do that expose on Police overtime.'

'Yes, him. They weren't claiming any. More to the point, he took a keen interest in his Fathers situation and had put together a story about the whole thing till Stanley – who turned out to be an absolute saint – talked him out of publishing it. It was a rocky ride though I don't mind telling you ... well, now Stanley's died and the son has been on to the director. Terry Towlyn's fallen over on holiday - it's therefore landed on my desk. Colin Clarke wants to meet.'

'So, just before my time, one day in 1999, this bloke was sectioned out of the blue by Barry Weatherall – why, was he causing concern down at the surgery?'

'No, he was reading the Daily Mirror.'

'So ... what happened?'

At this point he caught Cindy's voice beyond then a knock on the half-open door. 'Hi, hi Alan, something's cracking off with one of Dr. Roses' patients, I'm just off down there while they're all about.'
'Right.' Said Val.' Give me a call if you need to.' Cindy shut the door fully on her way out and Val turned back to Alan. 'So, let's get back up to speed with yourself, there've been one or two events on your caseload – you know about Bob Prince?'

'No but there was something in my box from Teddy.'

'Yes well, Mr. Prince died, apparently quite peacefully in his sleep, but it was a bit of a mystery how it happened. They eventually tracked it down to some sort of tiny cardiac complication no one could have known about. The daughter was heartbroken but I gather she's had some effective support from Nav.'

'Not a bad way to go I suppose.'

'No and his prognosis was dire with him dementing so young – they were spared that. I'm coming to see Nav in a new light you know.'

Keep your eyes peeled, thought Alan. 'Much else I should know about?'

'I gather that Mr. Clayton's made a big hit with social inclusion – he suggested they start a dog walking group, gets an old mate from the council kennels to bring three or four down for some exercise and off they go. They've all ready re-homed one. I went along with Cal one week but some of those rescue dogs are very nervy ....'

'A bit like some of the rescue people.'

'Yes I suppose so. There were a couple of new cases you'd picked up before you went off, I think you'd only just assessed them, needed to be farmed out again. Oh and nutty old Mr. Norris locked himself in again and started posting letters out through his front door every day. Two weeks before anyone noticed – most of them were addressed to Princes Fergie of Stretford but the more recent ones were to Whispering Willie, who turns out to be you. We managed to get topside of him without admitting but I think he'd like to see you, have a word with Roger from Rehab. The people you were seeing for supportive counselling have either got worse or better but I don't think any of them have come to my attention – I guess you'll chase them up.'

This last bit seemed to sum up a neat critique of the 'therapeutic' work he and some of his colleagues fancied they were doing; people either got better or they didn't and it might or might not have something to do with whatever you said to each other. At any rate Bill Clayton was on the mend and he ought to give himself some credit for that, oughtn't he? 'Bill Claytons pups parade sounds good.'

'Yes but you wouldn't believe the palaver we had – dangerous dogs act, Councillor Bishop putting his oar in, were people clued up about rabies? Oh and that precious twit from psychology asking was it fair to encourage a level of intimacy which could be cruelly snatched back, and this was in relation to the dogs. I mean honestly, what's it coming to when the separation anxiety of a West Highland terrier comes before the pleasure of some lonely old men?'

He felt there was nothing he could add and steered them towards the topic of an appropriate workload. Val had mapped out a limited three-day week then back up to full power by late summer – had he much holiday to take? – so he could play himself back in gradually. There was a pause while she searched for some elusive form or other and he sensed anxiety in the air. 'Alan, that business I was telling you about before …'

'That business with Stanley Park and the Daily Star.'

'Stanley Clarke, and it was the Mirror – the Daily Star we might have got away with. No, our old friend Barry Weatherall sectioned the wrong man but it was all supposed to have been squared off and forgotten about, well now it's re-surfaced and I think we need a level headed, experienced social worker to do some trouble shooting. You know, familiarise yourself with the circumstances, work closely with the family, oil on troubled waters or even a bridge over. It could be very interesting and you're ideally placed – Graham and Cindy have quite a bit on at the moment.'

Alan felt a bit miffed at that bit but there was nothing he could say. 'You say the son is some sort of big cheese in the papers, is he after some big why-oh-why type of story? Can we stop it? Sounds like a proper balls up to me – you say they never sued or anything at the time.'

'No and that's where we've some elbowroom. Mr. Clarke senior was remarkably forgiving at the time; knew the difficulties we faced, these things happen etcetera'

'Well that suggests he might not have been all there after all. What's this Barry like?'

'Well I dare say anyone looking into this now would need to go and see him, do some discreet digging. It would be like

ASK ME NOW

that John LeCarre book – 'Tinker Tailor Social Worker'. Can you see yourself as George Smiley Alan?'

He thought about as likely as you being taken for Carol Smiley. Did he have a choice and would it involve furtive flights to Eastern Europe? 'The family live locally you say?'

'There's the daughter and the son comes up to visit – Stanley's widow's in care at that private place near Bacup, 'Lavender Mists' is it? It should be straightforward enough to see the main players and you'd be doing the service a big favour.'

'Whatever the outcome?'

'Oh yes, we're not in the business of buying them off besides it's Barry's head on the line.'

'Fair enough, have we got plenty of documentation to hand?'

'Excellent, yes there's a box with all our stuff in – letters between the director and Colin Clarke and sundry papers, I'll get it to you today.' Then the phone went and Alan worked out that it was Cindy calling from the Rio Grande with news of what was cracking off. 'Oh dear.' Said Val. 'Not the telegraph.' He gathered up the pots and left.

He could see why Graham was amused by all this but it was beginning to appeal to him, he was always more likely to be Alec Guinness than Brad Pitt and he was still a way off taking on any difficult work just yet. It was getting on for noon so he gave himself an early lunch and took a brisk walk up to town where he bought his Indie. from Smiths and his dinner from PastiesRUs (cheese and onion though he could have had apple and custard if the fancy had taken him). He found an empty bench by the bus station but he was too tense to enjoy his hot lunch and trying to read the paper at the same time only made him more so. He told himself this was normal and especially so for him that it would disperse sometime between two and three, helped on its way by purposeful activity. Just another bit of the rough, he'd get out if he just kept chipping away. Or reshape the shit in his head and push it around to a place where it wouldn't bother him so much. These thoughts returned him to Howard Green, Greenie of the salty wit and reckless chutzpah, his mentor and role model for life's challenges.

He remembered when a notorious playground bruiser had asked 'soft Alan' if he was taking the piss, Howard had asked in a general sense whether you could take the piss out of shit as he passed. Even though the thug hadn't really grasped his pals' use of irony he did get a firm grasp of Howard's neck and a legendary roughhouse for three soon kicked off. Alan also remembered that the fight and subsequent detention had brought the three of them together for some time after and done wonders for his own street credibility; such, such were the joys of his schooldays at Spennymoor Road Secondary. He couldn't be sure if this had a message for him now but it helped lift his mood slightly. He put down the rest of his pasty and caught up with the latest 'boardroom brouhaha' at Newcastle United – 'boo boys back boss' according to a fans spokesman. He got off his backside and walked about in the light. Let it go, he thought, up and out through the top of your head to float off into space like Mr. Dick with his kite of dull cares.

The only other luncher he could see was a young man with a can of pop and a mars bar so he took himself off for a walk around Wilkos. The place was full of dawdling shoppers and the panic he began to feel took him back to his worst days when being home was awful but going out was worse. He bought some batteries for his cassette player and did some deep breathing in the checkout queue, the surly girl at the till gave him a mucky look but he still felt better for it and took the scenic route back to work This took him by an area of reclaimed industrial land tarted up with some naff sculptures,

ASK ME NOW

wrought iron seats and a hard wearing children's play ground. He circumnavigated the place a couple of times but thought he'd better not hang around the playground doing his deep breathing. The first morning over with then, he looked forward to seeing Cindy after work. He'd been glad to feel he was looking after her a bit the other day when she'd got upset over her Mum. She'd told him all about it at length, and that hadn't bothered him either. He couldn't see her car when he got back to work.

Back in his office he put the batteries into his cassette player and eyed up the sturdy box that had appeared by his desk. It looked to be half full with at least one large multi-disciplinary file and a couple of smaller buff folders. This was the hard copy documentation of an unknown corner of the Stanley Clarke affair, not in the same league as Watergate but not bad to be going on with. As Chet Baker crooned softly in the background Alan began to learn the appalling story of how a sane and blameless member of the public had been forcibly detained under the mental health act. After he'd sorted the material into a rough and ready order he began noting a few broad themes. The main plank in the services defence was that social worker Weatherall had acted in good faith and, apart from admitting the wrong man, had followed procedures, guidance and local codes of practice and could therefore be defended by the department. Any further reckoning would therefore have to come via the family lodging complaints and, incredibly, this hadn't happened largely due to Stanley's amazing levels of tolerance and understanding. The file had been shamelessly retouched in a way the Kremlin might have blushed at so unless you knew what you were looking for you would struggle to find it.

The larger picture showed itself in the other folders holding the correspondence with the family, hospital managers and the GP's practice manager. Also, some arse-creeping communication to the nearest relative of the person

Mike Pearson

Weatherall should have been seeing that day, a Sidney Smith who had eventually presented himself later on at Accident and Emergency with detailed plans for his brother-in-laws abduction. He had been taken uncomplainingly up to the admission ward for assessment but the brother-in-law had visited the next day and taken him home on the basis that 'he was always saying that.' The most revealing document was a copy of the minutes for Barry Weatheralls informal disciplinary meeting with the then director, Bob Burns, and Val Meating; here the facts were to be seen in all their jaw dropping diversity.

Barry had been alerted to the need for an urgent assessment at the Parkside practice where a disturbed patient had been seen staring at 'the mirror' and saying that someone had 'had it now' then giggling in a high pitched and menacing manner. Barry had felt the need to 'act swiftly' as 'the risk profile was quite evident' and had thus set out for the surgery with the intention of coordinating events as they unfolded from there. Things took a left turn at this point when he confused the Parkside practice with the Southside surgery where he came upon Stanley Clarke chuckling to himself over a story in his newspaper. Apparently concerning the incumbent England managers job following a bad result on their summer tour of Papua and New Guinea – 'he's had it now' Stanley had said quietly to himself, but Barry heard him and that was enough. He had somehow talked Stanley into his car, telling him he was off to 'somewhere were he'd be properly looked after' and the rest seemed to flow frighteningly smoothly from this point. He knew himself how the momentum for an admission built itself from within the assessment process once the approved social worker decided what was going to happen. He wondered how the health trust would view the admitting doctor but really the patient would have had very little room for manoeuvre by this point and Stanley's seeming passivity would have worked against him because you could generally persuade yourself this showed insight and you were therefore correct to admit them. If they cut up rough of course that

ASK ME NOW

meant the converse but you were still doing the right thing banging them up. In reality Stanley had been to see his doc. about his arthritic hip and talk about his holiday jabs. He'd taken too many painkillers with his Wincarnis and was consequently quite amenable to Barry's 'offer of help' or, as Barry interpreted it 'inappropriately elated, possibly manic and no doubt unpredictable – possibly dangerous.' Alan read on then closed the file, someone had pencilled 'When Barry Met Stanley' on it and that seemed to be how it had come to be seen after the fuss and carry on began to lie down.

Now that it had found its legs again Alan puzzled afresh as to why on earth the family had stayed quiet. Maybe there had been some shame over the pills and booze also, Barry did have a nice way with him people said – no force had been used and he'd come quietly, which could explain Barry's failure to interview him in a suitable manner, let alone check names, surgeries or streets. Thank goodness he'd gone to the right hospital, it might have been worse. Well now it was and if he was any judge the department was in for a right rollocking. Val was obviously hoping for some damage limitation so he'd best make sure he got the right man when he met the family. He sorted through the rest of the stuff licking his thumb and forefinger just like George Smiley, enjoying himself more as he went along. There wasn't much else to come though apart from his discovery that the admitting doctor was called Todgers, but this turned out to be more slap dash work from Barry, the SHO had been a Dr. Rodgers – T. for Ted. 'You couldn't make it up could you?' Said Graham when he returned. 'Not if you were in your right mind.'

'That's the point though isn't it. That soft beggar decides he's got his man and everyone goes along with it. It's frightening and he'd been around for years, experienced and all – some sort of wise acre wasn't he?'

'I wouldn't go that far, felt to be pretty sound in his day. They shouldn't have tried to train him up really, just let him lapse then place him somewhere out of harms way.'

'It's amazing though Graham, they really thought it would all fade away.'

'Everyone thought it had, it took more than one mention of Colin Clarke getting in touch before it clicked with Ina. And now she wants you to help her shovel the brown stuff.'

'Well ... I'm not sure it's quite like that.'

'You'd better be sure with this one Dickie, no margin for error here.'

It being four twenty they shared a pot of tea and discussed the latest goings on at the Labour group. Sue Hubbard had moved in with Dave behind the bar but as the beer had gone off since then everyone was trying to reunite her and Fred. Nav had taken Briony away for a weekend in Southport and the monthly talk was due to be given that night in the upstairs function room by Shay Willis. It would concern itself with some lesser known byways of the local trades councils noble history, under the heading of 'Those Golden Threads' he promised to draw together a rich historical cloth – did Alan fancy coming along? He'd think about it. Graham washed the pots while he set the office to rights for the next day. On his way out Alan noticed a man by the entrance to the car park cleaning the lens of a camera but thought nothing of it.

He drove to Cindy's house and felt a spasm of anxiety when he saw her kitchen light on. 'Hi.' She said as he let himself in. 'How did it go?'

'Okay, not bad really. How'd it go for you, you got lumbered with something didn't you?'

ASK ME NOW

'Oh much ado about nothing.' She moved across to hold him. 'So that's the worst bit over with – well done.' He immediately felt better and prolonged their embrace so he could savour her familiar smell and warm his hands on her. He sensed her responding and they shared a speculative snog till the micro-waive pinged. 'Baked spuds.' She announced as they disengaged. 'What do you fancy with them?'

He toyed with the idea of saying something teasingly suggestive but thought better of it. 'Got any of those nice sardines from Sainsbury's?'

'Mmm ... you sit down while I slap it together.'

This is very nice, he thought, one spud at a time though. He appreciated that Cindy's kitchen coquetry was very much a feature and served to undermine a cultural role she appeared to enjoy while being opposed to in principle. It was all the same to him, a chaps tea tasting much the same whether it was served with gusto or irony. It mattered to her though and he'd begun to wonder if there were other areas of their life together, which stirred up ambivalence. The other day she'd popped out somewhere and suggested he might take a look at her guttering while she was gone. It had come across in her playful wife addressing a slothful husband manner but he sensed there might be more to it. Anyway, he'd walked all around the property looking carefully at the pipes without seeing anything obviously out of place. When he reported this she took it well enough and nothing more was said. There was no alternative way to maintain the plumbing or love someone, and this was the real thing all right. During his convalescence there had been times when the depth of his affection and regard for her had brought a lump to his throat, now of course it was bringing about a lump somewhere else but that wasn't really the point. Cindy had been there for him and now he was determined to do the same for her 'How did your Mother get on at the hospital today?' He asked as she dealt with her last wodge of rocket salad and potato.

'Oh I don't know, I'd have to phone to find out.' She replied flatly. 'I was a bad girl not to take the day off to go over with her but they'll have to start sorting things out for themselves over there – I'm not going back to look after them all.'

'Did Age Concern come up trumps?'

'That was my understanding, anyway, do I ring now and miss The Archers or later and forego Corrie.' Wetherfield won out over Ambridge where nothing much was happening anyway; Kenton had been to a night club in Felpersham and Clarrie had taken in a stray cat. The general view was that no good would come from either venture. Alan did the washing up and locked horns with Cindy's new percolator as she played the dutiful daughter. By twenty past seven she was off the phone and flopped down in the armchair by herself. 'I'll have to go over again this weekend, she's in a right state. I'll need to phone the social worker too – and my fucking brother will have to get his arse into gear.'

Alan had kept her coffee warm and passed it across to her. 'Thanks.' She said. 'Why can't I have a brother like Ken Barlow ... or Dev. even.?'

'What's he like then?'

'Steve McDonald without the sense of responsibility.' Soon enough the genuine article appeared and they watched the evening's episode in silence. Cindy laughed briefly when Hayley had to use Roy's favourite cardic to douse a fiery chip pan but gave nothing of her feelings away otherwise. 'Do you mind if we have the telly off?' She asked when the credits came up.

'Yeah sure.' He said and got up to switch it off.

ASK ME NOW

'Thanks.' She said and then sat quietly for about ten minutes. 'I can't do it.' She said eventually.

'Can't do what Cindy?'

'Look after my Mother. I feel terrible about it but it's not the answer, not for anyone.'

'Is that the message you're getting?'
'One way or another. Last time I was over she was laying it on thick 'what's going to happen to me you can sort things out?' – the rest of them are just standing about waiting for me to give in. I think the social workers got the picture though but lets face it we both know it would suit them as well if I did the decent thing.'

'Would it suit you though? That's the point and is it realistic anyway – to take it on I mean? It sounds as if she's becoming quite confused, maybe marking out a boundary will make something happen with the local services. They've got your brothers number if something happens haven't they?'

'Yes.' She said without much conviction. 'I can see the logic of that from where you're sitting but I just feel so bad about the whole thing – pissed off, scared – and it's so awful seeing her like that.'

Alan smiled and said. 'Well come across to where I'm sitting and see how it looks from here.'

She said nothing but got up to join him on the settee where they talked about old Mother Watson and Alan explained his mission of mystery. 'Yes well, just be clear with Val what she wants you to do. I sometimes think her air of harassed integrity is a bit contrived, she's a survivor is old Valerie.'

'Do you think she might be dumping something on me?'

'Nothing as crude as that but just make sure she knows what's happening and tell her if you think its going bottoms up.'
'Has she talked to you or Graham about it?'

'No she hasn't but I'd heard the story a while ago – I just assumed it had become greatly exaggerated at the time then forgot all about it. But it wasn't and now people want to know the full story?'

Alan decided he didn't want to talk about it anymore and held Cindy closer, which seemed to be the right thing. They lay awkwardly until cramp set in then Cindy put on her CD edition of 'Hunky Dory' and made them a more comfortable arrangement by the fire with some free standing cushions, by the time her breathing had deepened against him he was feeling happier than he had for a long time. He forgot his head and he was free.

Next morning brought the heebie-jeebies back but he managed to get up first and put in a solid effort with the instant coffee, reluctant kettle and special treat wagon wheels. By the time he'd served breakfast in bed and had an all over wash he was as ready as he was going to be. Outside it was pissing with rain so they scuttled off to separate cars. He had to smile after he'd switched on the tape and Ivie Anderson came on warbling 'Stormy Weather', Cindy's baked potatoes were a fading memory though. When he got to work Val was waiting in the team room – generally a bad sign. 'Alan, things have moved on a bit with our special project, have you been able to go through the documentation?'

'I've made a start. There's some odd sounding stuff ... '

'Yes, yes I know. Listen the son is upping the ante, you know he's a big noise in the media, well that naturally makes him a bigger one with the local people and he's been on to Jacky Charlton at the Echo. We'll have to be proactive on this one,

ASK ME NOW

things shouldn't go plum shaped. I know you'll come through on this one Alan – you'll have to talk to all the players and keep me onside, with regard to this one. We can't afford a replay.'

He could tell she was properly rattled in regard to this one because she was talking bollocks, presumably her unfocussed footballing analogy had caused her to confuse Jacky Charlton with Jenny Chilton, the editor of the local paper who was not generally known for advertising Shredded Wheat or shooting pheasants. 'I suppose you want me to tackle Barry and Colin Clarke?'

'Yes, if you could kick the director off the ball too.'

Alan liked Val and didn't like to think of her being knocked about by the sinister suits over at Halitosis Hall. 'I'll go through the main bits again this morning and take notes – I could see Weatherall this afternoon. I suppose I ought to start with him.'

'Yes. Ring him this morning though and tell me what you've arranged.'

Alan found Weatheralls number and called him straight away. The answer phone came on taking forever to notify him that there was no one there. Two points to interest him did emerge though; Barry's mobile number and his accent – he was from the northeast. He decided to try again in a bit and returned to the world of Stanley Clarke in the mean time, making notes of the less obvious anomalies. At one point Cindy showed her face and had her coffee with him before setting out to see Mrs. Brestbohn whose confidence she had won. Alan tried the landline again then the mobile. Barry answered directly. 'Aye.' He said after Alan's intro. 'Thought that might come up again, I heard about old Mr. Clarke.' They arranged to meet at his house at two, Val pronounced this to be excellent news and felt sure they'd get on.

The end of the morning brought his mid-day melancholy. He resolved not to walk up to town alone and instead join in with the loose café society to be found in the small group room, which he'd made a bad decision to avoid yesterday. He marched across to the nearest corner shop selling rolls, newspapers and also some of the tackiest top shelf porn he'd ever noticed in passing. He wondered that if this stuff was deemed fit for public display what on earth was available to the connoisseur? He looked away from that months 'Still Swinging' to claim the last Indie. and order a cheese and onion roll. The Indian lass who served him looked about fourteen, she smiled when she gave him his change and he wondered if she would have to face the men who came in for their 'Asian Babes'.

Back at work Dilly from psychology was asking Daz from social exclusion about a referral to the gardening group and Nav was having a crack at the Mail prize crossword. 'Aright cousin.' He said as Alan sat down next to him. 'Gizza hand eh.' Alan loved them all at moments like this. Why shouldn't Nav go out with Briony Prince? Who cared if Dilly was an unregulated narcissist? They were all human; everyone had something wrong with them – nobody's perfect. It was said that Daz had a spent conviction for football hooliganism, well what of it? He helped Nav do his puzzle as he ate his roll and it was agreed they would split the £25 if his name came out of the hat first then Tommy Smith came in to entertain them with a barely believable account of his weekend at the 'Gestalt Therapy Made Simple' conference – 'apparently it's all in the mind'. He tried to ease into George Smiley mode as he got ready to go out but decided that anybody sane would want to be George Clooney, or even Rosemary, and put it all to the back of his mind. Barry Weatherall lived over in Bury and the journey across coincided with the sun coming out. By the time he reached Aylott Avenue it was a bright fresh afternoon with enough wetness left to hold light in the

ASK ME NOW

pavement. All told he felt he wasn't doing too badly really.

The place was on a new build estate, barely five years old he guessed, and he was early so when there was no answer he sat in the car and caught The Archers. He was just about to learn who'd been tampering with the sausages when he started at a tapping on the car window. 'Mr. Duright?' Asked an older man in a baseball cap. Alan nodded and as his companion stood he could see he was also wearing a denim jacket with red drawstring cargo pants. The cap was bright mustard. As an aging British jazz musician he'd have carried this off with cool aplomb, but as a public servant he looked a twit. The effect was mitigated a little when he learned that Barry was on leave and had been for his 'power saunter'. Alan had never set much store by first impressions anyway. The first time he'd clapped eyes on Cindy she had been dancing the Macarena in a car park, she hadn't done it since.
Barry's house, like Grahams and his own place, was shaped to the needs of a man living alone; here the tell tale detail was the compilation of Inspector Morse DVD's set out by the computer. A woman about the place would have had them in the correct order but Barry's were filed every which way, some upside down. There was a large shelf full of books though no sign of musical appreciation but an informal photograph propped against the books caught his attention. It was of Barry with a younger man at some sort of party and Alan thought he recognised the younger man who was looking to Barry and laughing, but couldn't place him. Barry came back down in some brown M&S cords and denim shirt to make some tea for them. 'So.' He said just like Inspector Lewis. 'Dear old Stanley's gone to a better place and his goody two shoes son wants to make mischief. Can't say I blame him really, have you met him yet?'

'Colin Clarke – the son?'

'Yes, smooth talker – watch yourself.' Alan felt his mood

slipping, this wasn't going well. He removed his glasses and polished them carefully with the cleanest wipe he could find in his trouser pocket. Barry sniffed then got up as the kettle clicked. Morse, thought Alan – real ale and Wagner, lives on his own, does the crossword, bit of a silly sausage with women. Maybe it was the trusty sidekick from Sunderland who interested Barry.

'I see you've got a full set of them.' He said nodding at the pile as Barry brought the tea.

'Oh aye, present from David – my son.' He nodded to the photograph by the books. 'Anyway this one will be the case of the careless admission I should think.'

Alan laughed at this. 'Well, the director wants the file on his desk and a result at the earliest.'

'Are you from up north then?' Asked Barry.

'Yes I was born at Stockton then we moved a bit further south when I was quite young.'

'Don't blame you. I'm from South Shields - Ridsdale seemed like a soft option. What brought you here?'

'College then a job – I like it here.'

'Aye, not a bad town like. Now, Stanley, there's no two ways about it, a monumental muck up on my part. What can I say, I acted in good faith, from where I was standing it all seemed to fit, I was mortified when it all started to unravel but it wasn't just me, old Ted Rodgers got it all round his neck at the hospital – I could tell you a thing or two about him if you like. Of course nobody was going to point a finger there, then it was time to shunt me off into early retirement … ' And so it went on, a predictable earful of self serving twaddle artfully sprinkled with enough earnest culpability to make it credible.

ASK ME NOW

It sounded a bit rehearsed a bit pat, a bit much. He realised he'd need to be more astringent with this genial chancer.

'I've got the facts as known down pretty clearly. What's required now is more in the line of a personal reflection, and of course anything new you can tell me.'

'I could of course tell you to fuck off.'

'You could but ...'

'It wouldn't be in my interest to.' Barry pulled in a deep breath and contemplated his mock Edwardian fire surround. 'That clever little twat's rattled somebody's tree. His Father was such a nice man too, a real gentleman and I was so sorry at the time. Nothing like that's ever happened to me before, I've years of experience, there's a tale or two I could tell you about community work and hospitals – you ever come across a bloke called Fred Hubbard? I could ...'

'What about the actual day it happened? My understanding is that a mistake over the site for this assessment began the chain of events bringing about Mr. Clarke's erroneous admission to hospital.'

The bluster left Barry abruptly at this and he lost his way. 'This is all very embarrassing but the thing is I thought I knew what I was doing but I didn't. It's this thing that sometimes happens to me under pressure.' Yes, thought Alan, that's one way to put it. 'There's a name for it.' Went on Barry in his new mode of penitent truth telling. 'Its called SIMON, I'm lucky really, I've got the simple sort.' Alan had to concentrate hard on one of the DVD cases to avoid laughing and spurting out a mouthful of coffee. The title of the DVD was called 'Fools Errand' and this did it, he collapsed back into his chair and a concerned Barry fetched a glass of water. 'I know it sounds a bit ripe but it's all true, the acronym stands for Stress Induced Misapprehension Or Neologism. Apparently it's a form of cognitive non-seqitur, you know – a logical fallacy where conclusions drawn do not follow from the premises proposed, I think that's right but how can one, I, be sure. If you see.'

Alan strung out his water sipping as long as he could and tried to see where they might be going. He composed himself sufficiently to ask for some general idea about the condition. 'Very little is known really.' Said Barry, brightening a little. 'It was first described in the early 1920's by a Hungarian doctor who'd been treating a celebrated conductor for the Budapest Symphony Orchestra. Very occasionally at a big concert he would lead them through a piece by Mozart believing he was conducting Wagner. There was nothing they could say to him and for a long time he would insist that these were performances of bold new music, full of challenging dissonance and rhythmic daring. It was all stress you see.' Barry let out a rueful chuckle and Alan was able to join in.

'You didn't say anything at the time though did you?'

'Didn't know. I had been working all round the clock that week so there was a general view that I'd been up against it, and then Stanley was so forgiving, and that was pretty well it.'

'Why do you think he was so understanding?'

'I could never work that out. At the time I was just so relieved, but you have to wonder. He seemed so out of it and Dr. Rodgers gave him a good looking at – we were sure we'd got our man. It's bad really how these things can happen.'

'But you're saying now that an undiagnosed condition was instrumental, on your part. When did you first learn you had it?'

ASK ME NOW

'Not too long afterwards. I'd been badly shaken up by it all and eventually went off sick. It was a bad time all round – my ex-wife was being difficult and our David wasn't speaking to me. Anyway, Sunderland were at Bolton for a cup game one Saturday so I thought I'd drive over. I set off and ended up at Brighton, who were playing Shrewsbury. I didn't twig till half-time when I heard someone asking why that Geordie cunt was cheering for Shrewsbury, who were two nil up by then. I mean, Brighton's miles away – I drove all that way because I'd decided I was seeing what I was looking for. As far as I can tell SIMON is all about the minds need for balance, with people like me there's a fault in the wiring somewhere. It's more complicated than denial and all that stuff – anyway it was lucky Shrewsbury got beat but it was still a long way home. I really thought I was going crackers you know, I was depressed but that was understandable, I had an awful Sunday and got in to see the doc first thing Monday.'

Alan was still taking in the implications of Simple SIMON and couldn't stop an unkind thought about Barry finding his way to the right practice that Monday morning. 'What did your doc make of it then?'

'I was lucky there, she's left since but my GP had heard of it so she referred me to a man in Manchester and he eventually diagnosed me – brain scans, blood tests, the lot. I had to keep a log, they even tested my pee – then I got out of social services so they didn't need to know and I've been all right since.'

'How do they treat it?'

'The key thing is to put together a personalised stress vulnerability profile then make appropriate changes in your lifestyle. I was also on anti-depressants for a while, which helped because I was, but they think there's a link to what happens to ones brain chemistry under pressure, but what makes the crucial difference to being SIMON isn't known. With the simple form it's pretty straightforward and treatment is pretty effective. God only knows what you do with the extended form – run for president probably.'

Alan didn't know what to say, it all sounded plausible enough and no dafter to his mind than attention deficit disorder, but was Barry simply finding symptoms for a more common condition known to visit people in trouble? Still, it could account for difficulties on the home front; women often struggled to understand men, had he been harshly judged there? 'You say it's unusual, have you ever come across anyone else with it?'

'Our David's got it.'

'Your son?'

'Aye, poor lad. It doesn't show itself till adult life then it's often misdiagnosed but he's got it all right.'

'I'm sorry to hear that – what does David do?'

'He's a lecturer over at TAT – does quite a bit of work on the social work course. David Bamber.'

Alan looked at the picture again. 'Dave Bamber?'

'That's right, have you met him then?'

'Yes, yes … we did meet. That's him in the photograph isn't it – I thought he looked familiar.'

'Took his stepfathers name after me and his mother split up, we're all right now though. Due round for his tea tonight.'

Don't bank on it, thought Alan then decided, for the sake of his own equilibrium, to talk about something else. After a

ASK ME NOW

playful natter about Inspector Morse ('you'd need to be up early to fettle him') and some improbable predictions of Newcastle Uniteds coming season Alan felt better able to return to the business at hand. Barry took him them through his story again with Alan noting key details here and there and asking for clarification along the way. They wound up their encounter with Barry's tall tales about some of the more colourful members of the local welfare community. He wondered if he really ought to be hearing some of the material or if he could believe anything this man told him about life the universe or obscure madnesses. The Dave Bamber connection rang true of course and this fortified him, it also reassured him about that placement – presumably 'Vic' had been Mick or Dick, or even Sally, and had been kicking their Doc Martens heels somewhere else in the North West that afternoon. He felt some sympathy for Barry, the department had obviously washed its hands of him as soon as they could and hoped he would sod off. He arranged to see him again the next week and set off back to base. The Ellington band was waiting in the car and bashed out an accompaniment to Ivie Anderson who chirruped 'Bi blip blip honey bang bang bang' which summed up his afternoon. He was feeling tired and edgy but knew he'd best show his face back at the office, he tried to remember what he'd agreed with Cindy. Barry had said he'd been depressed, what if I get SIMON he thought? She'd definitely said for him to come round for his tea and he knew that she preferred their evenings together to unfold round at her house. This seemed fair enough to him, his kitchenette was damp and she'd recently bought him a present of some fresh bathroom towels – one of the old ones had been there when he moved in though he'd washed it often enough. She'd complained that it scratched – what a girly. He'd told her she was too used to central heating and that she therefore didn't need to use towels as much as he did – this had only made matters worse and she'd gone home. Still, they were rowing again which he reckoned boded well..

When he returned to Northfield he found a message from Val asking him to call Colin Clarke on a London number, she was nowhere to be found. He sat at his desk to look at it, this was his biggest test since the comeback, sometimes the returning of a phone call was the hardest thing. Barry Weatherall had told him the son was a smooth operator. He knew that if he didn't make the call now all would be lost, he might as well pack up and go home, and stay there. He'd heard that fortune smiled on the bold but was fate in a pleasant mood? Dr. Wallace floated past the doorway like a better fed Cordelia, outside the sunlight played against the water tower. He picked up the handset and tapped in a number. It rang for a while and he hoped his gutsiness would be rewarded with an answer phone – the best outcome all round. 'Hallo?' Said a confident voice from London. 'Colin Clarke here, who am I I speaking to?'

Nobody yet thought Alan chipily. 'It's Alan Duright here, I'm just returning your call.'

'Oh Alan, thanks for getting back to me so quickly. Listen, I gather from your Mrs. Meating that you're working on this regrettable business over my late Father. I'm glad the authorities are doing something now – can we talk? If we can get this sorted out with the minimum of fuss so much the better. I'm going to be up later this week – could we meet?'

'Yeah that would be fine. Where would you prefer to do it, here or somewhere more neutral?'

'Could we meet at my sisters place? I'll be staying there and she's like to be involved if that's okay.'

'Yeah yeah, that's fine.' Said Alan. Clarke gave him an address and they fixed a time for Friday which would leave him two days to get his phased introduction airborne and more time to get round 'this regrettable business'. He tapped into his computer and got into the mercurial shared

ASK ME NOW

information terminal, it was all ready past home time but his firm way with the telephone had emboldened him and he could stop off for a drink on the way to Cindy's. He found a number of Clarks but only three with an e and a Stanley. One was 25 but the other two had died within the past twelve months, he needed to be very careful not to get the wrong one. The first late Stanley had died at the hospice from cancer after a lifetime of schizo-affective disorder. One of the CPN's from the elderly team had been involved so it was unlikely to be his Stanley. Poor sod, he thought, life couldn't have been much of a minestrone for him or his family. He brought up the details for the other Mr. Clarke; there were the basic details but nothing else he'd been only 66 when he died and the address was a local one. The GP was entered as Dr. Nadgett from the Southside lot so there was a connection but nothing entered in case notes, episodes or scanned into correspondence, which clinched it for Alan. Patient record BO/ 85567321 was his man but, as yet, there was no sign of a leaking biro.

He sat for a solemn ponder, the only sounds came from the distant cackle of cleaners – a dreadful set of out-sourced wasters who sat fagging it in the waiting room before they emptied the paper bins then went home – and the radiators pinking. He felt sure that Dr. Wallace would be in her office but she generally had a nap before the traffic eased so wouldn't emerge just yet. It was now or never. At 5.41 he left his office to slip next door to the medical secretaries room where he collared the master key from its hiding place in the hat stand. At 5.44 he let himself into clinical records and by 6.17 was back at his desk holding a whiffy old file and a sense of having set in motion events that might wreck his sanity and bring forth the breaking of nations, or at least a modest second division community mental health team. He smiled and placed the file at the bottom of his drawer without looking at it. He could always put it back without looking.

Mike Pearson

Alan stopped off for a bottle of Rot at Key Largos and dully presented himself at Cindy's for 8.00. She looked pale and tense, he thought she could have been crying too. Poor Cindy, but he knew she didn't like that so he just smiled and put his arms around her. 'Your Mum?' He asked.

'Yes but it's my brother that's done it – God he's a selfish sod. Would you believe there's a band that wants to record some of his songs so he has to be away from tomorrow till the weekend. He's going and he thought he'd better let me know because Mum's taken a turn for the worst. After I'd told him to fuck off I phoned her – I'll have to go over on Saturday and get something sorted.'

'What about your brothers girlfriend?'

'Oh she's away as well, something to do with her job, which explains his movements. I bet she knows nothing about it.'

Although he quite liked what he'd read of Adrian's songs and wished him success, Alan could see that his timing needed working on. Perhaps he'd write something for their Mother. He stoked her hair and maintained close but careful contact, She held on and wept into his shoulder. They stood together for a while buttressed by Cindy's compact work surface, he felt full of ardent concern for his deliquescent princess, in his head Rita Coolidge sang 'Help Me Make It Through The Night'. They stayed put for long enough for their breathing to synchronise then she kissed his neck and pulled away to sit down at the kitchen table. 'Have I to make us some tea?' He asked.

'There's not much in.' She said. 'Shall we have chips?'

'Yeah that would be nice.' He took her order for curry sauce, peas and chips and joked that he'd decide once he could see what the days special was. Tapscotts Chippy was only a couple of blocks away across Pogson park near the end of

ASK ME NOW

Water Lane where he joined the early evening queue. As immediate gratification went fish and chips were as reliable as it got, better in that regard than sex and streets ahead of fresh air and exercise, once you got your hands on them. Tapscotts was manned by an oldish man in stained wellies and once white caterers coat assisted by an unpromising looking youth in a white cap. The lad worked capably enough though and soon had the customers ahead of Alan satisfied and off home with their teas. When he reached the top of the line the older man announced that chips would be five minutes and tossed several battered fish into the glass cabinet ahead of him where they glistened on a metal grill. Alan felt himself salivate and looked around the shop, the vernacular landscape of chippies had often caught his eye while he waited for the goods. This one was reassuringly idiomatic; bizarre cut outs in lurid pink signalling specials, a fixture list plus football team photo, cards for taxis, builders and person centred counselling, also a cannily placed notice for the local weight watchers. The best thing though was a large soft-porn poster conflating sex and chips and rock n' roll; an attractive couple were posed in an old American car eating haddock and chips, he was feeding her with a wooden fork and she was sitting forward to suck off a chip. Her shapely hooters spilled over a skimpy top. A likely story thought Alan as he took a closer look at the dashboard.

'Have you had yours mate?' Asked the man in the wellies.

'Eh? Oh no.' Replied Alan as he tore himself away from the fish and tits to put in his order.

He wondered about those wellies on the way back, were they a humorous touch meant to suggest that he'd been out to Fleetwood for 'today's catch'? He certainly went about his work seriously, well in control of bucket and batter. He'd ridden the controls of the ancient fryer with nonchalant aplomb. The youth seemed to know his stuff too, no doubt they were second and third generation Tapscotts steeped in the ways of a dying tradition. He would talk of this to Cindy as they ate and enjoyed himself enjoying these reflections. She'd warmed the plates so they set to in front of the tele. Sandy Tucker was taking them through the local news when Alan began to gag on a chip. 'Look.' He coughed. 'It's Northfield.'

'My God.' Gasped Cindy and turned up the sound. The reporter was talking to camera in front of the big blue hospital sign; questions were being raised about the treatment given to a man by mental health services who had died recently. A cover up of poor practice had been alleged and a full inquiry was being demanded. Cut to a closer view of Northfield and short statement from Colin Clarke – 'the well known investigative reporter with local roots' – who was absolutely clear that 'shoddy work' involving his late Father must be exposed and lessons learned. Then it was off to Merrylegs pony club where some very junior members had been going through their paces.

'Bloody hell.' Exclaimed Alan. 'They made it sound as if the death and the bad practice were connected and our local cleverarse didn't help matters – absolutely clear, I'll bet. I had no idea this was going to be on the soddin' tele.'

Cindy left the room and returned with the local paper. 'I haven't looked at it yet but it'll be in here if Sandy Tuckers got wind of it.'

'Now I come to think of it Ina was mythering on about the media today but I didn't think anything of it at the time.' Said Alan.

''Yes well, if it's a battle between our lot and the media they'll wipe the floor with us. Lets hope it doesn't make the nationals.'

ASK ME NOW

'You don't think it will do you Cindy?'

'If sniffer Clarke's on the case it might. I mean it's a good story and you can see where he's coming from.'

'I'm supposed to be seeing him on Friday.' He said. They sat for a while in silence pushing at their chips, deep in a dream. Neither had made a move to open the Echo. Eventually Cindy said she thought it was unfair of Val to land this on his desk.

'I don't know – all she's asked me to do is talk to a few people, get some feedback.'

'Yes well, just make sure that's all it is' you know how things can snowball.'

Alan hadn't a clue how these things snowballed and started to fret. What if this was too much for him? Was that what she was getting at? 'I spoke with Barry Weatherall this afternoon.'

'He's the social worker who sectioned Stanley?'

'Yes, he's all ready cleared up one mystery.' He told her all about SIMON and how Barry had been badly knocked about by it and how it involved Dave Bamber. He also explained that the process of concealment looked to have taken on a momentum of its own without anyone person being personally responsible.

'Well.' She sighed. 'That last bit sounds right enough but do you believe this brainstorm fit of the vapours type thing?'

'Well it explains dodgy Dave and his strange ways.'

She thought about this. 'Oh I dunno. I'm past caring. Isn't the real mystery about why this bloke never jumped up and down at the time?'

'Well, I've tracked down an old hard copy file which isn't referred to in our record.'

'What's it say?'

'I dunno, I haven't looked yet.'

'Well let's open the paper anyway.'

It was a short feature on page three beneath a picture of Northfield. Alan picked out Dr. Wallace's car and some stray figures walking near the entrance, none of who could be recognised. It left him with a bad feeling, were they watching you all the time and could they do this whenever they wanted. The write up did at least get the facts as known in the correct order but, to Alans mind, still linked Mr. Clarkes death with the earlier miss deeds. They might be right for all he knew. He left the rest of his chips so Cindy finished them off. 'Look Alan.' She said mopping up the last of her curried mush. 'I can't see that this whole palaver is worth getting too bothered about. It's not your responsibility and if what Barry Wazzockfeatures says is true … well who's going to point a finger?'

'He told me he'd been to see a specialist, cited a well known conductor who had it in the twenties – somewhere in Eastern Europe.'

'In the twenties, in the soviet bloc was it? God knows what they diagnosed there if your music wasn't right, more likely to get Stalin than SIMON. You'd be an enemy of the people.'

'Well that does bring us back to state powers and Barry's behaviour doesn't it? You've never heard of it then?'

'No but that's hardly conclusive – I'll ask Beth tomorrow, if

ASK ME NOW

she's never heard of it then that'll settle it.'

Cindy seemed to be in a good mood despite all this and clearly didn't want to talk about her Mum anymore so they settled together on the settee to watch the ten o' clock news with Nicholas Witchel who made no reference to monkey business with the mental health act in Ridsdale. The regional news just repeated its earlier piece which seemed innocuous enough second time around. He reflected that the bad thing here was that people expected this kind of stuff in the public services and took little notice unless they were directly involved. 'Will you stay tonight?' She asked him.

'Yeah, been a long day one way and another. I'll clear away if you want to go up first.'

'Thanks Alan.' She said and kissed him on the neck again. He went about his tasks with a will and soon had things in apple pie order. She hadn't finished in the bathroom so he sat in the quiet room with the main light on, there was something sad about it; growing cold, settling into a repository of traces – paperbacks bearing signs of reading, plumped cushions, left chairs. He felt a bit cold then heard the bed creak as she settled into it the bath water rattled through the pipes. The spare warmth of her bathroom lifted his mood and he enjoyed his Spartan strip wash. He was tired that was all, he'd done too much – two days off and he'd be back on track.

'What were you singing?' She asked as he got in with her.

'I don't know, I only know some of the words.. 'I'm just a soul whose intentions are good' tralala. It's the Bachelors isn't it?'

'The Animals.' She said as she stretched to switch off the light. He'd all ready noticed that she didn't have her nightie on, now her left breast pulled into a beautiful soft sphere as she moved, parking her elbow next to him for balance. She turned back towards him and kissed his neck where she had earlier then stroked his hip leaving her hand there as she parted his lips with her tongue to give him a lovely smackeroo. They fell into an extended snog and feel-up during which he was glad to find himself in working order, he could feel her rubbing her fanny against his thigh then she lay back to direct him south of the border with her hands kneading his shoulders. He loved her no-nonsense approach to their sex life and licked his lips in anticipation. Then the phone rang. Cindy cried 'shit' and shot out of bed. Alan's response had been more muffled.

He layback determined not to fiddle in the breach and tried to catch what Cindy was saying downstairs. He'd picked up an impassioned 'Oh no' then 'they'll have to now' but apart from sundry 'emms' and 'oh yeses' most of the detail seemed to be coming from the other end. She'd be off the boil by now anyway, he hoped she'd put her coat on, his own state of arousal had fallen off but he found the whole thing to be quite a pleasant experience and rolled over onto Cindy's side to keep it warm for her.
'Alan.' She said. 'You'd better get up.'

'Eh?' He coughed, then. 'What ? Oh.'

'Get up it's eight o' clock.' She was sitting on the edge of the bed fully dressed and looking stressed. He caught sight of a mug of tea steaming beside him on the bedside table.

'How long have you been up?' He asked.

'I haven't been to bed.' She said.

'There was a phone call wasn't there.' He said reaching for the tea.

'There was a phone call.' She replied blandly.

ASK ME NOW

'About your Mother?'

'About my Mother, from the woman next-door God bless her. She heard a crash from my Mothers side and to cut a long and sorry story short, Mum's in hospital – fractures and concussion. I'm going straight over.'

'Cindy are you okay to drive, have you slept at all?'

'Yes and no.'

'I'm off today, I could drive you over.'

'No Alan, thanks, but I'd rather go on my own, in fact I'm going now – let yourself out and I'll phone you tonight.' And she was off.
He propped himself up to finish his tea feeling guiltily relieved that Cindy had declined his gallant offer then he managed another little nap till nine fifteen when he phoned Val Meating to let her know about Cindy. He also debriefed her over his findings at Barry's. There'd been a silence at her end when he'd finished then she said. 'I'll ask Dr. Wallace about this – you say you're seeing Colin Clarke on Friday, I'll talk to the media lot and try to make some time for you before then. Give Cindy my love and me a ring tomorrow.' Then she was off too.

Alan sat in more familiar surroundings with another mug of tea trying, at a point near lunchtime, to make some sense of his ever-changing world. It was at such times that a man looked for guidance from 'The World Of Jake Thackery' where rude wisdom could be found but he couldn't find his old vinyl copy and settled instead for 'The World Of Cecil Taylor' where fixed and settled truths were in shorter supply. It was the sort of serious stuff he loved when he could give it the attention it deserved but was hopeless when the windmills of his mind were on double time. He took it off and put on George Benson whose thought for the day was 'love and be loved in return' – fat chance he thought. He spent the rest of Wednesday sitting around at home in a way he hadn't been able to for quite a while. He cried for a bit in the afternoon and wanted to be with Cindy but he went for a walk and it was all right. He found that passing through the entrance hall seemed to be difficult but once he was back up he spent half an hour writing down some reflections concerning the Clarke affair.

She phoned him at seven o' clock. 'I can't speak for long, it's been hell on wheels over here – Mums pretty bad, the fall's shaken her badly and her hips knackered ... '

'How are you anyway Cindy?'

'Oh all right if I keep busy. I don't think she'll be coming home Alan.'

'Well ... what have they said?'

'Not a lot ... not a lot they can say. I'd better go, I'll phone tomorrow, hopefully I can get back for the weekend.'

'Love you Cindy.' Then she was gone again.

He got straight up out of his chair and set out for a long walk past the roundabout and under the bypass to a new estate called Burnaps Field. It reminded him a little of his Fathers place in Northallerton; a bit more down market, fewer trees but there was a large expanse of green space in the middle with footie pitches and some swings. He sat down on one of the benches by the field and was buoyed to learn that if he wanted a shag he should call this number. Elsewhere on the seat he was told that Mr. Harris was a 'peedo' and Thommo a gay boy. Nothing changes, he thought, the graffiti was as 'traditional' as the carriage lamps outside 'The Burnap'with

ASK ME NOW

its roadhouse exterior and farmer on the sign. Three boys were pulling branches from one of the trees and he had half a mind to say something but this was just the kind of blameless pursuit golden lads and lasses both would have enjoyed uninterrupted in the days before social workers. Also, he didn't want to be thought a peedo so he went for a pint instead.

The pub was a nice surprise with wide screen football and gentleman's club chairs to sit in, he ordered a pint of 'Weavers Answer' and made himself comfortable. The match turned out to be the usual premiership fare; lots of throw ins, protracted 'injuries' and theatrical stuff with the officials. Somehow one of the teams managed to score two goals so they were each shown half a dozen times. The 'Weavers' wasn't bad though so he had another and pushed the boat out with a packet of crisps. By nine thirty the place began to fill up so he tottered off home, stopping off for a piss and sit down in the park. He remembered the strange afternoon when he'd ended up round at that lady's house on Gas Street, what had he been playing at? He should go back and apologise but not just yet.

By tea-time the next day he'd been able to shepherd thin hope through another cycle of time via his jog, the library and a nice natter with Steve from downstairs whose girlfriend Sandy had called round while they were talking of Tennyson. She seemed very nice and he resolved to get some kind of foursome set up with Cindy, who rang earlier than she had on Wednesday. 'I'm sorry I was so rushed yesterday – there was so much to take in one way and another. All a bit of a shock really.'

'Where are you staying, how is your Mum?'

'Not good really, I'm staying at the house. I'm sure she can't come back – she fell all the way downstairs you know that night, it must have been about tennish, thank goodness Mrs. Minerva heard through the wall, she's not too clever herself.'

'You said about fractures.'

'Yes. An arm, her hip and a couple of ribs, then there was the concussion and the shock. They're keeping a close eye on her.'

'Is Adrian there?'

'Yes, he is now – had the effrontery to tell me she shouldn't have been left alone. Alan, I hit him.'

She sounded shocked and he remembered what a punch she'd packed before. 'You haven't put him in the next bed have you?'

She tsked softly and said. 'He might be looking for one soon, I think Bodi could be about to boot him out, he can come round here and make himself useful.'

'Really?'

'Oh I don't know. I can't understand any woman taking him on I suppose. How are things at your end?'

'Not bad really. I was tired on Wednesday so I didn't do much. I've been thinking about how to take this thing with Colin Clarke tomorrow, jotting down some thoughts. How are you bearing up at your end, it sounds pretty bad?'

'It helps me getting so cross with Adrian – I'm going to stop feeling so responsible for them, he knows how to press that button though. You might bear that in mind tomorrow, it's not down to you to sort it all out.'

Cindy's mode of brisk stoicism alerted him to weed out the

ASK ME NOW

sort of soppiness he was sometimes prone to. It also cautioned him not to fish for any soft soap over the phone. Cindy needed tough love at a time like this, he inwardly flicked up a collar and lit a cigarette. 'Is Adrian facing up to this, I mean he must know he'll have to sit down with you at some point?'

'Yeah, oh yeah I know he will.' She fell silent so he waited. 'Basically we both feel guilty about not wanting to take her on.'

'But you have taken it on Cindy, it's you that's had it all to do. You're the one they phone.'

'Yes but look at all the wailing I set up, poor old Mum doesn't deserve any of this. I'd better go; my little brother has just arrived. Can you ring me tomorrow, I'm not sure what I'll be doing? Good luck with doodah.'

'Yes, of course, Take care then.'

'Bye Alan.'

Mike Pearson

ANY MAJOR DUDE

'Oh hallo, you must be Alan – come in.'

The man, who Alan thought must be Colin, held a mobile phone to his left ear and beckoned him indoors with his free hand, which he then cupped around the phone to say to his visitor. 'One of the Features people, they get the jitters if you don't spell things out for them.' He took his hand away and spoke smoothly into the phone while rolling his eyes conspiratorially in Alan's direction in the manner of one used to dealing with simple folk. Alan couldn't help but be impressed by this effortless authority and parked himself on the new looking IKEA sofa. Very nice, he thought and hoped the phone call might go on for a bit longer the better for him to gather his thoughts following his briefing with Val. The main advice had been to give the ball away as little as possible and not to stray off side, Clarke being well known in the ways of referee intimidation. His manager had been badly rattled by the local press coverage and, according to Graham, spent most of the previous day cloistered in her office with Linda Harvey from Media and Communications. Linda had been a journalist in a former life and could therefore be trusted in these matters, he'd also learned via Dr. Wallace that something like SIMON was believed to exist on the fringes of psychiatry; it wasn't in the current Diagnostic and Statistical Manual proper but was grouped with other poorly understood conditions under 'Factitious Diseases Not Otherwise Specified'.

'Yap, yap.' Said Colin to Features. 'That'll do nicely and remember to give the photographer a credit, he's going to be the next Martin Parr – I know, wonderful isn't it.' He turned to his guest. 'Sorry about that Alan, now my sister should be back any time so I'll make tea if you'll mind the shop.'

A smooth talker Barry Weatherall had said, not to be trusted –

ASK ME NOW

but who was he to talk? Colin looked back in from the kitchen. 'How's your department reacting to the Mental Capacity White Paper?'

Alan stepped up to the plate. 'I think your Fathers case has caused some hard thinking.'

'I was thinking more about the Bournewood ruling though I can see a connection – the absent-minded almoner. I gather you've spoken to Mr. Wherewithal.'

'Yes, well, I need to talk to the main people involved.'

'I quite understand. Tea or coffee?'

At this point Colin's sister arrived behind an obese black Labrador that fixed its good eye on Alan and made a stately beeline for him as soon as his heavy chain was slipped. 'Sabre.' She said. 'Heel – he's very friendly really. Do you like dogs?' Before he could answer Sabre presented him with a soggy paw then gassed him from both ends.

'Perhaps Sabre would like to see what's happening in the garden.' Suggested Colin. Tea for three was then served while the dog gave disgruntled snuffles from outside. Colin got up to close the door into the kitchen and nothing further was heard from Sabre. 'Now, have you two introduced yourselves?'

'No.' They said more or less in unison.

'Okay, Alan this is my sister Helen Chadderton, Helen this is Alan Duright from Northfield.'

'Yes.' She said evenly. 'Were you directly involved in all that business with my Dad?'

'Not directly but I'd like to help in any way that I can now.'

'And how do you think that might be, now?'

'Helen.' Cut in Colin.' We're looking for what Alan would call closure here; at least someone has come to see us. I assume you've been lumbered with this from higher up, obeying orders as it were.'

Alan paused then said. 'Yes.' This seemed to help.

'Fine, so nothing personal then.' Said Colin. Helen was looking out of the window, she looked pale and tense, and Alan reminded himself that it couldn't have been that long since Stanley's death. He wondered about her life; the house gave away no signs of children – she'd probably been closest to their parents while Colin got away and did things. He'd sometimes wished for a sister, he thought about Cindy and her troublesome brother; had Colin done any better?

'I'm sorry about the local rag.' Said Colin.

'That's all right.' Said Alan. 'We won't be kicking up about it.'

Helen laughed sourly. 'That's big of you, but then you didn't at the time did you?'

'Yes, yes. Your Father was remarkably ... tolerant is the word I suppose.'

'My Father was an ironist Alan.' Explained the son as to a fellow sophisticate. 'His view at the time was that by not complaining he was marking himself out as truly mad.'

Alan was getting fed up with being Alaned all the time and she hadn't got started yet. 'So why didn't he make more of it at the time?'

ASK ME NOW

Helen turned round to face him and Colin sat back. 'There are a number of reasons.' She said and Alan felt bad because he all ready knew what one of them might be. 'My Father was a tolerant man as you say, it was one of his many qualities – but it wasn't just that. There was the condition he was in that morning, pretty well stoned on tonic wine and chemicals – and he was also very frightened.'

'Yes.' Said Alan. 'I think I can understand that.'

'I wonder if you do. You see he'd been through it before – been sectioned – and thought it would go against him if he objected, then when it all started to unravel as it did … well he was just so relieved when you let him go.'

'You'll see now why we made so little of it while he was alive.' Said Colin.

'Yes.' Said Alan. 'I know what happened from before; I mean there's a brief record from the Mental Welfare Officer. It was quite a while ago wasn't it?'

'I remember it.' Said Helen firmly. 'Colin was too young to.'

'I had no idea my Father struggled with depression until I was a teenager.' Said Colin. 'And then I can't honestly say there was anything out of the ordinary, I suppose I was pretty well shielded from it all. It was worse when Helen was little.'

Alan took his time. 'It was 1968 wasn't it, under the old 1959 Act it would have been – to St. Cuthberts.'

'You've done your homework.' She said.' What else is on this file?'

'There's a report from the social worker and a later note

concerning discharge and follow up.'

Helen asked if they could see the file and he said of course deciding that he'd just bring it over if it came to it. 'You'd have been five and I nearly two.' Said Colin. 'Poor old Mum. You can recall it then Helen, do you mind?'

'I can remember the day. He was crying in bed and said he couldn't get out. I had to go to school and he wasn't there when I got back, I'm pretty sure you went with Mum when they took him off.' She spoke as she poured the tea and Alan got an image of a little girl getting through her day at school then coming home to look for her Dad. He began to see how it might have been for them when it started to happen again. He felt like pulling the plug on Barry. Some of this must have shown.

'Sad story isn't it.' Said Colin. 'That was as bad as it ever got though wasn't it Helen?'

'Yes, nothing as bad as that.'

'Till he went along that other morning.' Said Alan feeling like a pious berk.

'And now we simply want to know how it happened.' Said Helen. 'And that lessons will doubtless be learned, procedures put in place so that it can never happen again blah blah blah.'

'So you know all about our old Dad.' Said Colin. 'What can you tell us about the licensed lunatic who tried to detain him all over again?'

Alan didn't bother to ask him how he knew about Barry or what else he was privy to, he felt so out of his depth with these two that he decided to stop flapping and see if the water would hold him up. He gave them an honest account of what he knew, Albanian conductors and all, laying great stress on

ASK ME NOW

the mysteries of SIMON and Barry's blamelessness. When he had finished they sat in silence for very nearly a full minute then Colin said. 'Alan that really is the most wonderful story and I can't not print it. You say it's in the DSS Manual?'

'It's DSM but it's not completely classified and you really should talk to our media section before …'

Helen then surprised Alan by forbidding her brother to do any such thing. 'We can't take the high ground over Dad then plaster it all over the papers, besides, do you believe it?'

'Not the point.' He said. 'These are issues we should pursue; how many public servants are unfit for purpose, what happens if …?'

'I should apologise for my brother Mr. Duright, I think he's raised enough dust as it is.'

So here we are then thought Alan feeling like a twat, ironising and apostrophising like billyo but unillusioned and seekers after truth now that old Stan's gone to that great back ward in the sky. He hoped St. Peter hadn't messed up the admission papers and that they could have a break, the balance of power being more nuanced and shifting than he was used to. He was also beginning to see why Colin Clarke might have gone into investigative journalism; for all his easy cynicism and sophistry he was just taking his own small punt at making the world a better place. He tried to remember what Stanley's occupation had been – something on the railways, self-employed? 'Was your Fathers work affected by his illness?'

'My Dad always worked.' Said Helen.

'He once joked about giving himself free shock treatment.' Added Colin.

That's right, an electrician. They gave everyone ECT in those days; trouble with it is that it seems to work. What really works though? What had worked for him? Had anything, how was he doing, really? The most reliable pointers were that the colour had come back on and Stan Tracey's piano sounded like an old friend – if Cindy's phone hadn't gone off the other night they would have. Had it just been time and changes and watching rubbish with Cindy? He was lucky really, that wasn't something you could prescribe. 'Will you really do something with this?' He asked Colin.

'Probably.' He replied.

'Will you?' Helen asked Alan.

'Well my role's quite straightforward really. I need to get peoples stories, feedback, make sure we're on the right track …'

'And that's quite straightforward is it, really?' Said Colin with some force. 'There's more irony there than you could shake a pink form at.'

Alan couldn't help but laugh at this as he thought he should steel himself for more of the old irony but Helen laughed too and the mood lifted. 'How long have you got Col.?'

'Less time than I thought – I need to get going by twelve now.'
'Okay.' She said decisively. 'Let's try to focus a bit.'

She put him in mind of a less bashed about Beth Wallace and he wondered what she did. He'd noticed that Colin deferred to her and it was she who had the main emotional investment in the story. Helen reached down into a magazine rack to pull out a blue file with Dad written on it. He and Colin sat quietly as she sifted papers and ordered her thoughts. Much of the material was familiar to him by now; well argued, polite

ASK ME NOW

letters from Helen, Colin or both, shamelessly round the houses stuff in return from the director, though he did notice VM on one of the references. There was also a small pile of notes in Colin's hand clipped under a sheet with The World Of Barry Weatherall written on it in the form of an old-fashioned playbill. Alan wondered if he might be able to enjoy himself here after all. 'As you can see we've had to do some research for ourselves.' He said.

'You had to.' Helen said pointedly.

'Look, I know how local government operates. Do you think our new friend would be taking tea with us today if I hadn't pressed the right buttons?' He replied scornfully.

Well, thought their new friend, if you know that much about local government you're wasted in journalism mate. He was a persuasive sod alright but then he needed to be. Had Barry made a bit of a prat of himself? Taken the field with a badly organised back four, conceded some soft goals on the break? It did seem to be his stock in trade. 'Look.' Said Helen you'll do what you want but you're not to drag Dads name through the muck. You'll be as bad as this lot if you do, worse at least Mr. Weatherall was acting in good faith.'

'You haven't met him.' Said Colin ruefully. 'In my view he's an unprincipled waister whose tongue runs away with him if you press him.'

Thought so, mused Alan. Perhaps he'd have to play daft, or dafter. 'If I understand this correctly, although you've had plenty of feedback what you want now is an explanation.'

'Yes.' Said Colin. 'And what you've told us this morning is quite incredible, though having met the man quite believable. I think I can probably get something out of this without mentioning my Father, would you like a credit on any feature

Mike Pearson

Alan?'

'No, no ... you shouldn't, erm – if your piece raises awareness about a serious but little known ...'

'Look Alan, you really ought to do something with this – we're always on the look out for good free-lance stories from the inside. You know, principled whistleblowers – no penny-a-line stuff either, I could get you a good deal, maybe a regular column if it all kicks off.'

Helen had been regarding her brother with a vinegary smile. 'It's principled whistleblowers now is it? Not malleable mugs who'll do the spade work, I sense Alan knows better.'

'Pity'. Yapped Colin and stood up. 'Time I was off.' This enabled Alan to get a good look at his baggy trousers and he felt his opinion of him slip up a notch; they were a wonderful example of gentleman's classics – thick bottle green jumbo corduroy cut capaciously with generous side pockets, pleats and two inch turn ups pegged to the ankles. They hung securely to within a half-inch of the floor as they flopped across a pair of brogues, which probably cost more than the settee. Alan knew class when he saw it and it was all he could do not to ask for the name of Colin Clarke's tailor.

'Don't mind my brother.' Said Helen when he'd gone. 'All mouth and trousers, do you want some more tea?'

'Yes please.' But what a pair. He heard her open the back door and some soothing chat to the dog who seemed content with his basket by the fridge when she came back with more tea. He'd expected her to turn to the main agenda once Studs Terkel had taken his leave but she seemed to want to digress. After some stilted banter about dogs and their doings she asked him if he enjoyed his job. 'Yes, by and large I'd say so.'
'I suppose you'd have to to do it.' She said.

ASK ME NOW

'Oh yeah, it's a job you choose, for whatever reason. I mean no one actually enjoys detaining someone under the mental health act but sometimes not doing that can be a real achievement. Then there's all the other stuff you know, that can be helpful to people.'

'Mmm, there's not enough quality control though is there? I don't doubt you do your best and you haven't said anything too fatuous so far but what about the man who mistook my Dad for a nut? Are there others like him and who regulates all this power?'

Alan sighed. 'Well this is one of the problems in any large scale organisation, you couldn't argue a case for everything that goes ...'

'Oh I know Alan, it's okay, I don't have a problem with social workers or the psychiatric establishment. In fact some of my best friends – do you know Claire Todgers, she must have contacts with your lot?'

Oh yes, he thought, she has contacts all over the place. 'Yeah, yeah I know Claire.' Helen was looking out of the window again and he found that her wilful vacancy was getting on his wick, or was it the seemingly inevitable introduction of the fair Claire. Cindy had been out for a drink with her the other week and come home in a disobliging humour.

Helen tore herself away from the weather in the street. 'A friend of mine went into The Lindens for a while, they seem to do a decent amount of good there. She just turned up on their doorstep actually and they took her in. Claire okayed it with the powers that be and she stayed till she got better. Do you deal with many families like us Alan?'

'How do you mean?'

'Pushy, middle class, inclined to ask you questions we all ready know the answers to.'

'A social workers lot in mental health tends to cover a wide range of demographics.' He ventured without being that sure if he'd said what he really meant.
Helen was dubious. 'But you're mainly concerned with the poor and the powerless aren't you? They might tell you to fuck off but they don't understand your organisational muscle, know where the power is. I'm sure my unbearable brother has put the wind up the right quarters.'

'Poor people aren't stupid.'

'No of course they're not but they see and basically accept that you're part of a force which shapes and regulates their lives. I've no doubt that without it things would be worse but it must be confusing trying to manage being a cross between policeman and nurse. People like me see this, the shifting sand you plant your flag on, can't help noticing how tangled it looks and uncertainly it flutters, I mean, can you tell me what social work is?'

Christ not that. He mustered a solemn chuckle and said. 'It's what social workers do.'

'Yes exactly, just so – anything goes, the good the bad and what happened to my Dad. They're all for giving social workers more powers so you can try to solve unsolvable problems – I'm all for diluting your existing ones. Give you a chance to get on with what you can do.'

This chimed dimly with a view he'd often come to but who'd be soft enough to take on their statutory duties instead? Why should he care anyway, wasn't this readiness to accept responsibility a sort of grandiosity, an outer ring of delusion, of madness? 'It seems to me that it was fear not magnanimity

ASK ME NOW

that made your Father so tolerant.'

'Yes and you didn't mind so long as he stayed that way. Can you honestly say that his record wouldn't have gone against him if he had made a stink? That the line wouldn't have been that Weatherall was spurred by serendipity to nip his recurring depression in the bud lest madness should ripen like rotten fruit?'

'I don't think it would have been put so well but I think I can see your Fathers position.'

She was visibly upset by now. 'It was awful, the whole thing was awful. I don't think he ever really got over the first time but what happened at the surgery shook him badly – he wasn't an old man when he died was he?'

'No, no he wasn't. I'm sorry, about the whole thing.'

She buried her head in her hands and howled as she stamped her feet on the rug. She gradually calmed but sat sobbing, he sensed Sabre standing beside him and she started again as the dog came forward and nudged her hand. 'I think you should go.' She said eventually.

On his way back to work Alan remembered that the 'Stanley Clark thing' had taken on a faintly comic hue to begin with; blundering Barry, hapless Stanley stoned but forgiving, the hospital happy to take anyone presented in a recognisable form. It seemed appalling to him now, much worse than what some folk liked to think of as 'Kafkaesque', more akin to Stalin's terror on a bad day. Helen Chaddertons grief and rage had shocked him and he was now ashamed to admit to himself that a small part of his preparation had been the hope that the family would see the funny side. He'd got that bit straight now. Barry was for it as well, he could see it now; Simple Simon says – a story everyone should hear, are social workers fit to be released into your community? He'd have to tell people at parties that he was an estate agent again.

He spent the rest of the afternoon jotting down reflections and savouring a pot of 'Floogie Boo' with Graham and Nav who brought them up to date with sundry goings on at labour club. This cheered them up no end and it was agreed that they should get along there again as soon as possible. On his way out he came across Dr. Wallace emerging from the med-secs. Office. 'Oh Alan, I gather you've encountered someone with SIMON. I'd be interested to hear about it.'

'Yes, well to be honest I thought this bloke was having me on it sounded so unlikely, and a bit convenient given his circumstances. You know, a bit like these men who murder their wives in their sleep then claim it was some kind of strange visitation they can't remember.'

'That would be unusual given what's known of the condition. It tends to boil down to a misapprehension of some detail within a sphere of activity which is otherwise understood and more or less correctly acted upon.'

'Yes I read about the Russian conductor.'

'Hungarian, Orsun Khaat, he was one of the earliest known cases. Then there was the pilot from bomber command who dropped a shell on Droylsden – all hushed up of course. I'll look you out some stuff over the weekend.'

'Is there thought to be a genetic link?'

'Yes but it's very difficult to pin down; if it's in the family it can be learned behaviour, like so many things.' She gave him one of her nice smiles then went off to her little office. Good old Beth, it was said that she liked a drink but her private life was basically a mystery, perhaps Claire Todgers would know. He considered phoning Cindy from work but decided to wait

ASK ME NOW

till he got home.

Alan braved the entrance hall of angst to take the stairs two at a time. There was a note pinned to his door with an envelope attached, the note was from Steve downstairs who had found the hand delivered letter and thought it might be important. He looked at it, his name was printed carefully in the middle in Cindy's handwriting, he felt his bowels shift and his breath shorten. As he barged his way inside the familiar smell of dormant gas fire and stale joss stick seemed terribly sad, seemed to say welcome back you sap, what else did you expect. No more sardines on toast for you lad. He sat down in the cold and looked at his letter, at least it hadn't lodged unseen beneath the doormat, then he remembered they didn't have one. Cindy had never written to him before so it must be big stuff; a Dear John or a meet me at the station with a one way ticket to the happier life. In the event it was pitched tantalisingly between the two and needed several readings before he could take much in; things at home much worse than she'd been led to understand – last few days a great strain – emotionally drained – brother a tosspot from Hades – think you know how I feel about you – (but) feeling mixed up about us. It came down to her needing to get away 'for a few days' where nothing would be expected of her, Claire had rented a place in Wales (no details) and she would go over with her today. She would see him next week – take care love from Cindy x.

He laid down his letter and drew the curtains, put on the fire, lit the soft lights and made a pot of 'Calcutta Cutie' . He read through it all again as he sipped his fine tea. After due reflection several points made themselves clearer; that he knew how she felt about him, that Ma Watson must be pretty bad, that Claire Todgers was becoming unavoidable and that Cindy's spelling was crap, which he put down to stress vulnerability. Old Mother Watsons state of health was surely the key factor and it could be that she was close to death, good old Claire was always there in a crisis and as for the first point, the knowing how she felt bit, well, if Tuesday night was anything to go by he was Claire Rayner crossed with Lancashire's greatest love machine. What more could a girl want? He could have done without that 'mixed up about us' though; it forced him to consider something he'd been not thinking about for a while now. Had she stuck with him out of a desire to help him through his bonkers time and now felt better able to dump him? He felt bad about this because it cast her in such a poor light, but it wouldn't go away. It was no good trying to blur the edges, deconstruct her meaning with a post-modern reading. This means you mate, us means you and her and mixed up means could go either way. But they were an us – they'd shagged each other silly, squabbled in Sainsburys, she'd met his Dad, he'd used her toothbrush and inspected her record collection. Was all this to be cast aside like so much driftwood on the shore? He folded the letter carefully and put it in his home organiser with the gas bills then poured a second cup of 'Cutie' the better to ruminate on loves mercurial ways. If this was it how would they work together and would he go downhill again? If this wasn't the long goodbye what was going to happen next? But he didn't care because just then he knew she was what he wanted, the full works; sex and shopping, watching the tele., giving each other space, spending whole days together, getting old together, maybe even .. ? Was all this what she felt so mixed up about? There was a knock at the door. It was Steve from downstairs. 'Awright mate, did you get that message only she said to make sure?'

'Yeah, thanks. What time did she come?'

'Bout three, lucky I was in really.'

'Yeah right, er, come in.' In the background loud explosions and screams came from Alans television.

'God.' Said Steve. 'Is that Beirut or Iraq?'

ASK ME NOW

'Eh? Oh no, Emmerdale Farm.'

'That was Cindy then.' Said his pal.

'Yes. How's Sandy?'

'Fine, well she was last week when I saw her.'

'Oh right.' Said Alan then, after a pause. 'Doing anything tonight?'

'Not a lot.'

'Fancy a drink?'

'Yeah.' Said Steve after another pause.

The nearest acceptable watering hole was The Slaters Arms, a tatty mausoleum on the Bacup Road where a man had been stabbed in 1965. They still closed on the anniversary of his death and his picture hung over the bar. Local folklore spun a tale of a man from Manchester and some stolen cigarettes, others told of infidelity and an affronted mill owner, either way it hadn't done the pub much harm and the beer was reliable. They also had live entertainment and they arrived just as the band was setting up, Friday night being music night. Steve got them in and they settled down with a pint of Robinsons, both agreed it to be 'an excellent drop' then wondered what they might talk about. ''Cindy seems very nice.' Ventured Steve.

'Yeah she is. Been down the 'Dale lately?'

'Off down tomorrow. Sandy's doing my head in.'

The band looked as if they would start soon so Alan followed this up. 'Things not going well then?'

'How should I know?' He said with a long-suffering sigh. 'Needed some space – fuck knows what's really going on.'

Alan felt a rush of fellow feeling for his drinking partner. 'I think that's what Cindys letter was about as well.'

'What, needing some space? Let's hope there's enough of the stuff to go round, it being in such demand these days. Ready for another?'

As they fell to hard drinking and weighty philosophising the band, a country and western group, tuned up as a few more punters shuffled in. Alan nipped up and back for their third round before the place filled up and was about to ask Steve if he thought male/female relationships were basically doomed when the band kicked off with 'Stand By Your Man'. They sat in silence through a better than might have been expected 'Wichita Lineman' – the lyrics bringing poignant thoughts to both – and a few more Cowboys laments then found themselves applauding with feeling. 'Good stuff.' Bawled'. Steve above the din.

'Yeah.' Said Alan as the musicians left the stage. 'Those songs aren't as daft as they sound are they?'

'Aren't they?'

'Well it must be hard to be a woman, sometimes – you know they only have two arms to cling to, most of them, but there are more of us trying to catch on, at any one time, if you get me. No wonder she wants a bit of slack.'

'And I need you more than want you.' Said Steve as he peered into his drink.

'How do you mean? Love will tear us apart?'

ASK ME NOW

'Appen – it's my round isn't it? All you can do is take it on the chin and give them just a little more time, eh?'

Alan remembered how quickly his last big night out had gone west and resolved to make his fourth pint his last, or at least make it last. When Steve came back he opened up another subject. 'Has there been much comment at the Echo about Northfield and the general hoo-haa?'

'Yes, I meant to tell you about that, not much interest in the story, as known, just another cock up in Social Services seems to be the general view. But everyone in the news room was wetting themselves over Colin Clarks visit – made me sick; home town boy made good tapping up the local gumshoes, what a cunt, sitting there in his stupid trousers treating the hicks to some metropolitan gossip – 'I told Hislop to watch that one the other week' – your Mrs. Harvey will have to improve on her performance over last years lego in the lasagne shock horror though. He's a total arsehole but he could make trouble.'

But you're not jealous, thought Alan. 'Media nous isn't one of our strengths.'

'I could smarten you up there, I know all the tricks of our trade.'

'I did hear that Linda was up for a job in Communication Networks at TAT – I'll keep you posted.'

'Yes, do anyway, how are your lot dealing with it?'

'The usual, done naff all and hoped it would go away, which isn't always the worst policy except that it hasn't so now we're on the back foot shipping water like 'Dales defence. I've been roped in to collate and clarify perceptions – to try and help mollify the family.' He paused to take a big gulp of his Robbos' then paused a bit longer and thought sod it then went on to give his pal a complete debrief. Steve had to admit it made a good story.

'But you weren't involved in the original fandango were you?' Steve asked.

'No of course not.'

'So why is it on your desk now?'

'It isn't really. I mean I'm just part of the process, essentially.' Said Alan feeling on the back foot himself.

'Mmm.' Said Steve thoughtfully. 'I should watch your step if baggy trousers is in on it.'

Then the band came back on with some interesting news; the first set had been their usual gig but for this one they would be doing their tribute to Steely Dan. Think of us as Nearly Dan said the singer, an aging swinger with a Lovejoy perm and dodgy complexion. The guitarist looked about thirteen but he tore into 'Reeling In The Years' like Frank Zappa. By the time the got to 'Bodhisattva' the joint was jumping. 'Fuckin' great.' Yelled Alan.

'Yeah.' Croaked Steve. 'That kids got a big future.'

Alan found this greatly amusing and likened it to the night Chas Chapman 'discovered' Jimi Hendrix. 'It was Chas Chandler you sarky twat.' Advised Steve.

'We're gonna cool things down a bit now.' Said the singer, Bob. 'This is one of our favourites so don't forget – when the demon is at your door in the morning he won't be there no more, any major dude'll tell you and these major dudes are about ready, are we boys? Yes, here we go and thankyall most

ASK ME NOW

sincerely.'

'What's that berk on about?' Asked Alan.

'Summat to do wit' song – ready for t'last one?' Steve was well pissed.

Last ones before them they listened as the song unfurled. It sounded to be a plangent minor key thing with vocal harmonisation and tricky rhythms. They'd obviously worked hard on it and Bob the singer, who'd shown himself a capable enough shouter on the rockier numbers, now reproduced an engaging Todmorden James Taylor, and they could hear the lyrics. They made him moisten and think about Cindy, something about any minor world that falls apart falls together again. He hoped she was all right, wherever she was.

'You enjoyed that one.' Observed Steve.

'Eh?'

'You were miles away.'

The rest of Alan's weekend featured three close re-readings of Cindy's letter, a trip to Spotfields with Steve (0-1 'sack the board' jeered the fans) and a difficult Sunday brought about by the last look at that letter. Earlier analysis had brought him reassurance that he was doing the right thing by getting on as normal and giving her the time she needed. However, Sunday's perusal had sent him into a tailspin of panic. What if the whole thing was a lovers test? A variation on Hans Christian Whatsisname where the handsome prince had to win his lady's favour by trying as hard as he knew how to befit her needs? She'd been called Cinders – was he the slipper who was leaving it all perilously late in the day? There had been a bit of a mystery a couple of weeks ago when she couldn't find one of her walking boots on their way out, where could it be? They'd had to abandon their journey. Now it seemed that he must find it and then find her then it would all fit. He spent about twenty minutes giving serious thought as to how he would gain entry to her house – another fairytale touch – look out the missing boot then take himself off to Wales. Cindy would see the funny side, the boot would be on the other foot and love would prevail because by giving her the means to walk away he could be sure she'd come back. But then he'd all ready done that anyway, any major doodah could have told him. He made himself go for a calming walk to Burnaps Field and back then distracted himself with the papers and a phone call to his Dad who asked after Cindy. Steve had suggested another pint but Alan demurred and was glad when it came to it, Heartbeat, Match Of The Day Two and bath night seemed like the right decision.

He lay in bed and thought about it all. Was the demon still at his door? He washed down his tablets with some cranberry type juice from Londis and flipped through his Hipsters Guide To Hot Music as Tommy Turrentine blew his trumpet on the tape player. He looked him up and found that Tommy had an allusive style just this side of threnodic which contrasted nicely with the entry for fellow brass man Bill Hardman where it was felt that never was such a plethora of notes used to imply a climate of such unrelieved austerity. Elsewhere he learned that Bryan Spring was mercurial, E.O. 'Poggy' Pogson capable of crepuscular notions and Big Jay McNeely a braying volcano of existential lust.

He settled down for the night wondering about Poggy – a phrase like that could make him search out one of the records. Whatever such notions were he wanted one. He rubbed himself half-heartedly and thought about Cindy but there was nothing doing. What's there to be mixed up about, he thought? Why do they have to make such a song and dance about everything? None of this was helping his mood so he flexed everything else he could from top to toe and concentrated on the random image of a piece of cheese tied to a stick hanging in the rain against a neutral background.

ASK ME NOW

When this didn't work he imagined a plausible story for why the cheese was there but when Claire Todgers appeared in the narrative he gave it up as a bad job and curled into a ball. He knew how things hung with Cindy of course, he had to be strong, and for himself, no matter how it panned out. They wanted ideal Mothers too, Mothers milk ... ideal milk ...... in a pan.

His dreamscape was a windy and troubled place. He was at various points caught up in a cardigan of many colours, adrift in an abandoned city of singing dust and, most troubling of all, trying with an exquisite sense of thwarted application to make love with Barry Weatherall. God knows what else had cracked off, he thought when he came to, but it was enough to be going on with. He was supposed to be seeing him later in the day, what if he asks me to make myself comfortable? He got up quickly and dressed for a short power walk to Londis for his paper. He picked up a scotch egg while he was at it and munched as he enjoyed the silver tongued lashing Sarah Montague was dispensing to some junior twit put up by the Health Secretary to field the week's care in the community calumny. Alan marvelled at the bare faced fatuity of his pitch; lessons to be learned, changes to be made, must never happen again – vast majority of local services delivering best practice effective locally tailored services te tum te tum etc.

The wily Sarah hadn't finished with him though; would he care to comment on the remarkable story the local press in Ridsdale was breaking concerning less than best practice under the mental health act? The man from the ministry batted it away deftly enough being unable to comment on matters of a local nature then it was time for Gary with the sport. It was also time for Alan to choke on his breakfast, as he coughed up his cold egg into the sink he almost hoped he'd finally gone psychotic, it being preferable to believing that the listening audience had also heard what he had. It wouldn't be that bad if he had, come to think of it – he could live at The Lindens and claim benefit, roll cigarettes and wear tracksuit bottoms all day. Cindy could visit him. But it would and he couldn't even if nobody really knew which way madness lay, even in Ridsdale. Well, that was it, a proper lash up and no mistake, but not of his making, that much was clear. So how had the sodding Today programme got wind of it?

Nobody said anything much when he got into work. When he mentioned it to Graham he'd missed it and seemed more bothered about Gary with the sport – 'is it me or is he an unctuous berk'. He also enquired after Cindy.

'Why?' Asked Alan.

'Well … she phoned in sick.' He said.

'Oh yeah, she's gone down with something, all this business with her Mother has worn her down.'

'Right – well, give her my best wishes eh?'

'Graham I'm way over my head with all this – what if it gets out of hand?'

His colleague gave him another puzzled look but before he could come up with anything his phone trilled and he became lost to a tetchy exchange with someone from somewhere asking him to account for not having done something. This settled Alan down, made him feel that this was after all the natural order of things and was the way most Mondays began. This could mean that he was getting better or compelled to relive the last six months of his life sequentially until it was all over. So what had changed and should he do things differently? He walked over to his manager's office and shouted at her. 'Are you going to tell me what's going on?'

She put her hand over her phone and motioned him to sit down. 'I'm on with Linda Harvey.' She said and gave him a

ASK ME NOW

funny look. Alan felt daft and sat down as she continued. 'Right, so nothings attributable – I don't know where they got hold of it, no of course it wouldn't, nobody would be that stupid, not even Barry – okay, well … yes, yes, okay well – look, get back to me as soon as you've heard from legal section. Listen, Linda, thanks for that – we'll talk soon, yes – bye.' Well that was unexpected Alan,'

'Yes I nearly did for a scotch egg when I heard Sarah Autocue this morning.'

'I meant you coming in here like that, please don't do it again eh.'

'Sorry Val.'

'Yes well, we're all going to need calm heads now it's got out.'

'That Colin Clarke wants seeing to.'

'Calm heads Alan. Your money's on him then?'

'Well who else?'

'That's not the point, at the moment. From what Linda tells me we may be able to put the bite on this before it gets any legs. If it has come via the Ridsdale Echo – which it almost certainly has – she thinks she can shoot their fox. In the meantime I want you to see Barry again, now in fact, before any more turkeys come home to roost in the woodwork.'

He could tell she was properly rattled. 'I doubt he'll be expecting me this morning.'

'Just go will you, please.'

'Trouble mate?' Queried Graham when Alan returned to their office.

'Got her Turkey In The Straw again.' Graham smiled and took his leave. Alan found he was staring at Cindy's vacant chair thinking about his night out with Steve. He decided not to and left for Barry's place with Steely Dan grooving through old tunes in his head, Lena Martell coming in this week down at number three. Any major dude they sang. He'd heard that Jim Naughtie was much nicer in person.

'Greetings.' Bawled Barry. 'I bring you untapped memories and a glancing wasp-like mind. Come across the chrome plated portals of destiny.'

Wonderful thought Alan, three parts pissed at ten past ten. Maybe I can admit him informally when he comes down, then the whole thing could resolve itself. Sealed off safely by a social worker at the top of his game, it couldn't be any dafter than the story they were trying to make stick. He followed Barry in. 'Right cousin, what's yours?'

Sod it, he thought. Why not? 'What are you on then?'

'Special cider from One-Stop, he gets it in special. I doubt it's seen many apples but it does the trick – William Tells.'

'I should think it does – go on then, just a small one.' Barry handed him a can from the plastic bag by his chair. The tight pouncing quality of the rustle told him there were plenty more where it came from. Alan enjoyed the graphics on the tin; a grinning hayseed lay beneath an improbably groaning apple tree with a couple of green 'uns bouncing off his head. He didn't seem to mind – at 12% who would? 'I take it you heard the Today Programme.' He asked before his first fateful sip. He then glanced at the small print to see if it had been brewed by Glaxo but it didn't seem to have been brewed by anyone.

ASK ME NOW

'Yes indeedy.' Said Barry. 'Hence my need for Adams ale – they didn't mention anyone by name did they – I mean I don't think they did?'

'No Barry, no names were mentioned, definitely. But somebody from this end has been on to them, but nobody knows how much they know – if you see what I mean.'

Barry didn't. 'Well I'll be buggered' He said wonderingly.

Alan had a hair trigger memory of something unorthodox – a faint echo of a faint echo of something unexpected involving Barry. He bounced them into something different. 'How's your job going?'

'It wouldn't be our David.'

'You've told him?'

'Oh yeah, I tell him things – he was round during the week. Called unexpected like you, I think he was supposed to be somewhere else, you know, but it was good to see him. Got himself a new girlfriend, lovely lass, Dad's on the council, something to do with waste and such – you ever come across a fellow called Hubbard, I could tell you a tale or two about him ...'

Yes, thought Alan, but would it be right? He took a mighty pull on his Tell as Barry blathered on. The strange brew wasn't too bad once it began to work its effects. 'I've got a nice new girlfriend.' He felt moved to tell his host. This led on to a topic he might have seen coming; the former Mrs. Weatherall. He had to spend a further twenty minutes and open another can while Barry cried up her merits. He heard that Ella had been a remarkable woman; quicksilver yet solid, vulnerable but strong, unyielding though soft where it mattered, a will-o-the-wisp, a diamond in the rough and a wonderful Mother (though David had had his troubles) and did Alan know what Barry's biggest mistake had been?

'Sometimes we make mistakes without realising – these things are seldom meant.' Mused Alan.

'What things?' Said Barry suspiciously.

'The things you were talking about.'
'Our David? I don't think it could have been him. My moneys on this George Knowall from London who's been seen about the town. Up and down the City Hall and round the Echo's offices.'

'Colin Clarke.'

'Yes, I can't really blame him. If it was me I hope our David would go to bat .. then again he might make things worse. Never trust a journo. Alan, they rely on people telling them things.'

'What things?' Asked Alan as he struggled to catch Barry's drift.

'You got any kids Alan?'

'No.'

'But a nice new girlfriend like our David – now if he ever took to adultery there'd be some reckoning up to do.' He tossed aside his empty can and opened another directly. 'They need space don't they – I need you to give me some space, only they don't say how much or tell you when they've found somebody else to help them fill all that space. I was a bloody fool Alan, don't you be. When it's space they want make sure you see the brochure, put your return ticket in a safe place and don't lose it.'

ASK ME NOW

Alan was beginning to think he could learn something from the older man, he could see he wasn't going to get anything of value about Stanley and he was getting bored with it anyway. Having spent enough time in his company he could just about believe Barry's account and, in his rough-hewn way, Barry was a survivor – Alan wanted to know how it was done. He asked Barry if he'd seen any decent Morse recently. 'Had one on last night, it's generally a surprise even when I've seen them before. He likes his drink doesn't he, no good without his mate though.'

'Which one was it?'

'The one where Morse cops off and there's some funny business by moonlight in a boatyard. She blows him out at the end and Lewis saves the day.'

This sounded roughly like every episode Alan had ever seen; there was usually a spot of bother in a boatyard or a brewery with plenty of evil doings under dreaming spires and John Thaw behaving like a twit with some posh bit of fluff. 'He doesn't seem to be very lucky in love does he old Morse?'

Barry sniffed derisively at this. 'Well what with his 'Ring Cycle' and his real beer I don't suppose they want a second helping.'

'You don't think Women like Wagner then?'

Barry looked ready to nod off. 'Eh – how the devil should I know. Need a piss.'

Alan did too and put the kettle on while he waited his turn. Barry looked in on his way back and said 'good idea' indicating via a disturbing mime that he had satisfied his needs and that the bathroom was now free. Alan enjoyed having a nosey and after he'd finished in Barry's bathroom – functional B&Q – he slipped into the bedroom next door. Here he saw another television resting on a very nice pine cabinet, some clean white curtains falling to within half an inch of the sill and an exercise bike taking up most of the space by the double bed. His bedside reading turned out to be Tony Parsons. 'Shall I make us some coffee?' He asked when he came downstairs.

'Yes I suppose so.' Said Barry without much enthusiasm. He then surprised Alan by picking up the thread of their conversation. 'In my experience when they say they want more space it usually means a part of their lives, the bigger part, without you and there's nothing much you can do about it. I hope I'm wrong in your case but if I'm not it might be very little to do with you anyway. You're not shagging her special friend are you?'

'No, nothing like that.' Said Alan feeling appalled at the idea.

'I was, what a Wally. Biggest mistake I ever made. Told me she regretted losing her bessie mate more than me.'

'Are you involved with anyone now?'

'Sue Hubbard comes round to see me now and again but I think she's got someone else on the go at the minute.'

Well whatever floats your boat thought Alan before he changed tack, sensing rocks ahead. 'I think I've got all I need really for Stanley.'

'Will you keep me posted?'

'Yes of course.'

Alan reeled as the fresh air hit him and he realised he wasn't fit to drive. He hadn't a clue where the nearest bus stop was

ASK ME NOW

and wandered off in the general direction of where he thought the main road ought to be but Barry's manor seemed to be shaped like a maze and he couldn't seem to get very far no matter how far he walked. The coffee and fresh air were sobering him down and his mood was taking on a meaner aspect. He stopped at the end of Deepdale and fished out his phone, there were no messages or texts he might have missed. This pissed him off further then he had an idea; he called Becky at work who gave him the number for a taxi, within twenty minutes it was dropping him outside the offices of the Ridsdale Echo. 'Is Steve Goodlad available please?' He asked politely at reception.

'I'll just see if I can locate him. Who shall I say is calling?' asked the lad at the desk. He put through the call but reported that Mr. Goodlad was tied up at the moment.

'Would you mind telling him that this is important?' Pressed Alan. The lad looked a bit uncertain but had another word with the busy Mr. Goodlad. He looked relieved when he was able to advise the visitor that he would be down shortly. Alan thanked him and took himself over to the coffee machine by an incredibly swish looking sofa and made himself comfortable with a scalding cappuccino and last months 'Lancashire Life'. He judged the sofa to be better than anything he'd seen Linda Barker draped across and wondered how they afforded such high living. He scanned the magazine but couldn't find anything about Stanley Clarke in it, the main feature was a glossy photo-spread taken at Lord and Lady Gravyface's estate which he was enjoying until he came to the Hunt Ball where Boy Gravyface was showing off his fiancée who was a dead ringer for Cindy with hair extensions. I'm slipping he thought, I am.

'Aright mate?' Said Steve.

'No I'm not mate – enjoy your cornflakes this morning?'

'Toast and Marmite actually. Have you come here just to ask me that ... what did you have in your Earl Grey this morning.'

'All right smart arse, and no I haven't called just to ask you that. Did you catch the Today Prog.? No? Well there was a mention of queer practices in Ridsdale under the mental health act, how do you think they got hold of that? You do know some big noise from Whitehall got put on the spot over it and ...'

'He wasn't a big noise, just some junior Herbert, that's how seriously they take mental health stuff.'

'Right, so you did hear it – so you must know how this came to happen. I thought they were going to mention names, I don't think I'll be able to face Scotch Eggs again.'

'Alan sit down, you're pissed. Listen, it'll all have blown over by tomorrow, nobody's that bothered. You know that show they've got on at the moment, you know fly on the wall thing ... 'He's A Nutter He Is' well Figgy Foster beat up that bloke off that thing with Kate O'Mara, that's the only mental health issue anyone is interested in. I know this bloke in Lond ...'

'Fuckin' 'ell man, are you soft or what?' Alan's fleeting Geordiesque menace turned a few heads.

'All right, all right.' Said Steve. 'Look I'll come round after work – I can see where you're coming from but it wasn't me, not directly.'

'God you're learning the ropes sharpish – what exactly does that mean?' Sniffed Alan contemptuously. 'Pictures in the local rag, mentions on the John Humphries show – what's next, Vanessa Investigates? You lot have no idea of the effect your actions can have on people.'

ASK ME NOW

'Well we could all say that.' Countered Steve reasonably.

'Poor Barry Weatheralls a wreck, a sinking ship, a shadow of a man, a dried up hulk ready for the breakers yard. Your actions have holed him on his plimsoll line but who cares, eh?

Steve had turned tactfully away during this last bit and was biting his bottom lip and frowning when he turned to face his accuser. 'What have you been on this morning, we could give you your own column at this rate?'

Alan stood up at this in the manner of a man who had done enough straight talking and had reached the stage for plain speaking, with implied supplementary action of a non-verbal nature. The effect of this was dissipated when he bumped into the low coffee table and fell backwards into the sofa. 'Straight round after work then.' Said Steve as he backed away and through some doors with a security pad. The lad looked across at Alan who assured him it was all just a passing cloud and picked up the magazine to have another look at the Cindy Watson look-a-likee and avoid getting himself chucked out. He felt an even bigger berk than he had after waiving his briefcase at Val, it really didn't suit him, people could tell. He resolved to treat with Steve, as would a Roman fellow with a duplicitous senator – all patrician affront and pianissimo denunciation, all the more deadly for higher motivation and subtlety. He would take another drink and prepare his case. Then his mobile went and the lad gave him a disapproving look as he left the building.

'Miss Meating needs to talk to you as soon as possible – you didn't sign out. Where are you?'

'Okay, look, I'm over at the Echo so tell her I'll be in by three.'

'It's not that far is it?' She asked.

'Oh look, I'm having to walk. Tell Val I'll explain when I get in.'

There was a brief hesitation then she said 'All right then.'
The light outside sapped his spirits again so he checked his messages - not a sausage. He wanted to be in bed with her, the pair of them dozing on the edge of oblivion through a dull weekday afternoon. They could get up at teatime to watch tele. – all the crap – then go back to bed and in the morning all this would be there no more. All he really wanted to do was go to bed, the lad on reception would have done just as well for warmth and support right then, he was getting a bit tired of thinking about Cindy really. He felt she could be having similar thoughts about him, then there was all that carry on with her family – he could hardly blame her for being mixed up – maybe she'd got SIMON? So, the wise course was to take it on the chin and see what came next. This turned out to be a man in a van yelling 'arsehole' at him as he slammed all on to avoid flattening him outside PC World.

'Sorry mate.' Said Alan.

'Twat'. Said the man. Honour satisfied he pulled off shaking his head as Alan veered across the road and into the precinct, a soviet bloc building housing a thriving indoor market with many a temptation for fools and their money. To reach the bus station he had to pass Papa Joes books and records which also served as the unofficial connection point for the areas gay community – liberal attitudes taking time to bed down in the town. Alan, of course had sorted out views on these matters, also, the place was usually well stocked with must-haves so he took himself in and perused pop 'n rock under S. He didn't find what he wanted but thought he'd ask Joe, a droll character with a ready knowledge of a fellows requirements.
Alan strode up to the till. 'Can't Buy A thrill?' He said.

ASK ME NOW

'Oh don't give up yet Sir.' Said Joe blandly.

'Steely Dan.' Said Alan with a smile.

'Is this my lovely day?' Came back Joe with fluttered lashes and hand on heart in mock swoon. 'They say a hard man is good to find.'

Alan paused but made an effort to keep smiling. 'I think we could be at cross-purposes.' He said cautiously.

'We could be but I think you're after a record Sir.'

'Yes, yes – by Steely Dan, 'Can't Buy A … well you know.'

'You'll find it on CD over there, cheaper than vinyl.'

'Thank you, you're a major dude.'

'Only a fool would say that.' Muttered Joe as his saucy punter made for the other side of the shop.

Alan located the record but couldn't see the track he was after. He eventually spotted it on a 'Best Of' compilation and went back to make his purchase. Joe looked forward to seeing him again when he had a better idea of what he wanted. He passed on through to the bus station; the nearest point for the route passing Northfield lay on the far side of the place. Alan hadn't been to the bus station for years, it was another world; old people and Mothers with unruly kids stood around breathing in diesel or sucking on fags, most of the children seemed to be involved in a furtive fist fight with each other until their Mums shouted at them. The old 'uns looked happy enough grumbling away, he was sure he saw one of them poke a passing boy with a manky walking aid. The whole area was marked by oil stains and tatty green paint. He found his queue and took his place behind a pair of aging Ted's and was relieved when his bus pulled in, also chastened when the Ted's helped an old lady with a surgical boot to board and assisted with buggies. He found himself a seat by the window and made himself comfortable then the bus seemed to shrug and the engine died, then the driver got out. He drifted off into a nice doze then fell awake as the bus got underway and out into the light. 'Who's a dozy twat?' A child behind him asked.

'Look at that doggie.' Came the hurried reply.

Alan looked and noted a smaller, cross looking version of Cal Meating parking its backside on the pavement and refusing to budge despite the best efforts of an old lady with a lead. This is obviously the time of day when they come out he thought, then began to wonder what Val might want him for and how he might account for his car less trip into town. He tottered off his bus halfway down Wilson Street and cut through the playing fields leading to the hospital campus. He felt sure that he wasn't obviously drunk but headed directly for the toilets for a modest wash and brush up. By the time he was busy at his papers he thought he might be able to wing it. Then his phone went and Becky advised him that Mrs. Briscoe wanted a word. He frowned and tried to make sense of this. 'Mrs. Briscoe?'
'Yes, Judith Briscoe. I think you saw her last year, anyway she'd like a word.'

'Right, yes – well put her through.'

Alan registered a tremulous hello then remembered; he'd only seen her twice then she'd cancelled and missed a follow up. 'Is that Mr. Duright?'

'Yes, how are you Mrs. Briscoe?'

'I don't know – can we get together?'

ASK ME NOW

At this point he became aware of Val hovering outside the doorway and nodded briskly to her in the manner of a busy team player who has his tasks well in hand. 'By all means – would Wednesday or Friday do, morning or afternoon? Val came over to him and cautioned that Friday afternoon should be kept clear. 'Wednesday at ten then – how are things going?'

'I don't know – not too well. I'll tell you on Wednesday

Val had waited until he'd finished. 'Come across Alan – you were with Barry a while, he must have given you plenty to think about. Listen, there have been some developments.' Alan sat down and she swivelled on her chair to face him with her hands on her knees. 'Well, whatever you said to Helen Chadderton had the desired effect.'

'Oh.' He said. 'Why ... what's happened?'

'They want to come in to talk to us, on Friday afternoon. You left a favourable impression on her – she's told Linda Harvey that Colin will do as he's told regarding the media but that the Today thing was nothing to do with them – apparently it's not very clever to go straight to the top with these things because it makes the beeb look daft if you can't make it stand up, as Linda puts it, and it also gives your opponent a moral advantage. Don't ask me why. So, whoever was behind that, and whichever clot told them, we can leave till later. The director has spent all day mollifying elected members and soft-soaping the local MP ... someone's for the high jump over this. What do you think?'

'Well these things are seldom intended, are they – I mean the way we live now and all that, hasn't Figgy Foster gone AWOL from that thing on BBC 2? People are much more interested in things like that ... I think, don't you?'

She looked at him carefully. 'Are you all right with this three days a week arrangement, I'm conscious that this unfortunate business has gathered pace?'

'Oh fine, you say they want to talk?'

She was still looking at him thoughtfully. 'Yes ... yes, she and Colin want to talk with you and I and Barry Weatherall. You and he seem to have engaged positively, what on Earth did you find to talk about today?'

'Well Stanley obviously, I think we've got him pretty well covered.'
'Good, that's essentially what we need.'

'And then general and domestic – Barry is an interesting man, he seems to be missing his wife also – you know who his son is don't you?'

'Yes, you told me. Barry's difficulty runs in the family, as for his marriage the general view is that she should have dumped him years ago ... I'm sorry, I can see you've taken a liking to him. Anyway, do you think he'll mind his manners on Friday?'

'Yes, I said I'd get back to him as soon as I knew more.'

'Fine, let's get that over and done with then we can root out our little mole. This really is like John LeMesurier isn't it?'

Alan laughed. 'Yes I suppose it is.'

Val continued and he tried not to think of Hattie Jacques. 'Well have a word with your man and produce him on Friday – if we're lucky we might just swing this one. You've worked well there I think, who was your call from?'

ASK ME NOW

'Oh a lady I saw briefly last year – wants to come in again, sounds like she's gone down bank a bit.'

'Ah, well next week we ought to look at building your caseload up a bit. I gather Cindy's not well?'

'No, it's all been a bit of a strain for her, what with her Mum and everything.'
'Well tell her not to hurry back – and well done Alan.'

He took his leave convincingly enough but once he was alone in his office it all came apart. He kicked his swivel chair then sank into Cindy's feeling blocked and bloated, self-disgust soured by slow drip misanthropy silted him up. The rest of his day looked pretty stale and unpromising, but how was he doing? Two months ago he'd never have managed all that, but was this a good thing? And how was he going to get home? He brooded anew on the sadness of his life then phoned Barry. All he got was the answer phone so he left a message about Friday and hoped Barry hadn't made a day of it. They'd both need to look sharp. He took another look through Stanley's old file which made him feel worse; listening to Helen had brought it all to life – the pathos, her anger and his own recognition of the other mans experience, here in the dull buff official file it was just another section baldly – and badly – written up with the minimum of expressivity or warmth. It could have been anyone, the paper clip had rusted on the report leaving an unpleasant yellow trace across the S in Stanley. Nobody expected Tony Parsons but they should be able to do better than that. He walked up the road and back for some air then it was about time to go, he headed for the bus stop and eventually caught a ride into town where he made directly for the Blacksmiths Arms to order a chicken tikka harvester with seasoned fries. Dave wasn't behind the bar but the lass who was advised him there'd be a wait so after a decent pause he asked for a pint of Pugwash and sat toying with the Indie' crossword till his tea turned up.

The beer was a guest ale – 'a hoppy session bitter with a salty aftertaste to shiver your timbers' and he had to admit that it slipped down nicely enough, certainly an improvement on the muck his host had served up earlier in the day. He felt his mood lifting and tucked into his tikka that turned out to be a traditional burger with some sauce, and none the worse for that. He got a couple of clues as he ate then decided to wash it all down with a small Pug that he upgraded to a pint at the last minute. He could walk home, plenty of time, sod Cindy – with any luck Claire Todgers would have a bad dose of cystitis and their holiday would be a washout. He continued with the crossword with the air of a man quite at ease with the world, enjoying his early doors pint, looking ahead with quiet anticipation to whatever the evening might bring.

'Have they moved you to the back pages now?' Scoffed an unwelcome voice.

'Eh?' Alan looked up, struggling to place it.

'Your lot at Northfield. Typical press coverage – make a right meal over that but ignore local issues that matter to local people.' Barry Bishop sat down beside Alan. 'Fifteen across is bemused, did it at lunchtime.' Alan looked at him quizzically. 'Bemused – like you and our mutual friend Barry Weatherall.'

'Ah, thank you.' Was nothing safe in this town and was Councillor Bishop a man of discretion? 'Well, I don't suppose the Independent will pick it up, do you?

'Hard to say, someone told me it was on Richard and Judy.'
'The Today programme.' Said Alan with crossed fingers.

'All the same. Anyway how did they get hold of it? That's what I'd like to know – Barry wouldn't blab.' He undercut this a bit by letting on that the other Barry had told him all

ASK ME NOW

about his connection with Alan at the last Labour Group social. 'He's all right is Barry.' Said Barry. 'I dare say they'll be wanting a scapegoat for it all, is your Mrs. Meating on the case?

'Val? Yes she is – we're hoping to draw a line through it as soon as we decently can then curve the learning procedure.. so to speak.'

Barry looked at him a bit gone out. 'She still got that great mutt?'

'You what?' Asked Alan with some feeling.

'Val Meating – has she still got her large dog?'

'Oh Cal, yeah – he's a great soft brush he is.'

'He's a dirty great shit machine that's what he is. A mate of mine on dog wardens nearly had her one night – he's got a little list, and she's on it.'

Alan felt glad of his second Pugwash. 'He's got a what?'

'A list of miscreants and muck spreaders – the dog shit in this town is disgusting. Why won't the echo get its teeth into that eh? Do you know the figures, the sheer tonnage of it all? And your Mrs. Meatings lovable old lion leaves his fair share be in no mistake on that score, I'd love to get my hands on …'

'I don't think you should be getting these issues round your neck like this. I know that Val takes a plaggy bag out with her, as do most responsible …'

'Doesn't always, been caught on camera. It's only a matter of time now, we're getting very close.'

Alan had swallowed the last of his drink and was getting ready to go but he nearly brought it back at this. 'You what, your mate is actually going out filming folk?'

'Only way to nail 'em, catch them and their adorable charges doing their business – it all goes through the proper channels you know, Police liaison are right behind us. We're going for a hard line name and shame policy soon.'

Alan was incredulous by now. 'You're having a laugh more like, the council would never …'

'Well actually they would, what's interesting about our Council is that they actually listen to what the electors tell them, what they feel passionate about.' Christ, thought Alan, not the things that people feel passionate about – in no time there'd be a UDI for the return of capital punishment in Ridsdale then a declaration of war with Wigan, were all Barry's bonkers? Was he fated to spend all day drinking with them. 'Time for another one? Asked the fiery Councillor.

This was to be a pivotal point in Alan's day, possibly his life. Barry Bishop might as well have been got up in a red silk body stocking with horns, cloven shoes and a large fork all set to tempt our daft lad. He thought about this but it was an easy one. 'Why not?' He said.

'Right, what are you one?'

'I've been drinking that Pugwash, it's quite nice actually.'

'Mmm, they do another one, Tarbrush. Fancy some of that if they've got it on?'

'Yeah all right.' So that would be one more after that to keep them on terms, he checked the time, it was six thirty. He checked his phone messages, dream on they said. He sought comfort in Val's good opinion of his work with Helen

ASK ME NOW

Chadderton and decided to tip her off about Barry's secret agent. He also wondered what else he might learn if he could get his new friend off dogs and their doings.

'There you are.' Said Barry. 'And good health to you sir.'

Alan realised straight off that this was a much stronger brew than the other one, practically a winter warmer. He put down his glass and smacked his lips like a conneosier. 'Not a bad drop, what did the write up say?'

'Eh? Oh there wasn't one just a skull and crossed bones on the pump – I think the strength of some of these real ales is over rated myself. A bit like the civic responsibility of pet owners …'

'Is there much undercover activity in other areas of the councils work?' Alan asked quickly.

'Rubbish.' Said Barry firmly and took a long drink of his Tar. 'Big stuff afoot there. There was this fellow used to fly tip down the canal, it probably took him more time and trouble than if he'd bothered to dispose of his household detritus in the correct manner, but no, he'd come out of his back door with it, all bagged up neatly mind, and lob it down the bank. What a dirty idle bastard eh?'

'So you staked him out and what, caught him at it?'

'It's not that straightforward, stakeouts are a piece of cake, no, what's needed is documentary verification but this was one botched operation and no mistake.' He took another thoughtful draught of Tar.

Alan was beginning to enjoy himself and reflected that it really was like John LeCarre with him as the patient spy master in some sleazy safe house near Finsbury Park plying a burnt out case, finding out exactly what did happen on operation botch up. Barry was the hapless placeman who'd seen too much pain and just wanted to be left alone with a bottle of Petrograd paint stripper, soon, very soon the questions would stop and Barrisov would sleep the sleep of redemption but first he must cleanse himself of what only he could tell. 'I knew it was going tits up when me and the photographer took up position on the tow path – some pillock had let his dog dump and with it being dark – anyway I was cleaning myself as best I could when we heard his back gate. I gave the photographer the thumbs up but the daft sod let his flash go off at me just as our tipper swung his sack. Of course he clocked what was going on and heaved it at me, I fell back in the shit and the cameraman got me. Swore afterwards it was a mistake reckoned the chap had been tipped off ha ha. Anyway the bloke had the nerve to call us a pair of weirdo's and threatened us with the Police. What a bloody caper – but I can't tell you how satisfying it is when you get it right.'

Alan finally thought of something to say. 'Do you get a hard wearing clothing allowance when you're in the field?'

'You must be joking, but that was one job when I really did need a debrief.' They laughed together at this and spent the rest of that pint sharing humorous tales from their various corners of public service. Alan took care to be more circumspect than of late but Barry was on cracking form when he began to break the thirty-year rule concerning Parks and Gardens.

'I suppose that shed should have its own preservation order.' Remarked Alan after a scarcely believable account of fast love in wartime. 'Shall we have one more for the road?'

'Go on.' Said Barry with mock reluctance. 'Another touch of the Tarbrush eh?'

Alan got them in and by the time they'd polished them off

ASK ME NOW

both were well gone. He was impressed that throughout their little session Barry Two had not raised anything concerning Barry One or tried to pump him in any way, as far as he could remember. They'd ended up talking the night away along familiar lines; national politics – Blair a twat, and national football – Sven a baldy twat - before agreeing to split a taxi home, Alan living roughly half way between town and 'Bishops Palace'.

Alan's psycho-chemical profile had been delicately balanced since his first taste of Tell that morning; by now it was a terrorist zone of bilious belligerence. As they set off he looked out of the taxi's window. 'Look at that arsehole.' He said to Barry and indicated a blameless pedestrian crossing the road. His fellow passenger didn't react beyond pulling out his paper and by the time he was ready to be dropped off Alan found himself wondering why you bothered trying to make conversation with some people. Barry bade him a fond farewell then Alan remembered another conversation he was keen to make with someone else. He marched through his main door with an air of bloated affront and knocked on Steves, when there was no answer he knocked harder and called his friends name. Then he shouted and knocked. 'I know you're in there you know so I'm not going till we've sorted this out – you devious sod – you took advantage of me when I was vulnerable – you knew I didn't know what I was doing you know, or saying (further loud knock) – you took me in and shafted me for your own (kick) amusement.' He felt his anger building and his stomach churning. 'Come out you using bastard, had what you wanted and now you don't want to (kick) fucking (harder kick) know. I'm gonna do you, you silver tongued shitbag – you've made a fool of me. Open this fucking door Steve before I kick it in (big kick).' At this point he became aware of a figure hovering behind him near the stairs. Right, he thought and wheeled round ready to apply maximum verbal violence.

Mike Pearson

'Hi.' Said Cindy. 'How're you doing Alan?'

Before he could speak the shock, Tarbrush, rubber chicken and all hit critical mass. 'bleuurrrrgfuckblarrrrke.' Vomited Alan, quite a bit over her bare leg. She went up a couple of steps and sat demurely while he crouched on the bottom one mewling and pewking some more.

Then Steve skipped lightly up the steps and in to the hall. 'What happened to you mate?' He asked.

ASK ME NOW

NEVER MET A GIRL LIKE YOU BEFORE

It was the early hours of the morning after the night before. Alan woke on a cold guilt rinsed world where there was a little man in dirty overalls pulling rusty cables around the inside of his head, his belly was bloated with graveyard gas from the year of the plague and Nigel Harding was chuckling with anticipation of the fun to come from this unexpected turn of events. Oh what a time there was going to be. Worse than this, he was able to recall most of what had happened after he'd offered up to Cindy the contents of his stomach. He had at least managed to ask after her mother once he'd composed himself; it seemed she was unlikely to see out the week and Cindy had been waiting for him to come home for about an hour. Steve had been all understated capability and not-to-worry as he'd busied himself with mop and bucket, thus nailing his guilt in Alan's eyes. He hadn't said anything at the time and wondered if he should now.

There had been a brief but encouraging time together up in his rooms for he and his troubled lover, leaving him with enough traces to build his hopes up; she'd held his hand and would probably have embraced him if it hadn't been so obviously out of the question, he'd refrained from blubbing lachrymosity and shown a proper concern for her difficulties and the need to get away with Claire. She'd made some tea and there'd been a fond farewell with a firm arrangement to get together after his big day with destiny. She'd kissed him on the forehead but held him at arms length; again, he couldn't fault her for that. She'd also said 'thanks Alan' and smiled enigmatically when she left. As with the letter, it didn't do to linger on the detail.

Alan managed to pull through his hangover but couldn't get her or Friday out of his thoughts for long during the next couple of days. He had Steve up for a pot of 'Cutie' and they'd come to an understanding about the medias fleeting concern with local matters, which seemed to have abated; it was best forgotten, Alan having more to lose than Steve, who hadn't really thought it through and as journalists were a misunderstood lot like social workers, just people trying to do a decent amount of good in a bad world, they should stick together and feel sadder but wiser. Also, now that Helen Chadderton seemed to have hosed down her brother, it looked as if they might get away with it.

So, he'd pondered at some point on Thursday morning, was he boxing clever? Was he Henry Cooper or Herbie Hyde? Ready with the big one or rolling on the ropes? It seemed to him he could go the distance but did he have enough points in his locker? An image of Cindy suggested itself – she stood facing him across an ill-defined boxing ring with a neutral expression and silk gown wrapped tight, she was wearing boxing gloves and looked uncertain about whether she was about to undo her gown or clock him one. He wasn't sure if she had kinky boots on and made an effort not to pursue this. At least he'd managed to push Nigel Harding to a place in his head where he couldn't hurt him so much but Nige was a sly beggar and Alan knew to keep a weather eye out for his old friend, but for now the mocking voice of his internal persecutor was stilled. It was a tricky one though; like many an old friend Nigel served his function well enough – the adaptive muscle of his existential anxiety, useful at times of uprooted tent pegs and great fear. Nigel might be horrible but he kept what could be worse at bay, just. And Alan knew that when things were at their worst there was always something worse, but maybe not at the moment. These reflections shocked him sometimes, he knew they were not unprecedented – in its extreme forms it might be what people called schizophrenia, and he'd been a bit mad all right – some folk hacked away at bits of their bodies, others did it with their thoughts. Could knowing why stop it? Would there always be something more to come? What was he so scared of? These and related questions occupied him for a while during the early evening as 'Fred Hersch Plays For Lovers'

ASK ME NOW

deconstructed familiar melodies in the background. Steve knocked on the door and said. 'Shall we dance?'

'Eh?'

'Fancy a pint?'

'You're not worried that people will say we're in love?' Said Alan deadpan.

'Very good, you could almost say I'm getting to kn .. '

'Yes, but then again you might not, anyway there's this new pub I've found.'

They walked out into the summer evening light and Steve laughed as their little rap reminded Alan of his recent encounter with Papa Joe and he related the whole thing now that they were mates again. After a couple of pints and semi-serious talk about those things of which a chap may not easily speak they sauntered back with many a chuckle along the way. He went to bed that night feeling that there were times when things didn't need to matter so much.

This was something he tried to formulate the next morning with Mrs. Briscoe as she took her seat in one of the interview rooms at work. 'I don't know why I've come really.' She said. He waited then asked her if she'd been feeling poorly again. She thought then said. 'No, not really.'

'But you must have felt you needed to come in again for some reason – did you find it helpful last time?'

'Yes, yes I did really. I can't remember much about it – you told me I must take the tablets.'

Alan hoped he'd said a bit more than that. She'd come along

twice then missed an appointment and phoned to say she was better. He'd dropped her a line three months later but hadn't heard from her and forgotten about it. He could recall a distant husband and a disabled Mother living nearby. Her daughter had left. They must have talked about that, something must have clicked. 'Are you still on medication Mrs. Briscoe?'

'I stopped them then I felt rough so I started them again.'

'Did you go to see Dr. DeParis?'

'No, he had me on a repeat prescription.'

'So, how've you been recently then?'
'I don't know – I'm all right really, it's just – I can't see the point anymore. It's not like I'm as bad as I was before – I think I should be happy but I can't see why. Have they got a pill for this?'

'No but that suggests the problem might be in the world, around you not in you, if you see what I mean.'

She sat calmly enough as he said this, then someone through the thin wall said 'psycho' then she said. 'You can't tell me what the point is can you, there just doesn't seem to be anything. I never used to be like this.'

He made an effort not to say the first thing that came into his head. In the old days Mrs. Briscoe would have gone to the local Priest, there would be an understood ritual of some kind involving wise counsel, confession and the promise of forgiveness if she tried harder to love a lousy husband and moany mother, and not miss her girl. Except that back then being stuck together like her lot weren't anymore would have been the norm so you wouldn't have felt that bad about it all and your children wouldn't go far away. Now we were all free of that and free to wonder what the point was. None of this

ASK ME NOW

would help her now – things were as they were and tended to evolve that way didn't they? 'Are you saying that the way you feel now isn't normal for you?'

'I don't know, I don't think I know what is normal for me.'

'Well perhaps it's normal to feel bad if what's been happening to you has been painful.'

'I used to be all right.'

'What do you think has changed for you?'

She looked at her shoe and her breathing grew faster. He felt like a prat, she fished out an old fashioned hankie and cried for a while. 'She never phones or anything now, I don't know what's happening to her. Why should she though? I never wanted her tied to me, I wanted her to get away – what if she has a baby? She used to make me laugh telling me the names she would call them all when she was little. They grow up in a funny way now.'

'How is your own Mother? I can remember you telling me about her, she was quite poorly, lived nearby.'

'We had to get her into a home – that was another bad do.'

'So at home now there's you and your husband?'

'Just me and Tex.'

He remembered now, how she'd sketched out a mans man with a peevish personality, a grafter, a bit on the mean side. Ran his own garage and went to the pub. Whatever conclusions a fly on the wall at their house would come to it was clear enough that he'd made her unhappy and that it seemed to have got worse. 'Does your husband know how you've been feeling?'

'He tells me I'll get over it then goes to work at seven 'o clock every morning. He doesn't know I've come here today.'
'How would he feel if he knew, do you think?'

'That it's all in my head, that I've got nothing to fret over, that I think too much. He hasn't much time for your lot, he thinks people are like cars – probably thinks I'm clapped out or just need a fresh set of spark plugs.'

This rang a dim bell for Alan but he let it pass. 'Well if something is in your head, in your thoughts, then it's in you isn't it? It's real for you – it might be frightening but it's normal …'

Mrs. Briscoe bridled at this. 'So you're telling me there's nothing the matter as well then. Should I count my blessings and look a little on the sunny side or should I tell you the next bus to Bacup's got my name on it and do you the coconut shake? Would you know what to do with me then?'

'No, no I didn't mean that. I was trying to normalise your experience, I mean that the bad things you're struggling with may be the result of a loss you've felt unable to bear – what seems to happen is …'

'I miss our Linda and he's no good at what he calls the lovey dovey stuff unless … and then he'll talk to me afterwards, but he still doesn't get it. He tells me she'll be all right – what about me? Some days I just sit.'

'Are you still at the library – I remember you used to like that?'

'No, I'm off work – not that I miss it. I can't see me back there in a hurry.'
'I hope you don't mind me asking, but have you lost weight

ASK ME NOW

recently? Also, has your sleep pattern been disturbed?'

'Well I'm not eating but I haven't bothered to weigh myself. I get off all right but I'm wide-awake by five and I can't get back off. That's the worst time.'

His stomach shifted in sympathy; metaphysical angst. How many fellow delicates were awake around the world then? Lying there with the collywobbles too scared to get up, terrified to stay put. Was there any comfort in this, the numbers, the weight of human suffering? A there's-a-lot-of-it-about line never really worked for Alan because he knew that there were always far more undepressed people about, so why couldn't he be one of them? Why couldn't Mrs. Briscoe? He knew of course; experience, what happened to happen – life as a game of dominoes, you did your best with the hand you got but if you weren't given the right little dots early enough in the game you were bound to struggle later on.

'Yes, that must be awful but I think we can help. There's no doubt that you're passing through a period of depression and that the medication will help you. I think it would also help if you felt able to think out loud about your feelings in a safe setting. Coming here could help that to happen, in a safe setting, with me or somebody else if you'd prefer.'

'Talk about my feelings? In a safe setting?'

'People often seem to find it helpful.' She seemed dubious but he put this down to the nihilistic affect of her condition – he shouldn't expect her to be too enthusiastic about anything, let alone talking to a social worker, but he knew she'd get better. 'I'd say it's about working out what your depression means to you and how to stop it hurting so much.' He'd honed his little homily over the years and it had proved serviceable enough at the shall we dance stage.

'I saw you before, I may as well see you again – saves having to tell the tale all over again.'

Fair enough, thought Alan, she couldn't see the point but she'd give it a go. Between them they might look out for hope. They agreed not to embark on the journey of discovery as mapped out by Alan today but between now and next week she could give some thought to what she wanted to say. The rest of their time together was taken up looking at how she was coping, practical measures and how much she'd withdrawn and cut herself off from the people around her. This took them up to the hour and they parted with him feeling that she thought she'd been taken seriously at least.

Graham had been screening a new referral that morning and Alan met him as they passed along the corridor. 'Ah Dick, how's tricks?'

'Oh, you know – got the Barry Weatherall road show this aft.'

Graham shook his head. 'Just seen a right one there. GP's refered him for the anger management group – the guy's up in court next week for laying out a policeman. Apparently there was a proper how-de-do outside the Four Horsemen the other week. You weren't involved were you?'

Alan ignored this. 'So, if he's connected to this place he must have issues so the court will have to adjourn for a report – nothing to do with him being a pissed personality disorder.'

'He told me they pushed him about.'

'Don't blame them – waste of everyone's time. Did he tell you he was on a learning curve and wanted closure?'

'He said it was doing his head in and he was shit scared of prison.'

ASK ME NOW

'Oh well, there's some hope for him.'

Graham looked sideways at Alan. 'You're uncharacteristically cynical this morning.'

'I'm sorry, it's this Barry business, it's doing my head in.'

'Do you fancy a drink after work?'

'No thanks, I'm seeing Cindy.'

'Oh right, is she better?'

'Yeah – listen, remind me to tell you about my happy hour with Barry Bishop sometime.'

'You can tell me know if you like, a happy hour with him should be worth hearing about.'

Then Val appeared to request 'just a quite word' with Alan. He followed her into the bunker and saw that she was doing a minimalist variation of the hidden scuttle. 'Alan, this business on the Today programme appears to have come via the Echo and we need to get something straight before this afternoon. Was it you?'

'Yes.' He said smartly.

'Right.' Said Val. 'Okay, fine. So what happened?'

'A friend of mine works there – some sort of rookie reporter – we got talking, I don't think it was him who ...'

'It wasn't. Linda Harvey managed to get to the bottom of it all and pulled a flanker in somebody's good offices so it's been put to bed.'

In somebody's good offices presumably. He didn't think he could decipher the rest of it but was glad he'd done his George Washington with the cherry tree bit, it being obvious that Val had worked it out anyway. 'Put to bed you said?'

'Yes, the Echo declined to verify the story because Colin Clarke got right up the editors nose and thanks to your other contribution to the proceedings the sister, who seems to be a fount of good news, has told him to wind his chin in – so that's all straight forward. You told your mate then?'

'Yes.'

'And he told someone else?'

'Yes.'

'Oh well, that's that then, let's see how we do this afternoon. How are you feeling anyway Alan? I'm glad you've been able to give your energies to this, it's turned into a right Fred Karno's and no mistake.'

Alan suddenly realised why Val's occasional malapropism had been bothering him of late. He thought she might be developing SIMON. 'Oh yeah, good – er, who is Fred Karno, is he in legal section or something?'

'Fred Karno ran a circus – my Father used to talk about him, same as Joe Baksi – he was a boxer.'

'Right. How's Cal?'

'I think he's depressed. He's got hard pad and struggles getting about.'

'He won't be getting out for his walk then?'

'No, has to go in the garden. He doesn't like it but it comes to

ASK ME NOW

us all.'

'Good, I mean it's good he's so well looked after – there are some funny people on the streets these days you know.' He said in his best thinking-of-you tones then Linda Harvey stuck her head round the door in the manner of someone at the BBC in the days of Joe Baksi, long before the Today programme was thought up. He'd never seen any pictures of Daphne Oxenford but just at that moment he thought she must have looked like Linda with her tight curls and red lippy. She smiled winningly and asked Val if she was ready.

'Oh yes, come in. Just need to clear a few things with Linda, Alan.'

He took this as his exit line and rejoined Graham in their office. Paul South from social inclusion was telling Graham something and Alan came in at the end of one of his amusing stories – 'got off with a bollocking from County Hall instead.' Southy was a terrible gossip and Alan couldn't help wondering why he was over at Northfield, he looked like Jack Nicholson but talked like Jack Shit, what was he doing cosying up to Graham?

'All right Paul, visiting the socially excluded?'

Graham stopped giggling. 'He's just been giving me the full SP on the mysterious affair at Woodcock's.'

'The what?' Said Alan

'That swanky health club by Dixon's, I'll tell you when you spill the beans on Councillor Bish.'

Their visitor took an interest here. 'Barry Bishop – the drinking mans John Prescott – what's he been up to?'

'Nothing really.'

Oh, right.' Said Paul. 'I'll get off but remember Graham, if you ever find yourself in the Jacuzzi at your local health club next to the directors daughter – just say no.'

'What a lad.' Said Graham after he'd gone. 'You couldn't make it up.'

'You don't think he does?'

'Not that one, and before you ask, I know nothing about Stanley, Barry or Uncle John Humphries and all, and no, he didn't ask. Probably too upmarket for Paul, he's strictly red top.'

Alan was too keyed up to be that bothered but he did remember what he wanted to ask his pal. 'Graham, what's domino theory about?'

'It's about how things fall against one another generating an accelerating process of chaos and collapse, scary really. Have you ever seen it done on telly – they line them all up and bingo.'

'Oh, right. Anyway I'm off for a walk before I fetch Barry.'

'Good luck matey.'

Alan's walk of preparation took him on a rough circuit round the playing fields then through a hole in the fence into Vernon Street, a well preserved plot of pre-war semis, the kind of place where you might find a my-pink-half-of-the-drainpipe arrangement though most of the runnels and guttering were black plastic. He saw this as a quieter sign of the times where individuality and self-assertion had retreated further indoors and out of sight. A man about his own age ran past in jogging gear, he looked so fit and determined making Alan aware of

ASK ME NOW

his fogeyish mullings and corduroy modes. He decided on a power walk to the chippy on Littleworth Street, if he hit top gear on the way back to work he could eat them off a plate then nip for Barry. He hoped his side-kick hadn't been to One-Stop that week.

The bloke at the chippy wore a glazed look as he dealt with a pack of feral school kids all swearing and gobbing on the pavement outside. Alan did his Roland Barthes bit with the stuff on the wall; this time the fish and chips equals a shag one was on its own – the couple were in bed and he was feeding her a sausage.

'Been to Jamie Oliver's then?' Quipped Becky as he passed through reception with his lunch in a flimsy blue carrier.

'Yeah, part of my fitness programme.'

'Keep fat eh, oh Alan, there's a message for you.'

As she passed him the slip of paper his bowels shifted; he knew it was going to be Cindy cancelling so he looked away from her. It was Barry saying he'd been delayed by something so could Alan call fifteen minutes later than planned. This made him edgy in another way. 'Was this all he said?'

'Yes, he sounded a bit muddled though.'

'Puddled?'
'No, just a bit ... distracted.'

This was less bad but Barry was a worry, Alan knew in his bones that he was going to raise a few eyebrows before day was done. What if all this stress had brought on some SIMON? He toyed with the notion that this could be turned to advantage if the Clarke's were to see for themselves the soft bugger in extremis, but this was foolish stuff, just the kind of nonsense social workers were apt to cling to in a crisis. It might wash but it wouldn't stick. He got himself a plate and tried to relish his spring roll and chips – it went down well enough then he found a spare can of coke in the kitchen fridge. Saint Jaime was all very well but he couldn't help sympathising with those fuckoff mums stuffing their kids with chips through the railings. Cindy had observed one day that he rarely mentioned his own Mother and he'd given the game away by getting arsey with her. Had this been part of their problem? Mothers were just there weren't they? He remembered now how she'd nettled him by asking him if he'd told his Mother how ill he'd been, and then, reasonably enough, why not? He'd muttered something ridiculous about their not having that sort of relationship. What sort she'd asked? He didn't feel like talking about it and made matters worse by asking Cindy about her Father who'd succumbed to cancer when she was in her second year at Uni. She hadn't needed to respond to that and didn't which made him feel like a stupid boy with Mummy. It must be about something about all that to have mixed her up, it had been as bad a scene as they'd had. Mothers just were, the hands that rocked the what sit and kept the planet going, the Saintly tribe that lived on a hill just off to the side of all the mess men made. He sat back and tried to stop thinking, if his darling could step inside his head she'd certainly catch something to talk to Claire Todgers about. He wasn't coping well with any of this; the place was quiet, even for a Friday afternoon. He imagined the Winter Palace had been like this on the afternoon Kerensky called round, or had it been Lenin, either way a terrible beauty had been born that Friday right enough and another one was hatching for this one, and no mistake.

He checked the time and set off, leaving a note on Val's desk telling of their delay. There didn't appear to be a soul in the place and Becky was in the back office telling one of the junior doctors about her bunions. At fifteen after one Alan pulled up the collar on his jacket and got into Chandleresque mode taking the straight route across town, by forty after his

ASK ME NOW

cold blue Citroen pulled up by Barry's place. As Alan hit the street sudden wind whipped up waste paper, had it been Small Change who got rained on and had it been Sidney Greenstreet who shot him with his own forty-five? Only the good die young, but these were not mean streets, Gatsby wasn't floating in the pond in Barry's back garden and he was ready at the door as soon as Alan knocked. 'Sorry about the delay.' He said.

'Something come up?'

'Oh nothing really, just got something back to front.' He replied airily.

'I've let them know we'll be late.'

'Not a good start though, they'll think I've gone to the wrong meeting.'

'I don't think it's going to be too formal you know, more clear the air and come clean, lines be drawn lessons learned type thing.'

'And administer Barry's bollocking – who's going to be there?'

'Us, the Clarke's, Val and Linda Harvey.'

'What's she coming for?'

'Linda Harvey?'

'Yeah, loopy Linda – they should have kicked me upstairs as well into a silly job to keep me out of harms way. Christ it narks me the stuff some folk have got away with over the years – I'm the victim here you know. Linda pissing Harvey, little Miss Do-As-You-Would-Be-Done-By –you know how she got that job don't you?'

Alan was spared any further briefing from Barry by a large grey mutt lumbering into their path forcing him to break. He thought he'd hit the dog and got out but the animal was crouched by the kerb with it's big ears flapping, it got up to wag it's tail hopefully at him then, as Alan approached, it rolled onto its back so he stroked the proffered belly and clucked. Then a breathless youth ran up to question Alan's sanity and parentage for knocking down 'our Sandy'. The stupid creature didn't help matters by staying prone with its paws aloft in submission until Alan could explain himself properly. Honour satisfied the youth stayed his hand and Sandy sloped off after him.. 'Honestly.' He remarked to Barry when they had resumed their journey. 'Did you hear him – I was only trying to help?'

'Barry sniffed and gave a sagely sigh. 'Aye – makes you wonder why you bother.' There was nothing much to say after this so he had a rummage among Alan's tapes in the doorframe. He pulled one out and waived it with a questioning look. Alan nodded so in it went – the tape was about half the way through The Glasgow Improvisers Collective Play Rogers And Hammerstien; the unchained melody of 'I Have Dreamed' could be just about apprehended within a sounds- cape of building site bally-hoo and orphic rumblings. Barry seemed to like what he'd heard so far and turned it up … 'I have dreamed of a tra la crash bang I have fwah screech pling and when lovers bang bang bang they can (rubbato crescendo). 'They're comedians this lot, our David likes this sort of thing you know, it's certainly different. Who's that fellow with the plastic bassoon?'

'You mean Ornette Coleman?'

'That's him – he's a funny one too, makes his own jackets.'

Does he wondered Alan. They weren't far from Northfield

ASK ME NOW

and Barry was happy to let the matter rest, tapping the dashboard speculatively to 'No Other Love' scored for bagpipe and massed glockenspiels. It was two twenty when they pulled in to the car park. 'Do you feel ready for this?' He asked Barry.

'Don't know – do you?'

By two thirty they were sitting in one of the interview rooms with tea, biscuits, the Clarke's and Linda Harvey. Val had been called away to a phone call so toothsome small talk was the order of the day. Barry rose to the occasion with a plaintive pitch around the theme of how much work still needed to be done in gaining public understanding of the realities of mental illness. Perhaps some of his piece grew a bit reckless when he opined that it would help if practitioners focussed on 'best practice' and took on board the views of service user movements. Helen and Colin listened politely though Linda looked anxious and tried to catch Barry's eye but he was more concerned with getting his hands on the last caramel shortbread before Val got back. He got it into his mouth and shut up, an uneasy silence immediately filled up the space and Val's voice could be heard beyond wondering where Graham had taken himself off to, what time he was due back and who else 'might be able to take this one on.' Helen and her brother began to talk between themselves so the three caring profs. knocked together a passable version of knowing what they were about as they chattered like seasoned hands about 'second recommendations' and 'the trouble with Guardianship'. Then Val joined them looking pained and flustered. 'So sorry about that – I've told them I'm in a meeting and not to be disturbed. Right, you've helped yourselves to refreshment, good, now I think we can start with Linda and the media aspect. I hope we can safely say that there's a line round this one now.'

Alan noticed Colin smirk, Helen gave nothing away. She

looked up and addressed the room with the kind of poised assertiveness that always worked on men like Barry and Alan. 'Well, from the family's perspective we are emphatic that no further coverage should seep out.' Colin nodded and Barry let out a sigh.

'Linda.' Said Val, perhaps you could lead off.

Linda made great play with the straightening of her papers then spoke in brisk and business like terms. 'The main issue here is the unfortunate leak to the 'Today' programme, it did look for a time as if this was going to blow up in all our faces. However, some deft fire fighting from our media people and good communications with the local press managed to damp this one down before it took hold. I understand that the beebs sole interest was in wrong footing the man from the ministry and that there was never any intention of following on with anything.'

Alan could feel himself colouring up then Colin decided to throw some weight about the place. 'You're actually quite right about that Linda, in my experience snippets like that are dead in the water if something else hasn't come through by lunchtime – damp squibs as you would put it. You must see though how it would have seemed to us, I mean, I won't deny my own hand in getting the local rag interested but I think you'll agree that it's generally the only way of getting you people to react.'

'Would we?' Put in Barry.

'Well anyway.' Said Linda. 'It was an obvious concern for us as to how far it went up the line.'

'I'll bet it was.' Said Colin who was beginning to enjoy himself. 'Nothing to do with me though.'

'No.' Said Linda cautiously. 'We've identified the leak and

ASK ME NOW

rest assured that it's been appropriately seen to.'

'That's all very well.' Said Colin. 'But what happens now? After all the press plays a vital role in these matters – I dare say you've squared off the people at the Echo but where doe's that leave us?'

You brass necked sod, though Alan, you bare faced poseur, you twat. Helen hadn't said much and seemed to be not much bothered with her brother's line of attack then she turned to Barry. 'What happened on that day then?' She asked him simply.

Barry looked at her and the rest looked at him. It was his big moment at their little party, the parcel was in his lap and he must unwrap and pull out a winner. 'I acted in good faith.' He began, Alan winced. 'I can honestly say there was no intention on my part to misinform or misdirect.' Alan wished he could metamorphose into a small winged insect and buzz blamelessly through the window into endless blue skies. 'But the truth is I made a proper lash-up of the whole thing. I mean, your Father didn't look well …'

'Well he wouldn't.' Said Colin. 'Being as how he was waiting to see his doctor.'

'Shut up Col.' Said Helen gently.

'Yes, I know.' Barry said quietly, and then went on to give a lengthy and affecting account of that day, something he'd given clear thought to, being unsparing with the shortfalls in his actions. 'As I say I was acting in good faith but not in my right mind so all I can really say now is that I'm sorry – I always was but, once your Father had been so understanding, forgiving really, I simply hoped it would go away.'

Helen sniffed decisively and said. 'Right, that's fair enough, that's all I wanted. Thank you.'

Val kept a straight face, Alan looked at her shoe and Linda busied herself with a puckish paper clip. Only Colin reacted. 'So that's it is it? The oldest trick in the book – some soft soap from our earnest buffoon here, an underdone apologia from our forgetful fool in office and that's it?'

Helen held up an emollient hand. 'Yes Colin, I think we've managed to generate enough discomfort all round and it wont bring Dad back.'

'Come off it Helen, what about this ludicrous neurasthenia type stuff, this Simpson thing? I've heard some things in my time but are we expected to swallow that?'

Val chose her moment. 'Oh I can assure you that Mr. Weatherall experiences transient effects from a mild form of a dissociative dysphasic condition which is known but little understood, so far. I have taken care to discuss this with a qualified authority – it can lay dormant for many years and sufferers lead normal and productive lives, also, it can be effectively treated. For example …'

'You people are incredible aren't you?' Snorted Colin. 'Any old tripe with knobs on plus a side order of fatuity … '

Barry, who had been silent and brooding, looked up at this. 'Hey you, watch your language and I can assure you it's not … what you said it was with a side order of your smooth talk.'

Alan spotted Helen stifle a smile. 'You must forgive my brother Mr. Weatherall but I think he's had his say now.'

Not quite he hadn't. 'Helen, we mustn't let them get away with this – people should know what happened – how many other instances – there ought to be an inquiry, at the very least

ASK ME NOW

a visit from Fiona Bruce, she'd liven things up.'

'I don't think your fantasies should cloud your judgement here Colin.' Said Helen crushingly and Alan knew then that that was going to be that. Barry was visibly upset by this point and asked if he could leave the room. Val agreed and suggested it was a good point to break. 'I don't think we need go on now.' Said Helen. 'Come on Col.' He stood up meekly and they left the room. Which left Alan, Linda and Val sitting and wondering if they would bounce back with second thoughts, then Barry shuffled back in and the tension slackened.

'You okay?' Linda asked him.

'Yeah thanks.'

'Well done Barry.' Said Val.

Alan nodded respectfully to him and suggested more tea.

'Good idea.' Said Val. 'And a bit of a debag.'

God bless her, he thought and collected up the pots while she chattered to Barry about the possibility of piloting some kind of SIMON network. Alan avoided his eye and took himself off to the kitchen where he washed, dried and popped the kettle on. He was trying to work out where the biscuits might be when Graham appeared and asked where Val was. 'In a meeting – hey I think she was looking for you, she's in the small group room, now's a good time to catch her … '

'No, I don't want to, I just don't want her to see me.'

'Oh Graham for heavens sake man – what is …?'

'It's too complicated to explain but it's basically an

assessment that's gone banana shaped as Val would say. I got misdirected and one thing led to another – I ought to lie low, I don't suppose you could …?'

But all Alan could do was run helplessly along the corridor towards the fire exit, burst out of the building without breaking speed or knocking over Dr. Wallace who was enjoying a smoke and come to a halt at the green mesh fencing off the playing field. She leaned against the doorframe and watched as she inhaled. From her vantage point he resembled Brer Rabbit stuck fast to the Tar Baby unable to do anything to pull himself free. 'You all right Alan?' She asked after a minute or so during which nothing else happened.

'Just needed some fresh air.' He said from over his shoulder.

'Mmm.' She said, stubbed her fag and went back in.

As soon as he was sure there was no one else about he brought his hands down to his sides and turned round letting himself be held up gently by the mesh behind him. Through the toughened glass on the door he was able to see Val moving towards the kitchen, he waited till she'd gone in then slipped back into the building then the small group room.

'Oh there you are.' Said Linda. 'Val's gone for the tea. Barry had loosened his tie and little beads of sweat showed about his forehead. Alan hoped he'd want his lift home soon.

'We seem to have established some good lines of communication with the Echo.' Observed Alan in Linda's direction in the spirit of a seasoned campaigner at ease with the other ranks.

She gave him a bland look and said. 'Yes, you could say that, careless talk not withstanding.' Then turned her attention to Barry. 'I think it's all done and dusted now, no more nasty

ASK ME NOW

surprises from the big bad media.'

Barry gave a rueful snort. 'Thought I'd finally lost the plot there – relieved when I found out he'd heard it too.'

Linda favoured Alan with a sharper look this time. 'I think we're all aware of the strain you've been under Barry.'

She's laying it on with a trowel, thought Alan – is there something going on, guilty conscience? Val came back with the tea; her demeanour suggested that Graham had seen her coming. 'Right, I'll be Mother, I think we've all deserved this.' Alan decided he should 'fess up to Barry on the way back then started to fret about Cindy. He wondered if he might be able to stay at Barry's house, he'd had enough of the heavy stuff for one day – when were things going to start going his way again? 'Well done Alan.' She said. 'Your contact with Helen Chadderton seems to have made all the difference.'

'Yes.' Said Barry. 'What did you say?'

'Not a lot as I can recall. She got quite angry – I don't think I said much at all really.'

'Probably the best course.' Put in Linda and caught his eye again. 'I thought you played a straight bat Barry, very well put I thought.'

'Yes, thank you Barry.' Said Val then she looked to Linda. 'What did you make of his nibs?'

'Colin? I think he's probably one of the good guys – doesn't always help himself with his hoity and toity though. His main subjects tend to be health and public services and from what I've seen his heart's in it. Did you know that he's very involved with a voluntary mental health group in Clapham?

Interesting – people are seldom all that they seem.'

She's definitely having a pop now he thought and tried to remember what Barry had called her on the way over. He looked over to him but he was tucking into shortbread from Vals special private stash and ruminating blankly at the multi-faith calendar on the wall. Alan wanted badly to get away with Barry, he had become aware of a kindling affection for the older man, he was also more keenly aware that Graham had hatched one of his specials and someone would be required to clean up after him. There was also the chance that Helen Chadderton might come back having changed her mind, but, most of all he wanted to be with Barry because Barry was bonkers but it didn't matter, personally or to others, apart from Stanley Clarke. Barry endured and inspired hope. Val and Linda were engaged in an off the record conversation about the councils Ridsdale In Bloom scandal; from what he could gather a nasty scam involving an artificial manure syndicate. 'Bad Smell Coming Up Roses.' Laughed Linda. 'You should have a word with your friend Alan.'

'What's she on about?' Asked Barry.

'Oh I don't know.' Said Alan holding up a hand dismissively. 'Do you need us any more Val?'

'Err, I don't think so do you Linda?'

Linda had had enough fun at his expense and let it be known that she didn't. 'Right, we'll get off then.' Outside in the corridor Alan indicated the fire door. A slight detour across the grass took them to the car park without hindrance and by four 'o clock they were speeding along Vernon Street with Barry cautioning him to hold his horses. 'Sorry, couldn't wait to get away, that Linda was getting on my wick.'

Barry said nothing and gazed out of his window. He could have been a deposed head of state en route to the station then

ASK ME NOW

permanent exile; the biscuits were eaten, the death warrants signed, Lotte and little Yuri were waiting for him, he would never look on his people again. 'I always had a lot of time for Val Meating.' He said quietly. 'She's pretty straight really.'

Alan nodded and they passed the rest of the journey silently then Alan's mobile chirruped as they turned onto Barry's estate. It was a text from Cindy; CU7atYRSLX. He was pleased when Barry asked him in and produced some more William Tell. 'I'll share one with you – one for the road, I mean half for the road. It'll have to be after last time.'

Once they were seated Barry took a drink from his glass. 'I should think about knocking this stuff on the head now that the worst looks like it might be over.' Alan mmmed. 'Val told me you'd been off for a while.'

'Yes, I've been quite depressed.' He said in the spirit of glasnost that was the order of the day. 'Pretty well on the mend now though.'

'It's horrible proper depression isn't it.' Said Barry, which was enough. Alan began to relax and then wonder about how much help Barry had had when he'd needed it, but then why should he or any of them get any? When he considered the transient 'interventions' that were all the best of them had to offer he wondered what help and support really boiled down to if you weren't able to get them at home. He'd once been told by a young woman living through psychosis that she felt like a tadpole in the ocean. They'd managed to stop her believing she was a secret agent but she still chucked herself in the canal. That these things happen only made it worse, if the most radical and envelope pushing risk assessments in the world can't stop them why bother?

He tapped his chair arm theatrically. 'So, does social work work?'

'It didn't for old Stanley did it?' Said Barry quietly as he half rose from his chair and looked about him before giving it up as a bad job and sinking back with a sigh.

Alan felt a bit of a twat. 'I didn't mean that – I was just thinking about my own doubts – I mean, you can't help wondering sometimes, you know.'

'Is it any use you mean?'

'Yes. Is it enough use enough of the time and without us would things simply sort themselves out anyway? I mean, you know, things happen, the worlds not a pleasant place, Gods a joke – you can't make people happy.'

Barry smiled. 'I noticed that nobody took that line with the Clarke's.'

'Well no, of course not but our existence made us responsible for what happened, our actions made it happen in the first place. Sometimes we create the problems we end up taking responsibility for – and nobody knows about the good stuff, the things we do right.'

'Well.' Said Barry. 'Isn't that just bad luck, one of those things that happens? We shouldn't expect applause for just doing what we're paid for, should we?'

'I don't know – what do you think?'

'What do I think? Well I think that if you go into social work and stay there you should be as honest with yourself as you can be about your reasons for doing so – as for whether it's any good … I'd say it depends on where you do it, what David would call the institutional context and how it shapes your practice, or some such piffle.'

ASK ME NOW

Alan laughed. 'That's another thing puts people off – the piffle and such like. What does he make of it all?'

'David spends a fair bit of time explaining things. He, of course, practices in a large and powerful institutional whatever so his stake in personal responsibility is correspondingly smaller, he's just one constituent part of a self-serving organism.' Alan saw that Barry could spin it with the best of them but was able to get a firm enough handle on what was being said. Barry reached his conclusion. 'As far as I'm concerned getting pushed out of the back door post-Stanley was the best thing that ever happened to me – I stopped being a social worker and started doing social work.'

'Right … go on.'

'What I mean is that I believe in social work – its ideals and principles, social work values if you like – you know helping folk, but not necessarily in social workers. Nothing personal but council run fandango's and gratuitous gobbledegook make a big difference for me, a negative difference. The set up I work for now isn't perfect but it's small, has no statutory responsibilities and people don't have to come to us. Perhaps the decent bits of social work are being picked up by other people who call it something else.'

'A bit like squirrels?' Mused Alan.

'What? Reliant on nuts for a living?' Laughed Barry.

'You know, red squirrels have given up and gone home but if you look closely enough at a grey one you'll see some red in him.'

'Yeees.' Said Barry uncertainly. 'Are you sure you don't want that other half?'

Alan made a show of looking at his watch. 'I should go.'

'You're new girlfriend?'

'Yes.'

'Good luck. Come round again, I'll invite our David, we can explore the moral maze. Could be interesting.'
Barry waived him off and Alan felt sure he'd be back. He'd wanted to ask Barry a bit more about SIMON and how he managed – his coping strategies and all the rest of it – but had thought better of it. At least he'd been able to not think of Cindy for a while, he noticed a few relapse signatures now though; gas belly, a hesitant way with the windscreen wiper and a rehash of the notion that it might be best if she binned him, bit of a relief really. He was struggling to remember how she looked beyond her long arms and legs and coal black hair. He thought her voice was sort of nasal and fluting and that the sex had been good but not available to any kind of clear recall. He could remember the last time, about seven weeks ago on a Saturday afternoon; 'Dale had managed to avoid relegation to the B&Q League with a last minute winner at Lincoln, he remembered it coming through on the radio as they dozed afterwards. Would his league status survive this evening's crunch fixture?

He didn't want to get home just yet so took a detour down an old looking road to pull over near a view of fields with moors in the far distance. A couple of old horses cropped at the grass. He knew what it was with Cindy, he feared that she'd only stuck with him because he'd gone a bit nuts and that now he was off the danger list she'd make her move. He also knew that if he put this to her she'd get angry with him; why was he so important and she so shallow, or some such. At some point she had referred to his grandiosity being part of his depression when he'd importuned her over some scratchy response he'd felt from her. He could therefore comfort himself with the knowledge that she wasn't one to pull her punches and would

ASK ME NOW

have marked his card by now if she'd been of a mind to. It was another twist on his familiar soliloquy; what's a nice girl like you doing in the open sewer of my soul? He watched the old cob look up, even from his position he could see that the horse was caked in shit and muck but it just tossed its flea bitten neck and got back to the scrub grass, it didn't bother him. What use was self-knowledge anyway, que bono eh, when you thought about it? All he wanted then was to be sitting on a settee – his or hers – with Cindy watching Hetty Wainthrop Investigates where nothing mattered and they were free in the moment. Fill your boots David Bowie, just forget your mind.

Friday was generally a crap night for telly – maybe they'd go to bed. This was another thing; Cindy showed no want of robust enthusiasm in the leg over department but she seemed just as keen on a plate of chips with curry sauce, in fact sometimes it seemed a close thing when it came to a choice. He had sometimes wished a man might be more like a woman in this regard – why should it matter so much? Were all blokes the same – tireless fuckwits anxious for their insert? Why was it so, why couldn't three good shags a year be enough? He needed Hetty Wainthrop just then, her aproned savvy and waggish with folks who weren't right in the head, she'd tell him. He knew what it was with Hetty as well, where the seductive fantasy led – he wanted he and Cindy to be Hetty and her husband (a doughty old josser in a Littlewoods cardie) safe in their snug little house, a world beyond sex and anxiety, a warm buzz that came on every evening with the curry sauce. At a less comfortable level he wanted to be in that house with Hetty and husband, to be looked after by them. Where on earth Cindy would fit into this scenario he wasn't sure – did he want her to be Hetty or Hetty to be Cindy? As with most things he wanted to have his chips and eat them.

Cindy had been through the ringer recently though and, as

Mike Pearson

Hetty might say; she'd had it all to do. The brother had shown himself a cloth eared Wally of the first rank and heaven knew what their local services were like. He knew he'd done the right things; been concerned but not pestered, asked after Mrs. Watson the night of his cocktail party with Barry Bishop. What had she made of all that? She'd worn a skirt and he remembered her washing sick off her leg in the bathroom, then there'd been that enigmatic farewell. He had to concede that, given the circumstances, it was the only kind he might have expected. He started the car and pushed in The Glasgow Improvisers, by the time they'd found the lost chord he was on the home stretch.

'Aright mate – had your tea yet? Asked Steve on his way out.

'Eh, oh very funny. Has Hetty been round do you know?'

'Who?'

'Cindy – has she been round?'

'Not that I know of. See you later anyway.'

He went up and was relieved not to find anything pinned on his door. He went in and set about smartening the place up, opened a window and sat down, it was six fifty seven. The last thing he wanted to do was listen to music but it was what he generally did so he pressed on the CD player without bothering to see what was in. It was Lester Young taking his secret pathway through the harmonies of 'These Foolish Things'. The music sounded remote, he was playing at being himself and Lester was a long way away. He put the radio on but by the time Tony Archer had found out where Pat had left their fondue set he wanted to take a baseball bat to Home Farm so he went out onto the landing and began running up and down the stairs as hard as he could. He went at it for as long as he was able then collapsed panting into his easy chair. Not very long after this he heard a hesitant knock at his door.

ASK ME NOW

'Hold on.' He gasped. 'I'm coming.'

'Alan?' Asked Cindy. 'Is that you?'

'Yeah, yeah – I'll be with you in a minute.'

He was still panting when he welcomed her in and his forehead glistened. 'Just been for a bit of a run.' He explained as he backed into the room. She didn't say anything and went over to the front window overlooking the street. He sat down in his chair, she seemed cool and distant. He didn't know how to reach her.

She spoke as she looked away from him through the glass. 'I've never noticed before that you can see the top of St. Cuthbert's church from here if you know what to look for.' He thought about following on with some pat stuff about finding St. Cuthbert if you knew where to look but fell into a fit of coughing as soon as he breathed in. 'You're not going to be sick again are you?' She asked flatly.

This and the awkwardness made him surly. 'No I shouldn't think so. Why don't you sit down and I'll make us some tea.' He went into the kitchen decisively then remembered that the kettle was back in the main room for some reason and had to go back for it. She was still at the window. Once he'd filled it and clicked it on he realised that there was no plausible reason for him to wait in the kitchen and went back in. 'How's your Mum Cindy?'

She sighed and he sensed the tension loosen a notch. 'Well she won't be going anywhere in a hurry, and then not back home, not at first anyway.'

'It must be pretty bad.'

'Could have been worse. They thought at first that she might have been dementing but now it looks like the fall and concussion upskittled her badly. She's pulled round a bit in her self anyway.'

'You said about not going back home.'

'Oh she can't go back home again.' She pursed her lips at the fireplace. 'Sheltered accommodation looks the best bet, certainly in the long term. Adrian's looking into it.'

'Your brother?'

'Yes – he's had quite a lot going on for him that I didn't know about. We had a good time together when he turned up you know.' Cindy's voice had been flat since the St. Cuthbert's business and now he looked he could see how tired she seemed. He heard the kettles muffled clack.

'I'll get the tea on, fancy a Wagon Wheel?' She nodded so he put together a nice treat for them on his period tea trolley and wheeled it carefully through. She didn't comment but went straight for a one of the tinselled goodies. He followed suit and after they'd munched awhile poured the tea. 'Shall we go out for a walk in a bit? I've found a nice pub on that new estate beyond the by-pass.'

'Yes.' She said carefully. 'I'm not much company at the moment though.'

'That's all right – it's just good to see you again, I'm picking up you've been through a rough time.'

'I don't know, seems to me I've made a bit of a meal of it all. It all seems to be working itself out – I feel more ashamed than anything.' Alan's instinct was to say nothing and, for once, he followed it. 'Anyway I'm sick of thinking about it, I can't be the first girl this has happened to. What's been happening here? How did your special mission work out?'

ASK ME NOW

He chortled as he reached for his cup. 'I don't know how but it looks like we've got away with it, the ghost of Paul Foot from downstairs not withstanding. All that high expressed emotion you happened across that night was to do with that – I'd told him all about it and the next thing is it's on the Today prog. Anyway, Linda Harvey managed to smooth it over at the Echo, to be honest me taking a sweetly reasoned roasting from the daughter and Barry's touching performance this afternoon seems to have done the trick. He's all right is Barry – what a carry on though, if they ever film it he'll have to be Bernard Bresslaw with me as Jim Dale. I'm not sure about Sylvia Simms or Barbara Windsor for Val.'

Cindy sipped her 'Cutie'. 'This tea's nice.' He gave up on his Pinewood fantasy and tried to amuse her with the supposed properties of 'this Queen among teas, specially picked and blended by our expert planters etc etc drawing on traditional blah blah blah.' 'Probably thrown together in Oldham.' She said. 'Tastes nice though.' She cupped her hands round the china even though it was a glorious evening and quite warm in the flat. Alan wanted to establish physical contact but could see no way of doing so without fast forwarding them from the hesitant intro they were still moving through. Cindy seemed so turned in on herself, she might have been aware of this when she remarked how still his room seemed without music. 'Can I hear that melodious clunk stuff?' Alan put on 'Miles Davis And The Modern Jazz Giants' with whom he was now back on good terms and felt her unwind to Monk's nursery rhyme solo on 'Bags Groove'. When it was over she said. 'They talk about musicians playing their instruments but he plays with his doesn't he?'

'Stan Tracey said that the piano was the best toy any one had ever given him.'

'Childs play I suppose – harder than it seems I should think.'

'Did you ever fancy playing anything?'

'I quite enjoyed the recorder at school but once I got in the county hockey team I gave up most of the extra stuff. Adrian was the musical one.'

'Oh, how did it go with his songs?'

'They recorded some of them – he was thrilled to bits.'

'What kind of stuff, the music I mean?'

'Grungy alternative folk stuff. There's some sort of collective over towards Hebden Bridge – painters, potters, and somebody who does things with a camera in their mouth. Not my cup of nettle tea I must say, Claire's probably been over and Adrian wants to move there but we've agreed he won't make any firm plans until we're sure about Mum.'

He'd heard all about Cindy's hockey days and knew from first hand experience how strong and well toned she was. She also had the most beautiful bottom he'd ever clapped eyes on, when she stood up to stretch then move back over to the window he knew it wouldn't matter if he never clapped hands on it again. Simply to have known her as he had would be enough, wouldn't it? This caused him to consider once more one of loves several ironies; the fraught business of loves object: its contemplation and consummation. He also wondered for the umpteenth time about those mixed feelings in her letter. 'How many clouds can you see?' He asked.

'None at the moment but come and look at the light on the brickwork' He joined Cindy at the window; it was the closest they'd been since she'd arrived. They stood together watching the sun pick out ancient chimneys then she asked if he was ready to go out. She picked up her bag and followed him down into the street. 'Which way?' She asked.

ASK ME NOW

'Down through the park then along some old fields next to the road – it's nicer than it sounds.' From street level the chimney pots were harder to pick out and Cindy looked lost again, swamped by the noise and traffic, cut off by the buildings. He began to feel worse than he had for a long time. They got to the park in silence but once they were through the gates he reached out to take her hand, she returned the slightest of pressures and held on. 'We come out at the bottom bit over there then it's open country for a while.'

'Do we need a guide now then?'

'Oh, I've been this way before, we'll be fine.'

'I'm glad one of us has.'

Was she taking the piss? This was definitely his least favourite side of Cindy – just say what's on your precious mind, spare me the heroic lost lady from across the seas routine, none of this was his fault was it? He was almost happy to let go her hand when they got to the single track and she tagged along behind him. He was able to manage some light hearted banter as they went on their way about crop circles, fossil fuel emissions and the adaptive possibilities of SIMON – in fact hadn't there been a hit once called 'Simon Says'? The 1910 Fruitgum Company hadn't it been? Cindy's reaction suggested it could just have well have been the 1812 Overture. They didn't know what to say to each other, he wondered if she felt as awful as she did about this. There was a bridge ahead of them which took the main road up and across to the coast while the other traffic turned outwards to the moors. He remembered their day out there, how bad he'd been and how she'd made him feel better for a bit. There'd been a bush bearing bloated condoms and the wind had blown her hair about her face, he thought she might have been laughing at the time.

As the track began to climb towards the bridge they came upon a torn bin liner spilling rubbish across the path. He sighed and tutted but she lingered to poke at the stuff with her foot separating out fag ends, a couple of soiled nappies, a tooth brush and some slimy bacon. Then something in the bag caught her eye and she bent down to gingerly pull out a bright red sleeve that turned out to be part of a childs pyjama top. She mmmed to herself then Alan crouched to turn the bag up and gather the spilled stuff carefully with a piece of cardboard before wrapping it in the red top and putting it back in the bag. He stood it up on its secure end and leaned it against the fence. 'You looked as if you were tucking a boy up in bed.' She said.

'How do you know it was a boy?' He asked.

'The top I suppose – it just looked like a small boy's.'

'He wouldn't be the smallest, the nappies might have been a girls.'

'He might have been old enough to ear bacon, but not smoke, I shouldn't have thought.'

'Or chuck rubbish.' Well, he thought, at least they were talking again. He spoke about his afternoon again then his encounter with Barry Bishop and the war on fly tippers. Cindy thought she might have met his daughter and this enabled Alan to bring Dave Bamber into the picture and amuse her with his Fathers notion of an adulterer with SIMON. She wasn't paying much attention but as they passed beneath the bridge she stopped and drew him towards her. He held her cautiously by the shoulders and after a pause she cupped her hands behind his waist to lean into him. He brought his hands down to mirror her embrace and she began to cry. This went on for about three minutes so he inched them back towards the tunnel wall where he could lean more

ASK ME NOW

comfortably and rub her back with his palms while scanning the framed view through the other end of the tunnel, after another couple of minutes a bin bag flew across the outlook to land with a rapid swish in rough grass. He closed his eyes and kissed her head, at this rate they could be walled in by tomorrow. She had stopped crying and tightened her hold on him, their breathing fell into a rhythm and they stayed put for a further ten minutes. Nothing at all was said. 'Shall we go on?' He said at last.

'Yes.' She said and pushed forward to kiss him chastely as they disengaged. He was bothered by those bin bags though, flying about the place like obese air borne Labradors. He'd also noted how bothered the split one had made Cindy for some reason and made sure he was first out through the tunnel making a great show of giving her the all clear. She gave him a wan titter but clearly didn't know what he was playing at. 'Can we sit outside at this place?' She asked him.

'Oh yes, there are some of those bench table type things you can buy in a pack.'

'Presumably we won't have to assemble one before we sit down?'

'No, you know the kind I mean B&Q knock them out.' It wasn't that funny but they were getting there and their time in the tunnel had stirred him so he let her walk ahead for a while so he could watch her safely; her hair fell back then upwards across her neck which clued him in for the sight of her bottom held firmly by stretched denim. Her natural walk described a sort of stately lollop and as she forged ahead he couldn't help thinking of Gary Lineker stalking off the pitch with magnificent contempt after gormless Graham Taylor had pulled him off in Sweden.

She stopped and turned around. 'What are you doing – we are

going in the right direction aren't we?'

'I was just enjoying the view – see how the sun picks out the old Gas Works.'

'Do you think those things were ever safe?' She asked as she frowned back towards the town.

'I think so, I've never heard of any explosions or leaks. I'll ask Graham, he knows about these things.'
Cindy seemed as if she couldn't have cared less but waited for him to catch up and reached for his hand again when he got to her. They were soon on the edge of the green with the pub in sight, the air brushed with the sounds of gardening and people talking out of doors. Two small girls approached them with a puppy skittering on a pink lead. One of the looked at Cindy. 'He's called Martin.' She informed her then they moved off. Barry's estate had depressed Alan but this one, just then, seemed close to a Barratt built Arcadia where shadows lengthened and children's eyes opened in them.

As soon as they reached the pub Cindy parked herself on one of the benches and asked for strong cider. Alan got himself a pint of 'Weavers' and once they'd taken their first sips and put down their glasses on the wooden table the earlier awkwardness returned with compound interest. He was about to break the silence with a more or less rehearsed account of an amusing story the elusive old man from next door had told him about frying eggs on a shovel when she reached over to stroke his forearm and say she'd missed him. 'Perhaps in ways I didn't expect to.'

Christ, he thought, they give you it with one hand then take it back with the other. 'I've missed you too – you mentioned in your note about feeling a bit mixed up, about us?'

'Yes.'

ASK ME NOW

'What did you mean?'

'I don't know.'
'Eh?'

'Well, as I said, I was a bit mixed up.'

Fair enough, don't make a fuss, it'll come out eventually. 'Did getting away with Claire help? I don't just mean about me but, you know all the complicated stuff at home.'

'Yes, yes it did.'

She didn't sound as if it was any big deal either way, he noticed himself getting a bit worked up. He'd never been any good at verbal footsie and thought he could do worse than stake it all on one throw, but not like he had at the bottom of the stairs. 'So, here we are trying to pick things up again and this is what I want so is it what you want, if you see what I mean?'

'Yes, yes it is.' She said without much in the way of enthusiasm, repugnance, what-you-on-about or expressed emotion of any kind known to him. She did reach out and stroke his arm again, with a touch more interest. 'It's all right Alan, and you're right – it wasn't just you. Actually, Claire and I fell out – she was doing my head in, you know what she can be like, and the last thing I wanted was to get into one with her. Apparently in some of the circles she moves in it's customary to settle disagreements with a fist fight.'

'Oh don't lets go there. What a performance you happened on the other night, it's just not like me. Maybe it's one of the life changing aspects of mental illness.'

'You seem to get on with Steve.'

Mike Pearson

She'd said this reasonably enough but something in her tone told him to shear off from his own troubles – which it was tacitly agreed were behind him at present – and be big. They managed to spin out a serviceable dialogue around sundry issues raised by his afternoons work then he went in for another round. When he came back out she'd buttoned up her jacket and asked if it was busy inside.

'There's plenty of space now, do you want to go in, it'll probably fill up later?' He said.

They found a seat by the window behind a synthetically weathered display board telling of the ways of weavers and the rich heritage handed down to our easier times. Cindy sniffed derisively and fell into a gloomy silence. Alan looked round the place – the kids had all moved on after their first couple of drinks and now the older lot were filing in for the mid-evening session. He recognised one of their number and stood up. Barry Weatherall saw him and sauntered over to their little bower.

'Hullo Alan, what's the strong cider like here?'

'Bit smooth for the connoisseur. Barry this is Cindy.'

'Pleased to meet you pet.' Cindy gave Barry her winning smile and invited him to join them. 'Has he told you all about it then?' Asked Barry. 'Our date with destiny? Listen Alan, I owe you a drink – I got the feeling that your interregnum with Stanley's daughter tipped the scales, spiked a few guns and generally squeezed us through in injury time.'

'He sounds a bit like a more focussed version of Val.' Said Cindy as Barry went to the bar. 'What's an interregnum?'

'It could be a neologism.'

'Which is a made up word, right?'

ASK ME NOW

'And part of Barry's problem.'

'Well it should be interesting to see what comes back with from the bar.' She frowned then said. 'Interregnum sounds Latin, sounds a bit like interlude which sounds as if it would fit. I suspect he's got it right – perhaps the daughter got that side of you …'

'What side would that be?'

Hercule Poirot by way of Alan Bennet played by Ant – or is it Dec.'

'What are you givin' it, I would never …'

'Here we are then.' Said Barry as Cindy moved over for him. 'I'd have got crisps but they've run short.'

'They didn't have any Dec powder did they?' Said Alan with his bland smile.

'Alan, it's been a puzzling couple of weeks one way and another.' Observed Barry. 'Don't go getting all enigmatic with me, there's no telling where things could end.'

Cindy inched round past Alan for the ladies, making a point of resting a warm hand on his knee. They both watched her go then Barry turned to Alan. 'That's that Cindy then – bonny lass right enough. She back from outer space then?'

'We're negotiating splash down – fingers crossed.'

'Ground control to Major Tom eh?'

Where were they going with this? Should he ask about life on Mars with Sue Hubbard? 'We did all right this afternoon though didn't we?'

Barry supped a manly mouthful and replaced his glass on the table with the air of a man who'd earned it. 'Aye, we did all right.' Then Cindy came back from the ladies and was as nice to Barry as she could be, listening to his stories and asking for more. They heard of his Cooksonesque boyhood in Northumberland with a widowed mother and older sister, early days of hand to mouth as he sweated through night school in Gateshead ('it was that or the pit') then his hair raising beginnings in Newbiggen as a mental health nurse where many a tale had been told by older hands which could scarce be believed, even now. 'And thank fuck we've left them behind.' He concluded.

Cindy took this in her stride and was genuinely interested, Alan could tell, in what Barry had to say about what had been lost and what had been gained in his experience. He tended to look at life from both sides now and felt this stood him in good stead for his current role which encouraged Cindy to talk at some length about her professional qualms and confusions. Alan noticed that no mention had yet been made of 'our David' or Barry's prior knowledge of her. He was all right was Barry; for all the pathos and bathos, the bumpy rides and crowded high streets, he hadn't ended up too badly. There could be worse fates then to be Barry, certainly at that moment. Cindy had begun to confide in him some of the troubles with old Mrs. Watson, Alan began to wonder when Barry was going to rejoin his other friends. 'Aye, I bet you're the one they phone when there's something needs seeing to.' She glanced at Alan when he said this but it took him a while to get it, then Barry clapped his thighs decisively and said. 'Anyway it's been nice to meet you – I'd best catch up with my lot. Give us a bell next week Alan, I'm off to One-Stop again soon.' And he was off across a crowded room. The noise level and alcohol left Alan and Cindy feeling a bit lost as they pulled over to let a younger couple wedge in. When the couple started snogging Cindy nudged him and they

ASK ME NOW

headed for the door. On the way he nodded to Barry but didn't recognise any of the people he was with.

'What's the deal with One-Stop?' She asked as they walked back over the green.

'A hellish brew called 'William Tell' mashed on an industrial estate near Nottingham – 12% proof cider. Barry swears by it – I was daft enough to try some when I went round there the second time. As a matter of fact a few stray particles may have found their way to your bare leg on Tuesday.' She made a dismissive noise through her nose so he put his arm round her. She eventually returned the gesture but it didn't feel right to him and he was glad when they reached the single track and had to disengage. She walked ahead again as they passed beneath the tunnel, without much traffic to distract him or light to see by he became more aware of the bad smell there. He'd been only partially aware of it as he'd comforted Cindy but now it claimed his attention via the back of his throat; a cold clammy whiff of piss with an aftertaste of something sinister and toxic. He spat and caught her up where she was kicking at the rough grass just beyond the abandoned rubbish on the other side. When he reached her she knelt and reached up a hand, after a pause he held it then she pulled him down beside her. He saw that she'd carefully spread her jacket on the ground then she embraced him and kissed him in a way that seemed to him like a sad parody of seduction. Her sweet cider tongue and ardent pelvis left him in no doubt - but none of this was Cindy. She pushed him down onto the jacket to sit astride him; she had her top halfway over her head before he could reach up to stop her.

'Cindy.' He said as kindly as he could. 'Are you sure about this, we're not that far from home.'

'I'd have thought we'd do better out here with no phones to bother us.' She said in her flat if-you-say-so tones. There was a puffed up, and overblown quality to all this and he felt happier when the fight suddenly left her and she slumped forward with her hands on his belly and her hair trailing forward.

He held her companionably by the hips. 'It's just a bit … unexpected, you know – I mean you know …'

'You don't have to get all precious with me – it's just a shag, or maybe you think we'll cause a late night pile up.'

'This isn't you Cindy. None of this is you – what's wrong?'

She sighed. 'What is me then? You've had a look in the shop window, maybe you should see under the counter as well before you go any further.'

For some reason this took him back to Lena Martell, hadn't she sung a mawkish song about a bargain store or had it been Joni Mitchell? 'Well, I don't think we should go any further here – one of us might catch a flying bin bag in mid performance. Those things are dangerous when launched, ask Barry Bishop.' This only served to darken her mood more and she slumped forward letting him draw her towards him. They lay together for a while. 'That bit about the bin bag seemed to bother you.' He said at last.

'It was the kids 'jamas. It's just over there isn't, I've had a miscarriage.'

Nothing more was said for a good while but after the shock began to disperse he saw that she was still there and that she was holding onto him with a fair degree of commitment. The next thing he noticed was the sound of a car pulling up somewhere above them then something bulky and plastic landing quite close to where they were lying. The fly tipping hour had arrived. The car took off at speed and she pulled in closer to him, he pulled her over far enough to pull the jacket

ASK ME NOW

free and lay it across her bottom half. He thought he might be getting a better idea of her mixed up state of mind and where he fitted into the overall scheme of things. He'd known there was something amiss; she'd barely mentioned home or work since she'd arrived and her offer of coitus amongst the cow parsley had set the cap on it. He was so glad he'd done the right thing there. He gave her a speculative stroke and she reached up to his shoulder. 'Will you stay at mine tonight?'

'Yes, but do you mind if we stay here a bit longer Alan?'

'Yes.' He said feeling alarmed that she'd started talking again; god only knew what she'd come out with next. He was dying to piss but determined to be heroic about this. They were lying like spoons now and he brought his knees up as far as he could without giving her the wrong idea but it was no good. He toyed with the idea of doing it there – jacket, Cindy and all, what did any of it matter? 'You'll have to excuse me.' He said eventually and stood up very carefully.

'I'll join you.' She said and wandered with him over to some sort of mutandis vulgaris blooming by the tunnel. She started before him and went on for some time after he'd waggled and zipped up. He knew that all manner of things were apt to happen to a woman post childbirth but the finer points of an early miscarriage were another country. He wondered how best to seek guidance. 'Would you get my jacket while I pull my knickers up?' A goose honked up above them. He was certainly getting a good look behind the counter now. He fetched her jacket and they set off in an awkward arrangement whereby he was obliged to walk a level down from the track on the edge of the field so that they could hold onto each other in the twi-light. She seemed more like 'his' Cindy again but what was a chap to do now? Stop and ask a few questions, run off into the night, sing something simple? But although this was happening to him it was also happening to her and she seemed happy to hold on as he tottered over uneven ground. He was shocked to think that there was so much about her he didn't know, so much of him she didn't. She'd known him when he was two sheets to the wind but that was only part of him. This thought offered consolation – things could only get better, couldn't they. He squeezed her and she returned the pressure as they reached the proper path. 'It was yours by the way.' She said as they passed into the bottom end of the park.

'Oh, yeah – yeah, I know.'

'I know you know.'

'Yeah, yeah.'

'Georgie Fame.'

'Yeah, ye ... right.'

'Full of surprises eh?' She said with another inflexion he'd not heard before; a variation of her more familiar ear boxing rhetoric with a salty, salutary edge to it.

He could sense the water works starting up again and pulled her over to him against an old conker tree. 'When did it happen?' He asked.

'The day after I called round – when you were tired and emotional.'

'Monday night.'

'Yes. The next morning, when I woke up, it happened.'

He wanted to know more but felt it would all be made clear in the fullness of time. 'Oh Cindy.' He said and stroked her hair where he knew she liked it. 'But that was barley three days ago ... do you want to sit down?'

ASK ME NOW

'Don't worry, it won't all fall out if I stand up for too long. My foot hurts though, is there a seat anywhere nearby?'

There was and they settled themselves so that he could deliver a fuller head massage and be stoical for a bit longer. 'I knew I was late before I had to go over that day, in fact I was certain I'd come on then – probably why I was so keen to get you to bed the night before. Anyway I kind of forgot all about it what with the whole shooting match over there so that by the time I remembered I was well overdue and with everything taking off like it was, well, I just felt I had to get away with Claire – I know you find her a bit full on but she's been a good friend over the years. I was able to sort out what I wanted, which was to tell you and she needed to be back over this way for something at work, so we drove over that afternoon. When you weren't in I decided to wait.'

'I'm glad you did – I'm sorry it wasn't really the right moment. Had you been waiting long?'

'Not that long and it's just as well it wasn't the time to tell you anyway was it?'

'I don't know – I suppose not. I have some fleeting memories of it all … but, that's about it.'

They stayed on the bench and watched the bushes for a bit. 'I came away from your place feeling a bit funny but I just put it down to all the excitement and chicken tikka then, on the way back to the cottage in Claries car we had to stop so I could puke then I got these terrible stomach cramps. Then I knew.'

'I'm sorry.' He said. 'It must have been awful.'

'It was.'

Mike Pearson

The moon was full and the pubs were kicking out, someone in the distance shouted 'piss flaps' and Alan's agitation got the better of him. 'What, I mean did ... what did you think when you tho... when you knew you were pregnant?'

'I wanted it.'

He suddenly felt way upstream and lost for directions, lost for words – sans compass, sans rudder and there were rocks ahead. The fabric of her jacket felt hostile to his touch so he held her a bit closer, the better to keep her from rearing up to rebuke him. She seemed disinclined to say much more but the position she was now in can't have been comfortable; leaning into him with her legs splayed over the end of the arm rest as he took her from behind like a local hero hauling someone to safety from deep waters. They made a few adjustments and stayed put, facing in the same direction looking across to the back gardens of houses beyond the green railings. Someone said 'arsehole' quite distinctly but calmly and was answered by a deeper voice that said 'cock', again in a bantering matter of fact tone that spoke of rough concord rather than conflict. It was odd and gave them something else to talk about. 'Is it some kind of game?' She asked.

'What kind?'

'Something to do with blindfolds and anatomy, drink fuelled and kinky.'

They listened carefully but heard nothing more except a back door closing in the house closest to them, then a light went on downstairs and a window opened. Eventually music drifted across. It can't be he thought, but it was; the narcotic brogue, the idiomatic arrangement, the fleet fingered guitar work as he flitted across someone's dreams with nets of wonder. 'What is it with Val pissing Doolican?' He asked passionately.

'Isn't it Doonican?'

ASK ME NOW

'Him too – hasn't this town ever heard of Van Morrison?'

'It's probably anal sex.'
Oh my godfathers, she's off again, no doubt the sensual Mrs. Todgers would feature in this next bulletin from behind the counter. 'What has Val Doonican got to do with anal sex – I mean, I know Delaney had a donkey but are you about to tell me it was in the biblical sense? I mean that man was Britain's top light entertainer in his day, he held down the Saturday night prime time slot for a whole generation. I'd never be able to sit in a rocking chair again.'

'No, listen, all that funny business in the garden – all we could hear for certain was cock and arsehole then Val Doonican crooning. I think it all connects.'

'Cindy please, I don't want to pursue this any further. My view is that that whole side of the doings is because some people just don't know the correct way of going about things – you know, a basic misunderstanding of the plumbing, what goes where.'

'Well, there's no excuse for us not knowing what goes where and what happens next.' She turned to face him and moved apart on the seat so that they were separate. 'What would it have meant to you if I had told you I was pregnant on Monday?'

'Well I suppose that we were going to have a baby.'

'And now we're not.'

Alan was keen to shift them away from the emotional issues and thought it would help if he showed some concern with the women's health type questions. He'd managed to dredge up some basic gyny knowledge since Cindy's bombshell, the normal complications and so forth. He decided to check a few points. 'Did you have to have a whatsit, a look and see?'

'D and C Alan – dilation and cuteledge, bit like a rinse out after the dentist. I was in and out yesterday morning.'

'But before – I mean by the tunnel after the pub … '

'Yeah?'

'Well you, you know – led me to understand … '

'And – my body I can do what I like with it.'

'But you didn't like – I could tell.'

She sighed and seemed cross again. 'Yes well, that's one of the reasons I'm here.'

They stood up together and held hands across the rest of the park, Cindy stepping in such a big pile of dog shit it should have been cordoned off with red lights flashing, luckily it wasn't her bad foot. As they passed through the last bit he drew her attention to the seat where he'd met 'Beeswing' for the first time and talked about his adventures on Gas Street.

Back in his sitting room Cindy sipped her tea and they talked about the 'Beeswing situation' some more. 'I don't see what harm it would have done, she might have found you a bit odd but you are – you returned her old mutt and generally showed a proper interest. I suppose going back the second time was the difficult bit, you both knew you wanted something from her. She got your number too by the sound of it.'

'I keep thinking I should go back round, put things right, but would that only confuse things more. What do you think Cindy?'

ASK ME NOW

She sipped and thought, Lol Coxhill tootled away in the background, Alan's tea had never tasted so good. 'Yes maybe it would.'

'Isn't it a bit sad though when a human contact throws up so much uncertainty and what's-it-all about?'

'Yes but it always does doesn't it. Can we have that David Bowie record on?'

He found the CD and put it on. As the cheesy synth kicked off 'Changes' he tried to imagine that generations view of the happier life; serious relationships, social sciences - communal houses flavoured by dope smoke and 'radical' politics. It might have been worse. 'I just felt I'd asked for more from her than I should have, it felt unclear, and not just because I was only just beginning to pick up.'

'No real harm done though, eh Alan?'

'No, I don't think so – it's just that it wasn't the kind of thing I'd do normally. I gave myself a vague kind of line about it would be a better world if we did this kind of thing naturally – talk about grandiose, at least when we do it at work we do it for money. Do you think that makes it better or worse?'

'It makes it more straightforward, I think.' She managed to make it clear that she'd had enough of this one so he asked her if she wanted to use the bathroom first. 'Mmm, yes – have you got an old shirt I can wear?'

'Oh yeah, sure.' He reviewed his spring collection of Oxfam shirts and picked her out a nice soft cotton one without a collar. She took it without comment and slipped off to the bathroom, which he'd cleaned up and set to rights the previous day. He turned his attention to the bed; the sheets passed muster but he turned the pillowcases to be on the safe side and fiddled with his bedside lamp to get a softer focus. He tried it in a few positions then the bulb pinged – if in doubt leave well alone, he thought, then had an idea. He went into the kitchen for a good root under the sink – tucked behind the toilet duck and similar fluids of fierce cleansing was an old cardboard box about the size of a catering pack of matches. He held it up to the light; it was dull red, a bit damp and bore an illustration of a lean and slippered old soul in a long night shirt skipping spryly along a corridor holding a brightly shining candle in a fancy holder. The flame gave off an unlikely degree of illumination and at the end of the landing, framed by an old style mullioned window, smiled the man in the moon. He'd discovered the little stash of candles when he moved in and left them there in the hope that he would find more evidence of past life; a mousetrap perhaps or some old coins – touch links of memory, shards of meaning but the only other find had been an ancient johnny mutating under the bed. He'd lost interest after that.

He found an empty bottle and pared away the candle to fit securely before lighting it from his cooker and trying it out on his mantelpiece. Cindy seemed to have been at it for a while, he heard the cistern go then the front door open and voices suddenly choked off as Steve opened and shut his own door. He lay back on the bed and tried to concentrate on the music, which told him that 'knowledge comes with deaths release'. This made him understand better the enduring appeal of Peters and Lee then the bathroom bolt went and Cindy stood demurely before him – she looked beautiful, graced by candlelight with his khaki granddad shirt coming down to just below her knees showing off her stout calves and lovely big feet. He thought himself a lucky so and so, and no mistake. She said. 'I'd better sleep on the outside in case I need to pee, my tits are sore as well, can we have David Bowie on again? 'He restarted the disc on his way to the bathroom and Cindy propped herself up in bed to do a candle meditation as she concentrated on the music.

ASK ME NOW

Alan got into the empty bath and lay back with a towel behind his head, things were happening fast, whether he wanted them to or not. Through the open window he could hear cats howling in slow motion and someone singing about the girl with the mousy hair, Cindy had been going to have his baby. All this had to mean something. When they'd lain together by the bin bags and the dog muck, where bind weed flourished and worms were at work, he'd felt something like love, some of what was reckoned to survive. He traced the cracks along the pelmet; a small spider scuttled out then froze on the wall. He got out, stretched then cleaned his teeth.

Cindy was lying down when he rejoined her but still awake. 'Can we have it on again, but with the sound down a bit?' He'd have preferred 'The World Of Derek Bailey' but saw that small sacrifices like this were what mattered. He pressed the right buttons and got in beside her. 'Shouldn't you blow the candle out Alan?'

'It's all right, you go to sleep. I'll stay awake till it's burned down.'

Outside in the overgrown back garden no one bothered with, a scruffy fox paused to look up at Alan's window. Dim light flickered and someone sang about changes. The fox went on her way, next door promising better bin bags.

Mike Pearson

THE COUNT STEPS IN

'What's it all about Alan - what's it all mean eh?' Cindy was leaning up against the wall swaddled in a quilt looking out over the back gardens. The view was a complete mess but as a slice of life's pointless and shifting pattern it seemed about right; lots of dead or discarded things but growth going on anyhow, hoping something might happen. Alan got up to join her, partly to shut her up - he had thought she might be about to sing like Cilla Black. She opened out the quilt and pulled it tightly round them so that they could stand together.

His back garden, like the others, belonged to no one. They were roughly partitioned off by stringy bits of wire, old half walls and lean-to corrugated iron petering out into an uneven cobbled lane. Similar arrangements stretched across to the backs of houses on the other side. 'Not a thing of beauty.' He said. She asked him if someone would do the whole block up so that people could live in them.

'People live in them now.' He said.

'Yes but you know what I mean.'

Alan knew what she was getting at; wasn't it time he found himself somewhere proper to live, somewhere the light bulbs worked and without draughts coming up through the floorboards on fresh mornings? She'd be organising his CD's next. He was enjoying the warmth of her bottom against his legs though and kissed the top of her head. At least he'd know where to find the Glasgow Improvisers. 'Quite a few of them over yonder are boarded up, squatters avoid them these days.'

Cindy looked up to him. 'What is it your landlord's called?'

'Arthur Astley.'

She bent forward laughing. 'That's it, I knew it was

ASK ME NOW

something daft. He's definitely not a music hall midget though is he?'

'Six foot five scouser, never had any trouble of us with the rent, nor does he sing 'nithangyou'
When he gets it.'

'Arthur Askey was dire wasn't he - nearly as bad as George Formby. People would laugh at anything then.'

'You must come down the Blacksmiths one night - some proper comedians get in there.'

They leaned into each other to watch the wind twitch things in the garden; bit's of newspaper, the odd mutant greenery he liked to see. A sudden gust shifted some black plastic to disclose a bin bag ripped open in the adjacent plot. He diverted her attention off and over to the far gardens where something seemed to be happening. An old bike appeared from over the top of a short wall. It looked to be floating slowly like seaweed in a rock pool until the cross bar appeared with hands to guide it. The hands released it to fall against the wall then a corpulent Indian man in a turban shinned up and over after the bike. He waited then another pair of hands passed over a large plastic bag, which he strung round the handlebars then cycled off towards the other end of the lane.

'I think the old guy next door's been here quite a while actually.' He said.

'He's given up on his garden as well though.' She said.

'Come to think of it I haven't seen him for a while. Perhaps Mr. Astley's waiting for him to rattle his clogs then there'll be some changes made.' He felt her stiffen as he said this and remembered her mother, as well as more from last night's learning curve. 'What do you fancy doing today?' He asked her.

'I don't know.'

'Well, Saturday - 'Dale could be at home, we could go shopping for light bulbs. Have you made any arrangements with your family?'

'I ought to go over really.'

'Shall I come with you?'

'If you want.'

The picture Alan had in his head of her mother was by now decayed but fixed; she was twitchy and gaunt - quite short, rattling round a faded semi grown too big for her with a troublesome back garden not far from a river. In his mind the interior would be in a similar state of decline, he imagined a wooden bureau stuffed with papers, the kitchen ticking over with ancient fixtures - the whole place limping on with a clapped out utility. House and resident going up the spout together. He thought she'd wear her hair short and dress in smart clothes, he caught a fleeting after image of a dark wood standard lamp and an expensive cardigan with brass buttons. Watery eyes, palsied warbles. The poor old lass losing her marbles. 'We could get a light bulb on the way.' He said.

Cindy repositioned herself and pulled the quilt tighter. His arms, holding it in position were cold and the overall arrangement was making him uncomfortable; her hair was irritating his chin and the window frame had begun to press into his shoulder. She seemed happy with it though so he determined to be stoicall. The Indian reappeared on his bike with two heavy looking bags hanging from each handlebar. He sallied down to the other end of the lane and turned out of sight, the sun catching his grey turban as he disappeared

ASK ME NOW

again. 'It'll keep his head warm this morning - do you think it helps protect against Alzheimers?' He asked.

'I wouldn't think it lets them off going ga-ga but they seem to get a better deal from their families when they do.' She said flatly.

He gave her a squeeze by way of apology and managed to shift his weight in the process and hitch up the quilt a bit further. He was beginning to feel as foolish as he sometimes did during sex and then reflected that this was sex really, part of the continuum. It just depended on how far you both wanted to go - it was nicer in some ways without the faff and bluster, the sadness of creaking mattress or ricked necks. He'd worked out over tome that narrowing something down to a boundaried function freighted it with more than it could stand, and did nobody much good. He thought of this as Durights first law of fun and held as good for a fuck as a football match. Basically you had to take the wider view, that way you'd see more. There wasn't much else happening outside his window. Cindy twisted round inside their blanket. 'You all right?' She asked.

'Yeah, how about you Cynthia?'

She squeezed his paunch with both hands and asked him when the baby was due. He smiled and disengaged, wrapping her back up before pulling on his jogging bottoms and extra large 'Free Tracey' (Barlow) tee shirt. She hopped over to the old armchair while he busied himself in the kitchen. He found museli but no milk and they'd polished off the Wagon Wheels last night - the tardiest bowerbird in the forest would have done better for his ladylove than these slim pickings. He explained the situation to Cindy and headed off for Londis while she took first crack at the bathroom.

He thought about on earlier trip to the shops on another

Saturday morning when he'd wept in the street. He felt like crying for himself there and then but it was all right, different, he was being to his sad self hereinafter kind, that he could walk on the ice, face Nigel Harding down. He was still inclined to be anxious tired and gloomy but he thought now that this was all right, that it was all right to be not all right. Whether it was the tablets, time off or Cindy or what, here he was on another Saturday morning in Londis and it wasn't like then. He collared the next to last Indie' then picked up some milk, real coffee and some fresh looking bread. He then dithered over strawberry jam, Marmite or what was offered as 'fresh Brie' in a plastic bag. Settling on the jam and Brie he went over to the old lady at the till who ignored him completely as she doled out his groceries into a bag with one hand while holding out the other for his money as she looked over her shoulder to scream 'Sangita Sangita' at a volume to drown out the Ellington band playing a loud number. He couldn't see any obvious problem and was relieved when she slapped down his change and he could go.

It all turned out better than he'd hoped; the bread was soft, as was the cheese, which mashed wonderfully with the strawberry jam. Cindy was well pleased and made a start on the crossword - 'we can finish it round at Mums.' The coffee caused him a few anxious moments but he managed to produce an acceptable cup by artful deployment of a small colander he didn't know he had and a pair of milk jugs. We should do this more often he thought as he sipped his coffee and went over again some of the stuff which had come his way in the last twenty four hours. It seemed to Alan that there was always so much more going on than you could ever know or guess at, most of the time it came to nothing and was invisible and so, in a way, never really happened. He thought about that tree falling in a forest - if no one was there to witness it falling did it really happen? He was fed up of this; it seemed a shame to have Cindy round then retreat into why are we here?. There was always plenty of time for that. 'What's going on in the world?' He asked her.

ASK ME NOW

'Eh? Oh, the usual - Debbie McGee's made Paul Daniels a happy man, it's magic says Paul - George Bush wants to build an Iraqland in Arizona and a mental health worker in Ridsdale has brought about a dramatic in practice opening the door for retrospective litigation and likely bankruptcy for local councils. It says here that Dick's law could spell unimaginable...'

'Gizit ... you're having a laugh - aren't you?' He had to look though. 'It would have been Barry's law anyway.' He said then provoked a playful tussle over the rest of the paper which caused her to hold on to him for balance then kiss his neck as she knew he liked her to. The stood like this for a bit, as he rubbed her neck his attention was caught by a headline on a page which had fallen open on the floor. Diki Gets Lucky it said and captioned a picture of a giant tortoise glaring implacably at a crowd of children and chuckling adults. The lugubrious beast put him in mind of Count Basie and his first instinct was to take Cindy on a slow jitterbug about the room so he could craftily conceal the piece. Instead he said. 'Maybe I have made it into the papers after all.'

'Eh?'

'Here look.'

They pulled apart then sat together on his little sofa to have a proper look. Diki the giant tortoise at Moscow zoo had found a mate - Ingrid a celebrated beauty from Belarus who it was hoped would bring him happiness and bare him children. The lucky so and so was felt to have a new spring in his step and Ingrid had accommodated herself skilfully to the ways of a notoriously anti-social reptile who had lived alone for too long. She had all ready got him to spend more time with his public, as the photograph showed.

Mike Pearson

'It's Debbie McGee and Paul Daniels again.' Declared Alan.

'I bet she's kicked him out so she can have her friends round.' Said Cindy.

The rest of the feature covered the difficulties in getting these animals to breed in captivity, especially in Moscow, the World Wildlife's campaign to outlaw shell poaching and the little known story of Stalin's tortoise imperative. 'His what?' Said Cindy.

'One of his little jokes.' Explained Alan. 'He used to reckon he could get them to reproduce faster than the workers in Leningrad could knock out locomotives.'

'Yes well, I dare say they were better looked after - what else does it say about Diki and Ingrid?'

'Her more extrovert personality will have a positive effect on her mate whose melancholic streak can usually be diluted when he forgets himself in company.'

They reclined and watched Count Basie on the wall, Cindy remembered something. 'There was another thing in the paper - that bloke's reminded me, Count Backwards is it?'

'Count Basie, one of the finest jazz musicians who ever ...'

'Yes yes, I get the picture but that's the point, his picture's in here somewhere.'

She leafed through and there it was in the review section, a grinning Count B. turning from his piano stool to face the audience while the band - the mid-fifties lot Alan thought - honked and clattered in the background. The image was part of a review called Happiness And All That Jazz of a book; 'The Meaning Of Life' by a bloke Alan had heard on the radio. The reviewer singled out the authors premise that living

ASK ME NOW

life in a certain way was an ethical construct which involved treating others as you wanted them to treat you, caring for those close to you, helping strangers and thinking long term. This led the author to arguing that the meaning of life was therefore like a jazz band; individuals engaged on a collective endeavour in pursuit of happiness through the mutuality of love. They both read this several times then Cindy said. 'I'm impressed, and I think I get it - a jazz band is made up of separate worlds but they manage to make something together.'

'Yes.' He said. 'Logically it shouldn't work, especially when you consider just how individual some of those individuals can be, but it does.'

'So, is that the meaning of life then Alan have you been right all along, it's organised chaos after all - the Evan Parker Big Band have a firmer purchase on reality than Wittgenstein?'

'Oh I should think so but then again, if Wittgenstein had played with Count Basie he could have learned philosophy from Lester Young.'

She turned to give him one of her grown up smiles. 'Shall we go then?'

Lightning Source UK Ltd.
Milton Keynes UK
01 December 2009

146936UK00001B/1/P